THE COMPREHENSIVE GUIDE TO IBUPROFEN

THE GOOD, THE BAD, AND THE UNEXPECTED

Aldrin V. Gomes, PhD and the Gomes Lab

Legal Disclaimer: This book is intended for informational purposes only. The authors and publisher have made every effort to ensure the accuracy and completeness of the information contained in this book as of the date of publication. However, they make no representations or warranties regarding the accuracy, completeness, or applicability of the contents and expressly disclaim any implied warranties of merchantability or fitness for a particular purpose.

The information presented in this book is the opinion of the authors based on their experience and research. It should not be used to replace professional advice. Readers should consult appropriate medical experts before taking any action based on the information contained herein. This book is not intended as a substitute for a physician's medical advice or help. The author and publisher shall not be liable for any loss of profit or any other commercial damages, including but not limited to medical, special, incidental, consequential, or other damages. The strategies and suggestions in this book may not be suitable for every individual and are not guaranteed to produce any specific results.

By reading this book, you acknowledge that you are responsible for your own choices, actions, and results.

Editor: Amelia Evelyn

Website: https://www.gomeslab.net/ibuprofen

Publisher: Mystic River Books

Printed in the U.S.
First Edition: June 3rd, 2025
ISBN eBook: 978-1-961460-06-5
ISBN paperback: 978-1-961460-07-2
ISBN hardcover: 978-1-961460-08-9

About the Authors

Dr. Aldrin V. Gomes leads the Gomes lab (https:www.gomeslab.net) at the University of California (UC), Davis, and is a renowned scientist and educator, and has made significant contributions to the fields of biochemistry and molecular biology. Ranked among the top 2% of scientists worldwide in his field and recognized as one of the top five all-time experts on Western blotting, Dr. Gomes has garnered numerous prestigious awards for his mentorship. These awards include the Presidential Award for Excellence in Science, Mathematics, and Engineering Mentoring, the highest mentoring award bestowed by the White House, the UC Davis Distinguished Graduate and Postdoctoral Mentorship Award, the College of Biological Sciences Principles of Community Award, and the UC Davis Chancellor's Award for Excellence in Mentoring Undergraduate Research.

His commitment to supporting students extends beyond academia through his authorship of "Whispers and Rainbows," a collection of uplifting poems, and "How to ~~Survive~~ Thrive in Graduate School," a guide for graduate students. Both books are available for free on the first day of each month on Amazon Kindle. As the founder of happiestlife.org, he continues to provide support for individuals facing adversity. A fellow of both the American Heart Association and the Cardiovascular Section of the American Physiological Society, Dr. Gomes has delivered many invited talks internationally. He resides in California with his family, pursuing diverse interests such as research, writing, photography, and painting, while his daughters playfully describe his singing skills as "dreadful."

Major Contributing Author

Ahmad Ikram graduated Summa Cum Laude from the University of California, Davis, with a Bachelor of Science (B.S) in Biological Sciences. He has worked on projects ranging from air quality modeling to studying the molecular effects of oxidative stress, as well as student learning in genetics education. Ahmad is dedicated to advancing scientific research and education, with a focus on making complex topics more accessible and impactful for diverse audiences.

Significant Contributors

- **Omnia Ali**, 4th-year undergraduate in Biochemistry and Molecular Biology, UC Davis

- **Maria Azmat**, B.S. in Biological Sciences & Public Health Sciences, UC Davis

- **Emily Barson**, 3rd-year undergraduate in Cell Biology, UC Davis

- **Priyanka Basu**, B.S. in NPB, UC Davis; currently a 3rd-year medical student at Texas A&M School of Medicine

- **Igor Bejenari**, B.S. in Human Biology, UC Davis; currently a Pathology Lab Assistant III at Sutter Health

- **Jillian Cellucci**, B.S., UC Davis; currently a Pediatric Vision Research Associate & Institutional Review Board Administrator at Smith-Kettlewell Eye Research Institute

- **Celeste Do**, B.S. in Biomedical Engineering, UC Davis

- **Ryan Dulong**, B.S. in Molecular, Cellular, and Developmental Biology, University of Washington
- **Daisaku Edwards**, B.S. in NPB, UC Davis; currently an EMT at Falcon Ambulance
- **Jaime Morales Gallardo**, B.S. in Global Disease Biology & B.A. in Chicana/o Studies, UC Davis
- **Emily G. Gartrell**, B.A. in Psychology, UCLA; currently a first-year medical student at Tufts University School of Medicine
- **Massie Gardizi**, B.S. in NPB, UC Davis
- **Timothy Gutierrez**, B.S. in NPB, UC Davis
- **Christina Jung**, B.S., in NPB, UC Davis; currently a research technician, Novo Nordisk
- **Cierra Hall**, B.S. in Cell Biology, UC Davis, Clinical Histocompatibility Scientist, Cypress, California
- **Tan Hua**, B.S. in NPB with Minors in Public Health Sciences & Sociology, UC Davis; currently an Assistant Specialist at UC Davis Health Department of Otolaryngology
- **Nicole Lonsway**, 4th-year undergraduate in NPB & Political Science with Minors in Psychology and Human Rights, UC Davis
- **Aparna Manoj**, B.S. in NPB, UC Davis; currently a 3rd-year medical student at UC Riverside School of Medicine
- **Natalie Nashed**, B.S. in NPB, UC Davis; Master of Science (M.S.) in Physiology & Biophysics student at Georgetown University

- **Rachel Nguyen**, B.S. in NPB, UC Davis; currently a 2nd-year medical student at Touro Medical School
- **Irene Park**, B.S. in NPB, UC Davis
- **Gabriela Del Toro Rivera**, B.S. in Biochemistry & Molecular Biology with a Minor in Psychology; M.S. in Physiology, UC Davis; currently a 5th-year Ph.D. student in Molecular, Cellular, and Integrative Physiology
- **Lauren Roehrs**, B.S. in NPB with a Minor in Public Health, UC Davis. Currently a Physician Assistant student at Tufts University School of Medicine
- **Siona Samanta**, 3rd-year undergraduate in NPB, UC Davis
- **Erik-Matthew Sario**, B.S. in NPB, UC Davis; currently a 4th-year medical student at California Northstate University College of Medicine
- **Gaia Soldano**, 2nd-year undergraduate in Systems & Synthetic Biology, UC Davis
- **Vanessa Su**, B.S. in Biotechnology, UC Davis
- **Isabella Tan**, Bachelor of Art and Sciences (B.A.S.) in Cell Biology & Sociocultural Anthropology, UC Davis
- **Jacob Tuazon**, 3rd-year undergraduate in NPB, UC Davis
- **Mackenzie Trpcic**, B.S. in Psychology, UC Davis; M.Sc. in Kinesiology (specializing in Exercise & Health Physiology) at the University of Calgary; currently a first-year medical student at the Cumming School of Medicine, University of Calgary

- **Tanishq Vaidya**, B.S. in NPB, UC Davis
- **Yael Vainberg**, B.S. in NPB, UC Davis; currently a 1st-year medical student at Stanford School of Medicine
- **Christina Vyvoda**, 3rd-year undergraduate in Global Disease Biology, UC Davis
- **Yue "Cynthia" Yu**, 4th-year undergraduate in NPB & Philosophy, UC Davis
- **Yuhan Zhang**, B.S. in NPB, UC Davis; M.S. in Biochemistry & Molecular Biology, Johns Hopkins University; currently a graduate student in Biomedical Sciences at UC San Diego

Consultant and Contributor

Qian Xu, M.D.; Ph.D. Rheumatologist

Figure Illustrators

- **Ahmad Ikram**, B.S. in Biological Sciences, University of California, Davis
- **Yue "Cynthia" Yu**, 4th-year undergraduate in Neurobiology, Physiology, and Behavior, & Philosophy, University of California, Davis

Free Resources

The webpage for this book https://www.gomeslab.net/ibuprofen offers additional resources, including a comprehensive list of commonly used names for ibuprofen across countries worldwide.

Table of Contents

Acknowledgments

We extend our heartfelt gratitude to the families of everyone involved in writing this book for their unwavering support, encouragement, and understanding throughout this three-year journey.

We gratefully acknowledge the University of California, Davis, for fostering a vibrant and collaborative research environment that empowers students to engage deeply in inquiry and cultivate critical thinking skills. This nurturing academic community has been instrumental in enabling their meaningful contributions to this book, transforming knowledge into impactful scholarship.

We also wish to acknowledge the invaluable contributions of former students who were part of our lab before this book was conceived. Their dedication and groundwork laid an essential foundation for this work. Thank you all for being an integral part of our collective achievement.

Abbreviations

AKI – Acute Kidney Injury

ADE – Adverse Drug Event

ADR – Adverse Drug Reaction

AE – Adverse Event

CDC – Centers for Disease Control and Prevention

CKD – Chronic Kidney Disease

CNS – Central Nervous System

COX – Cyclooxygenase (enzyme inhibited by ibuprofen)

COX-1 – Cyclooxygenase-1

COX-2 – Cyclooxygenase-2

CF – Cystic Fibrosis

CYP – Cytochrome P450 (enzyme family involved in drug metabolism)

DILI – Drug-Induced Liver Injury

ED – Erectile Dysfunction

FDA – Food and Drug Administration

GI – Gastrointestinal

HSP70 – Heat Shock Protein 70

IBD – Inflammatory Bowel Disease

IBU – Ibuprofen (common abbreviation in clinical use)

IV – Intravenous

OTC – Over-the-Counter

NO – Nitric Oxide

NSAID – Nonsteroidal Anti-Inflammatory Drug

PDA – Patent Ductus Arteriosus

PGE2 – Prostaglandin E2 (mediates inflammation and pain)

PGH2 – Prostaglandin H2

PGI2 – Prostaglandin I2

PGs – Prostaglandins

RA – Rheumatoid Arthritis

ROS – Reactive Oxygen Species

SJS – Stevens-Johnson Syndrome

TEN – Toxic Epidermal Necrolysis

TXA2 – Thromboxane A2 (affects platelet aggregation)

mg/kg – Milligrams per Kilogram (dose calculation based on body weight)

WHO – World Health Organization

Introduction

The real danger of overusing or misusing ibuprofen isn't just in its ability to relieve pain, fever, or inflammation; it's in the illusion of wellness it creates. Pain is not the problem; it's a messenger, signaling what the body truly needs. When we focus on masking symptoms rather than addressing the root cause, we fall into the trap of temporary relief at the cost of true healing. There are no shortcuts to recovery, only a deeper understanding of what our bodies require.

- Aldrin V. Gomes

This idea of masking symptoms rather than addressing the root cause is particularly relevant when it comes to ibuprofen, a drug that mutes the body's signals of distress without necessarily resolving the underlying issue. Few over-the-counter drugs are as widely recognized and frequently used as ibuprofen. This small pill has become a household staple, relied upon by millions to relieve pain, reduce fever, and combat inflammation. Yet, despite its accessibility and overall safety, ibuprofen carries risks that are often overlooked. Behind its convenience lies a complex story, one of medical innovation, scientific discovery, and the body's intricate response to pain.

Since its introduction, ibuprofen has become a cornerstone in pain and fever management, providing effective relief to millions of people around the world each year. Additionally, it is commonly used to alleviate swelling and inflammation. However, over the past two decades, research has linked ibuprofen to an increased risk of stroke, heart attack, kidney damage, and other serious health complications. Yet, many remain unaware of the correct dosage, timing, and best practices for safe use, including proper dosage intervals and potential drug interactions. How often do we even think to mention ibuprofen when listing the medication(s) we take? While healthcare providers emphasize the importance of disclosing prescription drugs, many people don't realize that ibuprofen use should be discussed with their doctor as it interacts with over 400 medications.

Despite its perceived safety, ibuprofen comes with a long list of warnings on its packaging and multiple advisories from the U.S. Food and Drug Administration (FDA). This is primarily due to the consequences of overuse or misuse, which can lead to serious complications—including gastrointestinal damage, kidney and liver disease, and an increased risk of heart attack and stroke. In some cases, ibuprofen may even mask symptoms of bacterial infections, delaying diagnosis and treatment. Additionally, emerging research suggests it may impact reproductive health by lowering anti-Müllerian hormone levels and impairing ovulation.

Yet, beyond these risks, ibuprofen also has surprising benefits that many may not realize. Studies indicate that prolonged use may help reduce the risk of neurodegenerative diseases such as Alzheimer's and Parkinson's, possibly due to its anti-inflammatory effects in the brain. Similarly, numerous epidemiological studies have associated consistent use of ibuprofen and other NSAIDs with a lower risk of various cancers. Research has also linked ibuprofen to a reduced risk of age-related conditions, including macular degeneration, gout flare-ups, and kidney stone recurrence. While these findings are promising, they underscore the complexity of ibuprofen's effects on the body.

So, why do we need a book on ibuprofen? Despite its widespread use, pain management education in medical schools remains surprisingly limited. Medical students typically receive only a few weeks of training specifically focused on pain-relieving medications. As a result, many doctors may not fully understand the nuances of commonly used drugs like ibuprofen, naproxen, and acetaminophen unless they actively seek out the latest research. Many new doctors are unprepared to evaluate and manage acute or chronic pain, especially in complex cases such as chronic non-cancer pain. Without up-to-date knowledge, healthcare professionals risk providing inconsistent care, delivering suboptimal pain management, and may overlook potential adverse effects.

This book is not just about the benefits of ibuprofen, but also about understanding its short-term and long-term risks. Backed by over 690 peer-reviewed references, including groundbreaking studies from our lab, it offers a comprehensive look at ibuprofen—covering its molecular mechanisms, common misuses, and how to maximize its therapeutic benefits while minimizing harm.

Understanding ibuprofen's effects empowers people to make more informed choices about their health, helping them balance pain relief with potential risks and avoid unintended harm from misuse or drug interactions. Our lab, the Gomes Lab, has dedicated years to researching the side effects of both ibuprofen and acetaminophen. Undergraduate and graduate students have played a significant role in this work, critically assessing scientific literature and conducting experiments to uncover a more complete picture of ibuprofen's effects. This book is a product of that research, designed to bridge the gap between scientific findings and public understanding. All contributors to this book were members of the Gomes Lab, with many going on to pursue careers in medical-related fields.

By the end of this book, you'll have answers to questions you may not have considered, such as:

- What are the potential long-term risks of ibuprofen use?
- Does it matter what time of day you take ibuprofen, and how can timing impact its effectiveness?
- Can ibuprofen affect your sleep or cause other unexpected side effects?
- Should you take ibuprofen with food? Are there foods that might interact with it?
- How does ibuprofen compare to acetaminophen in terms of effectiveness and safety for children?
- Does ibuprofen raise blood pressure, and if so, how significant is the risk? When should you consider these risks?
- What alternatives can be used to reduce the amount of ibuprofen used?

Whether you occasionally take ibuprofen, are a medical professional, or are simply curious about how this drug works, there's much more to this everyday medicine than meets the eye. So, as you hold this book, perhaps with the same hand that has reached for ibuprofen in times of need, let's explore the science, benefits, and risks of one of the world's most widely used pain relievers. This book will provide the knowledge needed to make informed decisions about its use.

Now is the perfect time to begin your journey of discovery into the fascinating world of ibuprofen. Let's turn the page and get started.

Chapter 1
Why Everyone Should Be Informed About Ibuprofen

Ibuprofen belongs to a class of drugs known as nonsteroidal anti-inflammatory drugs (NSAIDs), which also includes aspirin, diclofenac, and naproxen—the active ingredient in *Aleve*. While ibuprofen is widely recognized for its ability to reduce fever, pain, and inflammation, many people are unaware of its additional benefits and potential risks.

How much do you really know about ibuprofen? Assessing your knowledge of ibuprofen before reading the rest of the book is important because it helps you identify some gaps or misconceptions you may have. This awareness makes you more likely to engage with the content and actively seek out information that can improve your understanding and safe use of this common medication.

Test your knowledge by answering the following twelve multiple-choice questions and assess your ibuprofen I.Q.!

Ibuprofen I.Q.

Please answer the following questions, then check your answers on the next page. Each question has only one correct answer.

Dosage and Usage

1. Although ibuprofen is an over-the-counter drug, a physician can also prescribe it. What is the average number of yearly prescriptions in the U.S. for ibuprofen?

   a) 1 million
   b) 5 million
   c) 10 million
   d) more than 15 million

2. What is the maximum dosage/day of ibuprofen an adult can take without a prescription?

   a) 800 mg
   b) 1200 mg
   c) 2400 mg
   d) 3200 mg

3. Which of the following is a surprising fact about ibuprofen?

   a) Ibuprofen at low dosages can decrease the lifespan of some organisms

   b) Ibuprofen can help treat certain heart defects that a child is born with (congenital heart defects)

   c) Ibuprofen can make you feel happy

   d) All of the above

   e) None of the above

4. You can use topical NSAIDs such as ibuprofen for migraine pain relief.

   a) True
   b) False

Side Effects and Safety

5. Which of the following is associated with long-term ibuprofen use?

a) Allergic reactions
b) Hearing loss
c) Anemia (lower number of red blood cells than the typical number)
d) All of the above
e) None of the above

6. Taking a single 400 mg dose of ibuprofen can increase the risk of which of the following?

a) Myocardial infarction
b) Stroke
c) Gastrointestinal (GI) bleeding
d) All of the above
e) None of the above

7. Which of the following are more common side effects when using ibuprofen?

a) Cloudy urine
b) Shortness of breath
c) Weight gain
d) All of the above
e) None of the above

8. Which of the following are rare side effects when using ibuprofen?

a) Broken bones
b) Memory loss
c) Seizures
d) All of the above
e) None of the above

9. Prolonged use of topical NSAIDs (such as creams) is associated with an increased risk for several body problems, including liver issues.

a) True
b) False

Drug and Supplement Interactions

10. Which of the following commonly used supplements and remedies might interact with ibuprofen and increase the risk of side effects?

a) Turmeric (a major ingredient in curry)
b) Fish oil (omega-3 polyunsaturated fatty acids)
c) Gingko Biloba (an herb used to enhance brain health)
d) All of the above
e) None of the above

11. Which prescription drugs should not be taken with ibuprofen?

a) Dicumarol (an anticoagulant)
b) Regorafenib (used for colon and rectum cancer)
c) Tinzaparin (used to treat deep venous thrombosis)
d) All of the above
e) None of the above

Special Populations

12. Which of the following could occur in athletes who take ibuprofen after long runs or moderate gym sessions?

a) Greater muscle loss than those not taking ibuprofen
b) Greater water loss
c) Less bone loss
d) All of the above
e) None of the above

Answers

1. d) It is documented that more than 17 million prescriptions for ibuprofen are issued annually in the United States. Yes, you read that correctly: millions of people are using prescription-strength ibuprofen daily.[3]

2. b) Without a prescription, the maximum dosage is 1200 mg of ibuprofen per day. With a prescription, the maximum dosage is up to 3200 mg per day. Why do you need a prescription to take higher dosages of ibuprofen? High dosages of ibuprofen are associated with more adverse side effects, including stomach bleeding, that a medical professional should monitor.

3. b) Ibuprofen can help treat congenital heart defects in children.[4] At low dosages, ibuprofen can increase the lifespan by 10-17% in organisms like yeast, nematode worms, and fruit flies.[5] Ibuprofen has been shown to extend lifespan in these model organisms through metabolic changes by depriving cells of amino acids, similar to how fasting can extend human lifespan. Additionally, it could alter mood by reducing social pain—helping some feel "less hurt"—though it does not induce happiness.

4. a) NSAIDs applied to the frontal head region help reduce the pain associated with migraines.[6]

5. d) Ibuprofen users are more likely to have intestinal bleeding, causing anemia, a potential side effect of these drugs.[7] Ibuprofen is also associated with many allergic reactions, which include a wide range of severity, from mild rashes to life-threatening anaphylaxis (a severe, life-threatening allergic reaction).[8] A study involving more than 55,000 women found that people who regularly used NSAIDs

over six years had a 10% higher risk of developing hearing loss compared to people who took them less often or did not use them at all.[9]

6. b) Unfortunately, even with the first use of ibuprofen, it increases the risk of gastrointestinal (GI) bleeding, myocardial infarction, and stroke.[10] However, occasional use of ibuprofen is safer than regular or long-term use. Additionally, the risk of serious adverse events is significantly higher in older adults, especially those with additional risk factors such as liver or heart disease.

7. d) Common side effects when using ibuprofen include cloudy urine, shortness of breath, and weight gain.[11]

8. c) Rare and serious side effects of ibuprofen include seizures, muscle tremors, and coma.[11] While the long-term use of NSAIDs when someone has broken bones seems to slow down the healing process, NSAIDs, including ibuprofen, have not been reported to increase the risk of fractures.[12] Currently, ibuprofen has not been shown to be associated with memory loss.

9. b) While topical NSAIDs are generally associated with a lower risk of systemic side effects, no studies have conclusively linked them to long-term health risks such as liver or heart disease.[13] However, it's important to follow medical guidelines when using them.

10. d) Unlike prescription medications, natural remedies and supplements are often not subjected to the same rigorous testing. In many cases, the FDA does not evaluate these over-the-counter products. Therefore, there is not enough information to say what, if any, natural remedies and supplements are safe to take with

ibuprofen. However, some supplements, have been studied and both turmeric and Ginkgo Biloba have been found to affect blood clotting when taken with ibuprofen, which can increase the risk of bleeding. This is due to ibuprofen having a mild blood clotting effect. Similarly, fish oil (omega-3 fatty acids) can have a blood-thinning effect and users should be careful if taking it with ibuprofen.[14-16]

It is recommended that you do not take these supplements within 4 hours of taking ibuprofen, and to tell your medical professional what medications you are taking, including supplements, vitamins, and natural products.

11. d) Dicumarol, Regorafenib, and Tinzaparin are all medications that can significantly increase the risk of bleeding complications, especially when used in combination with other drugs that affect blood clotting, such as NSAIDs like ibuprofen. These drugs interfere with different aspects of the coagulation pathway.[17-19]

12. c) Some athletes use ibuprofen to prevent sore muscles or reduce joint inflammation. However, several studies suggest that under some conditions (such as after a run), NSAIDs may increase bone density and delay bone loss due to inflammation.[20-23] These effects may be due to the anti-inflammatory action of ibuprofen, which can help reduce the inflammatory processes that lead to bone resorption (the breakdown of bone tissue).

Now that you've tested your ibuprofen knowledge, let's look at some exciting factors related to ibuprofen.

Recent estimates suggest that more than 20% of adults in the U.S. experience some form of chronic pain.[24] Many rely on NSAIDs like ibuprofen for relief. However, numerous studies indicate that high doses or long-term use of ibuprofen can significantly increase the risk of severe side effects, including internal bleeding and stroke.

Findings from our research studies in mice show that ibuprofen, even at moderate doses, can significantly alter liver enzymes and metabolic pathways, with some effects differing between males and females. However, while these results suggest that ibuprofen may have more complex impacts on liver function than previously recognized, further research is needed to determine how these findings translate to human health and whether similar sex-specific effects occur in people.[25]

Additionally, recent publications reinforce the need for greater caution in ibuprofen use. While ibuprofen is effective in treating pain, fever, and, to a lesser extent, inflammation, its potential side effects, ranging from mild to severe, are closely tied to dosage and duration of treatment.

Fun Facts About Ibuprofen:

- The inventor of ibuprofen first tested it on himself to treat a hangover-induced headache, marking the first time it had ever been used for headache relief.
- Ibuprofen works by preventing the synthesis of certain prostaglandins, which are responsible for making nerve endings more sensitive to pain.
- In some countries and for children with Patent Ductus Arteriosus (PDA), ibuprofen lysine, a faster-absorbing form of ibuprofen due to its improved water solubility, is used instead of regular ibuprofen.

The Hidden Risks of Ibuprofen Misuse

One of the biggest concerns about ibuprofen is that its widespread availability has led many to assume it is completely safe. However, millions of teenagers and adults misuse it, often unaware of the risks. A 2018 study of 1,326 ibuprofen users revealed that 11% exceeded the maximum recommended daily dose.[26] This excessive intake was linked to poorer physical function. While occasional overuse may cause short-term side effects, this type of use is less likely to result in lasting harm if corrected promptly. However, chronic misuse, which involves consistently exceeding recommended dosages daily for extended periods without medical supervision, greatly increases the risk of serious health complications, including GI bleeding, kidney and liver damage, and cardiovascular problems.

In 2022, over 17 million ibuprofen prescriptions were issued in the United States, with 59.3% of those being for 800 mg tablets or capsules.[3] Disappointingly, more than 11% of prescription users reported taking more than the prescribed dosage.[26] While not classified as an addictive substance, ibuprofen can lead to psychological dependence in some users, particularly when used to manage chronic, non-specific pain. Warning signs of dependence may include increasing frequency of use, escalation of dosage, and continued use despite negative consequences.[27] This phenomenon, known as ibuprofen-use disorder, is uncommon but occurs when people struggle to stop taking ibuprofen despite negative consequences. Studies show that exceeding the maximum daily dose of ibuprofen is even more common than with acetaminophen.

Ibuprofen and Athletes: A Common Yet Harmful Practice

As noted above, despite its benefits, ibuprofen has important risks that need to be understood. This is especially true for athletes who misuse ibuprofen, often taking it preemptively to reduce pain and inflammation before or after exercise. However, research suggests that this practice not only provides no benefits but may actually be harmful. A study on long-distance runners found that ibuprofen use led to increased inflammation, rather than reducing it.[28] This was due to endotoxemia, a condition in which bacteria from the gut enter the bloodstream, an effect that ibuprofen appears to worsen. Instead, athletes could try physical therapy, mindfulness techniques, or acupuncture.

How is ibuprofen absorbed?

Many students we surveyed thought that ibuprofen is mostly absorbed and broken down in the stomach. However, the majority of ibuprofen is absorbed in the small intestine (**Fig. 1.1**). Any ibuprofen that is not absorbed moves to the large intestine and is eventually excreted in feces. Once in the body, ibuprofen is metabolized in the liver, where it is broken down into byproducts, that are then excreted in urine.

Fig. 1.1. Absorption of ibuprofen taken orally

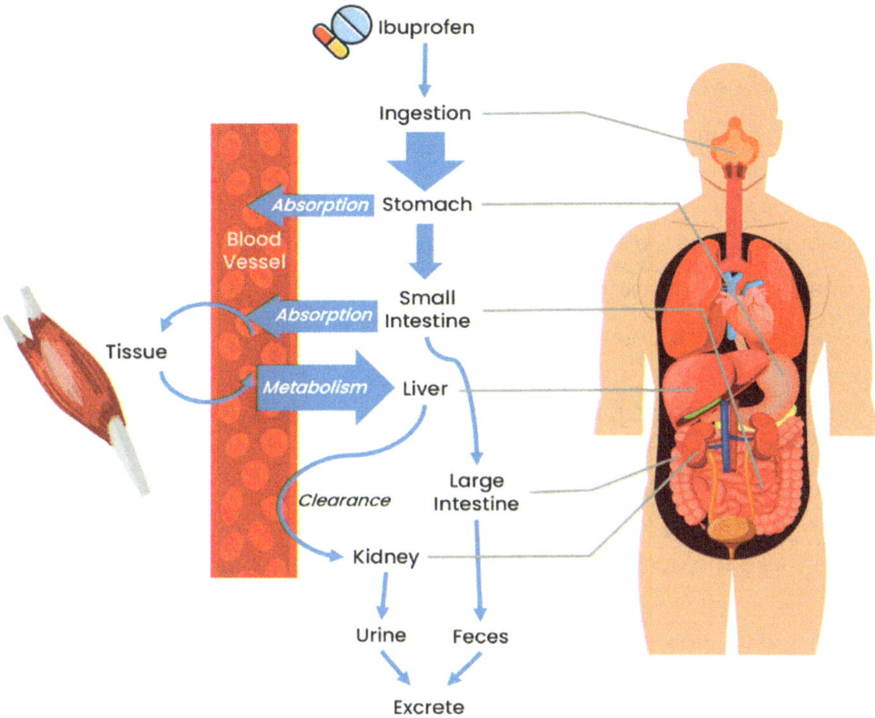

Common Side Effects of Ibuprofen

While ibuprofen is widely used, it has side effects that occur in at least 1 out of every 100 people who take it. Given the number of ibuprofen users in the U.S., it is estimated that millions experience at least one of these side effects each year. Although considered common, these effects can be distressing and significantly impact daily life.

Common side effects (> 1 in 100 people) listed by manufacturers of ibuprofen:

- Bloating
- Diarrhea
- Dizziness
- Gas

- Headaches
- Heartburn
- Indigestion
- Irritability
- Nausea
- Nervousness
- Reduced appetite
- Vomiting

Warning as seen on a bottle containing ibuprofen:
Stomach bleeding warning: Because this product contains an NSAID, there is a risk of severe bleeding in the stomach. The chance is higher if you

- take more or for a longer time than directed
- are aged 60 or older
- take a blood-thinning (anticoagulant) or steroid drug
- take other drugs containing prescription or nonprescription NSAIDs (aspirin, ibuprofen, naproxen, or others)
- consume three or more alcoholic drinks daily while taking this product

Let's take a closer look at some additional, less common, but more severe risks.[11] These occur in less than 1 in 100 to less than 1 in 10,000 ibuprofen users.[11] The mechanisms behind some of these effects are discussed in other chapters of this book. **The sheer volume of less common and rare side effects listed may be overwhelming, but it is included for users to realize how varied the side effects could be.** These include:

- Abdominal cramps
- Agitation
- Back, leg, or stomach pains

- Bleeding gums
- Blistering, peeling, and loosening of skin
- Blood in the urine or stools
- Bloody, black, or tarry stools
- Blurred vision
- Burning feeling in chest or stomach
- Change in vision
- Chest pain
- Chills
- Clay-colored stools
- Coma
- Confusion
- Constipation
- Cough or hoarseness
- Crying
- Dark urine
- Decreased urine output
- Depersonalization
- Depression
- Difficulty breathing
- Difficulty swallowing
- Dilated neck veins
- Discouragement
- Dizziness
- Dry eyes
- Dry mouth
- Dysphoria
- Extreme fatigue
- Fast, irregular, pounding, or racing heartbeat or pulse
- Feeling sad or empty
- Fever with or without chills
- Frequent urination
- General body swelling
- General feeling of tiredness or weakness
- Hair loss, thinning of hair
- Headache
- Hives or welts
- Hostility
- Impaired vision
- Increased blood pressure
- Increased volume of pale, dilute urine
- Irregular breathing
- Irritability
- Itching
- Joint or muscle pain
- Lab results that show problems with the liver

- Lack of appetite
- Lethargy
- Light-colored stools
- Loss of appetite
- Loss of interest or pleasure
- Lower back or side pain
- Mental depression
- Muscle twitching
- Nosebleeds
- Painful or difficult urination
- Pain in the stomach, side, or abdomen, possibly radiating to the back
- Paranoia
- Pinpoint red spots on the skin
- Puffiness or swelling of the eyelids or around the eyes, face, lips, or tongue
- Quick to react or overreact
- Rapidly changing moods
- Rash
- Red skin lesions, often with a purple center
- Red, irritated eyes
- Redness of skin
- Runny nose
- Seizures
- Severe abdominal pain, cramping, burning
- Severe and continuing nausea
- Sleepiness or unusual drowsiness
- Sleeplessness
- Sneezing
- Sore throat
- Sores, ulcers, or white spots in the mouth or on lips
- Stiff neck or back
- Stomach soreness or discomfort
- Stomach upset
- Stuffy nose
- Stupor
- Swollen or painful glands
- Tenderness in the stomach area
- Thirst
- Tightness in chest
- Trouble concentrating

- Trouble sleeping
- Unable to sleep
- Unpleasant breath odor
- Upper right abdominal pain
- Vomiting of blood
- Vomiting of material that looks like coffee grounds
- Wheezing
- Yellow eyes and skin

Still wondering why it's important to understand the risks of ibuprofen?

A 2016 study of 89 ultramarathon runners found that those who took ibuprofen had a higher risk of developing acute kidney injury compared to those who did not.[29] Acute kidney injury occurs when the kidneys suddenly fail or sustain damage within hours. Research, including our own studies, suggests that ibuprofen increases oxidative stress by triggering the production of reactive oxygen species (ROS) in tissues. ROS are highly reactive molecules that can damage cells by oxidizing lipids, proteins, and DNA. Excessive ROS production leads to oxidative stress, which disrupts normal cellular functions and triggers inflammation. This process can result in long-term damage to organs like the kidneys.[30] Although the human body has natural antioxidant systems to counteract ROS, excessive oxidative stress can overwhelm these defenses, leading to significant cell and tissue damage.

Severe Health Risks and Unexpected Reactions to Ibuprofen

While ibuprofen is a widely used and effective pain reliever, understanding both its benefits and risks, especially when taken over extended periods or in high doses, is essential. Although the body's natural defenses are typically effective at reducing reactive oxygen species (ROS), certain external factors, such as medication use, can exacerbate oxidative stress and its consequences.

In very rare cases, ibuprofen has been associated with the sudden onset of severe health conditions, including:

- **Stevens-Johnson Syndrome (SJS) and Toxic Epidermal Necrolysis (TEN):** A 22-year-old male developed these life-threatening skin and mucous membrane disorders after taking three 400 mg doses of ibuprofen at 8-hour intervals for eye pain.[31]

- **Reye's Syndrome:** A 56-year-old woman developed this rare but severe condition, affecting multiple organs, most notably the brain and liver, after taking ibuprofen for headaches.[32] Laboratory tests revealed she had influenza A, which, when combined with ibuprofen use, led to acute liver failure.

Although these severe reactions occur in fewer than 1 in 1,000,000 cases of SJS and Reye's syndrome, they are both important to acknowledge.[32,33] Importantly, SJS—though exceptionally rare, can sometimes develop even after a single dose of medication.[33]

Additionally, ibuprofen is known to interact with hundreds of medications, which may lead to moderate or severe health consequences when taken together or in close succession.

- **Case Study:** A 55-year-old woman was found unconscious at home and diagnosed with a coma caused by critically low sodium levels in her brain.[34] She had von Willebrand's disease, a lifelong bleeding disorder, and regularly took desmopressin before dental procedures to help with blood clotting. Two days before a dental extraction, she took desmopressin as usual but also used ibuprofen for pain relief. The combination led to dizziness, vomiting, and ultimately a coma. Ibuprofen can interfere with blood clotting, which increases the risk of bleeding or other complications when combined with medications like desmopressin.

These cases highlight that, even when ibuprofen is taken within recommended doses, unexpected and severe reactions can still occur. The risks increase significantly when ibuprofen is consumed at higher-than-recommended amounts.[35]

Symptoms of Ibuprofen Overdose[11]

- Bluish lips or skin
- Difficulty breathing or not breathing
- Drowsiness, confusion, or disorientation (including coma)
- Dizziness or fainting (especially when standing up)
- Hallucinations or mood/mental changes
- Muscle tremors
- Rapid, deep, or irregular heartbeat
- Restlessness
- Stomach cramps
- Sweating
- Enlarged liver

Now, let's explore some general questions about ibuprofen that few people think about:

Is Where You Store Ibuprofen Important?

Did you know that where you store ibuprofen could impact its effectiveness? Many people unknowingly store their medications in places that could reduce their potency. Like many other over-the-counter drugs, ibuprofen typically includes a label recommending storage in a dry, room-temperature environment (between 68°F and 77°F) and protection from light.[36,37] However, many people store their medications in bathrooms, often due to the convenience of built-in medicine cabinets. The issue with bathroom storage is that the environment is often humid and experiences temperature fluctuations. Studies suggest that nearly 50% of the population improperly stores their medications.

A 2020 study monitored the active ingredient in ibuprofen stored in a bathroom. The recorded temperature ranged from 59.9°F to 86.2°F, with an average humidity of 63.2% (ranging from 29.2% to 100%).[38] This study also investigated whether improper storage led to the formation of 4-isobutyl acetophenone, a toxic breakdown product of ibuprofen. Researchers tested three commercial ibuprofen tablets (200 mg each, from Brands A-C) and three ibuprofen suspensions (100 mg/5 mL each, from Brands A-C). The good news: no toxic breakdown products were detected after 12 months. However, the potency of ibuprofen tablets dropped to 73%, and the suspension strength fell to 83%. Hence, while toxic products weren't detected, the reduced potency still compromises the effectiveness of taking the drug.

Fluctuations in temperature and humidity can cause the active ingredients in ibuprofen to break down faster, reducing its ability to effectively manage pain. To ensure ibuprofen remains effective, it should be stored at room temperature in a dry location, away from heat, humidity, and significant temperature changes.[38]

Could You Store Ibuprofen in the Fridge?

Storing ibuprofen in the refrigerator is unnecessary as it is a stable compound that does not degrade significantly under typical storage conditions (68°F to 77°F). Storing it in cold temperatures is likely to influence its physical characteristics. The active ingredient in ibuprofen might crystallize when exposed to low temperatures, potentially impacting the drug's dissolution and absorption rates. A refrigerated environment might also expose it to excess humidity, which may affect its stability.

Can You Break a Tablet and Take Half?

Swallowing ibuprofen tablets whole is essential, as many are coated to protect the stomach lining.[39,40] This coating, often an enteric or gastro-resistant layer, prevents the tablet from dissolving in the acidic environment of the stomach, thereby reducing irritation, ulcers, and gastric pain commonly associated with NSAIDs like ibuprofen. Instead, the coating ensures the tablet remains intact until it reaches the more neutral pH of the small intestine, where the drug is safely and effectively released and absorbed.[39,41]

Breaking or chewing ibuprofen tablets can damage this protective coating, exposing the stomach lining directly to the active drug, which increases the risk of stomach irritation and ulcers. Moreover, if the tablet is formulated as a time-release (also called extended- or controlled-release) preparation, breaking it disrupts the carefully designed mechanism that controls the gradual release of the drug over time. The result is that more of the dose is released at once, which can lead to uneven absorption, increased side effects, or overdose.[42-44] For safe and effective use, always follow the manufacturer's instructions.

Does Ibuprofen Affect Birth Control Pills?

While some sources claim that ibuprofen does not interfere with birth control pills, research suggests that ibuprofen can alter potassium levels and increase the concentration of contraceptive hormones in the body, potentially raising the risk of blood clots.[45,46] This risk is particularly concerning for individuals taking birth control pills containing drospirenone. Ibuprofen can raise potassium levels by reducing kidney excretion, and drospirenone can also increase potassium levels.[46,47] When taken together, they further elevate potassium levels, increasing the likelihood of dangerous heart rhythm problems and blood clots.[48,49] In contrast, acetaminophen (*Tylenol*) does not appear to cause these effects.[50]

How Long Do the Pain-Relieving Effects of Ibuprofen Last?

Ibuprofen bottles typically indicate that its effects last between 4 to 6 hours. However, while ibuprofen's pain-relieving effects typically last between 4 and 6 hours, studies suggest that the therapeutic benefits can extend up to 8 hours, depending on individual factors such as age and liver function. It's important to clarify that the pain relief wears off before the drug is completely eliminated from the body, which can take up to 24 hours due to its half-life of about 1.9 to 2.2 hours.[51,52]

Individual variability in the duration of ibuprofen's effects is influenced primarily by liver function and age because these factors affect how quickly the drug is metabolized. In children, ibuprofen is metabolized more rapidly, with a half-life similar to adults, approximately 1.8 to 2.0 hours. However, overall clearance may be faster due to more efficient liver enzyme activity.[51] Conversely, in individuals with impaired liver function, metabolism slows down, leading to a longer half-life and prolonged effects, which can increase the risk of adverse effects.[11,53,54]

Age also plays a significant role. Older adults often experience altered drug metabolism due to decreased hepatic (liver) blood flow and reduced enzyme activity, which can prolong the half-life and effects of ibuprofen.[53] This may partly explain why elderly users of ibuprofen experience increased health risks from taking ibuprofen compared to younger individuals. Overall, dosing should be adjusted accordingly to minimize side effects and ensure safe use.

How Long Does Ibuprofen Stay in the Body?

After a single use, ibuprofen stays in the body for up to 24 hours.

- 9-12 hours for children
- 12-24 hours for adults

These values depend on the absorption and metabolism of ibuprofen. Drug absorption is the process by which a drug moves from the site of administration (such as oral or skin) into the bloodstream, influenced by factors like the route of administration, drug formulation, and chemical properties. Metabolism refers to the body's breakdown of drugs, primarily in the liver. This process converts drugs into more water-soluble compounds, which can be inactive or active metabolites, enabling elimination via urine or bile. Many factors, including genetics, drug interactions, and disease, can influence how quickly or effectively a drug is metabolized. Absorption determines how much of a drug enters the bloodstream, while metabolism affects how the drug is processed and eliminated, both of which are crucial for the drug's efficacy and safety.

Does the Dosage Form Affect Ibuprofen's Action?

Yes, the dosage form does affect ibuprofen's action. Ibuprofen in tablet form tends to have a longer duration of action than in chewable forms, and chewable forms generally last longer than liquid forms like suspensions. The liquid form of ibuprofen appears to work faster than tablets or chewables because liquids do not require dissolution in the stomach, allowing for quicker absorption into the bloodstream and faster relief of symptoms.[38,55-57]

Duration of Action: Tablet > Chewable > Suspension
Time to Peak Concentration in Blood: Suspension > Tablet = Chewable

Is Ibuprofen Safe to Use After Its Expiration Date?

Ideally, all medications should be used before their expiration date. However, taking recently expired ibuprofen does not seem to be harmful, as it does not typically break down into significantly toxic substances after its expiration date. Always consult your healthcare provider before taking expired medication. If ibuprofen has been appropriately stored away from high heat and humidity, its effectiveness in reducing pain and inflammation gradually decreases after the expiration date. However, if it has been exposed to unfavorable storage conditions, its potency may decline even sooner. Using ibuprofen that is significantly past its expiration date, such as beyond 2 years, is not recommended.

Do Ibuprofen Products Contain Other Inactive Ingredients?

Yes, ibuprofen products often contain inactive ingredients that vary by brand and formulation. These may include carnauba wax, colloidal silicon dioxide, corn starch, hypromellose, lactose anhydrous, microcrystalline cellulose, polydextrose, polyethylene glycol, red iron oxide, sodium starch glycolate, stearic acid, and titanium dioxide. While labeled as "inactive," some of these ingredients have been linked to adverse reactions in sensitive individuals (**Table 1.2**). Therefore, it's essential to check product labels and consult a healthcare provider if needed.[58]

Table 1.2. Three "inactive" ingredients in some ibuprofen tablets and their potential adverse effects.

Ingredient	Potential Adverse Effect	References
Lactose monohydrate	GI issues like bloating, gas, stomach pain, cramps, and diarrhea in individuals with lactose intolerance	59
Polyethylene glycol	Allergic reactions, GI upset (nausea, diarrhea)	58
Titanium dioxide	Possible GI inflammation, rare allergic reactions, and potential concerns in those with irritable bowel syndrome	60

Is It Better to Have a Healthcare Team Administer Ibuprofen?

Most people can safely take ibuprofen on their own for short-term relief of minor pain or fever, following the directions on the package.[61] However, collaborating with a healthcare team can improve patient outcomes when ibuprofen is used for chronic conditions, higher prescription doses, or in combination with other medications. Medical professionals can provide guidance on the safest and most effective use of ibuprofen. For instance, in cases of acute pericarditis, ibuprofen is often prescribed alongside colchicine for more effective symptom relief.[62] A healthcare provider can ensure the correct dosage and monitor for potential interactions or side effects.

Can Animals Take Ibuprofen?

Yes, but only under the supervision of a veterinarian as ibuprofen has a very narrow safety margin in most animals.[63,64] In general, moderate doses of ibuprofen and other NSAIDs are toxic to animals, including cats and dogs. Even a small dose (>5mg/kg/day) can cause severe health complications.[63] This is partly due to ibuprofen being metabolized more slowly than humans, leading to a higher risk of toxicity and adverse effects in animals.

- **Cats:** Ingestion of ibuprofen tablets can lead to vomiting, diarrhea, hematochezia (bright red blood in stool), regurgitation, and apparent abdominal pain in an adult cat.[65]

- **Dogs:** Doses greater than 50 mg/kg of ibuprofen are highly toxic to dogs, potentially causing vomiting, diarrhea, hematochezia, regurgitation, and apparent abdominal pain, as well as pollakiuria (frequent urination), tachypnea (rapid breathing), and tachycardia (elevated heart rate).

- This means that a single 200 mg tablet would be toxic to small and medium-sized dogs 4 kg (8.8 lbs) or less.

- **Other Animals:** High doses of ibuprofen have been linked to comas and fatalities in animals such as ferrets, birds, hamsters, and potentially for reptiles as well.[66-69]

- Overuse or accidental ingestion by animals can lead to serious health problems, including stomach ulcers and GI bleeding, kidney damage or failure, and neurological effects such as depression, seizures, coma, or even death.[65,70]

For these reasons, ibuprofen should never be given to pets or any other animals unless prescribed by a veterinarian. If accidental ingestion occurs, seek immediate veterinary care.

Summary: Ibuprofen Overload!

While ibuprofen is a widely used and effective medication for humans, its misuse—whether in pets or people—can lead to serious health risks. More than one in ten adults take excessive amounts of ibuprofen, often without understanding the risks.[26] Overusing ibuprofen can lead to GI damage, kidney injury, liver issues, higher blood pressure, and increased risk of heart attack, stroke, and other heart complications.

These risks are especially pronounced in older adults, people with a history of ulcers, heart, liver, or kidney disease, and those taking other medications. As such, high school students should be educated on the maximum safe dosage per dose and per 24-hour period, as well as the importance of starting with the lowest effective dose. As students become older, they will be better aware of the risks of ibuprofen overuse.

As a society, we must strive to reduce unnecessary use of ibuprofen and other NSAIDs to minimize the risk of avoidable health complications. Athletes, in particular, should avoid taking ibuprofen preventatively. Research has shown that it does not reduce muscle soreness or improve performance, and may actually increase health risks.[71] Additionally, public health campaigns and clearer labeling should help reduce unnecessary NSAID use and prevent avoidable health risks.

Key Takeaways:

- Over-the-counter drugs are still drugs, just like prescription medications, and all drugs have side effects.

- Every teenager and adult who uses ibuprofen should understand when it is appropriate to take it and the risks of improper use.

Chapter 2
IBUPROFEN:
Common Uses and Practices

Ibuprofen is widely known for its effectiveness in reducing pain, inflammation, and fever. Among cyclists, it's even humorously referred to as "Vitamin I," due to its frequent use for muscle soreness, both before and after long rides.

In its pure form, ibuprofen appears as colorless crystals, with the chemical formula $C_{13}H_{18}O_2$ and a molar mass of 206.28 g/mol. While it has low solubility in water (only about 21 mg per liter at room temperature), it remains highly effective in small doses. The compound has a melting point of approximately 75-77°C, and a boiling point of about 157°C, though you're unlikely to encounter it in these extreme states outside a laboratory.[52,72] These parameters are important to ibuprofen's stability and effectiveness.

What's in the Name?

Ibuprofen's name originates from the three functional chemical groups that make up its structure:[72]

- Isobutyl ("ibu")

- Propionic acid ("pro")
- Phenyl ("fen")

Fig. 2.1. Chemical structure of ibuprofen

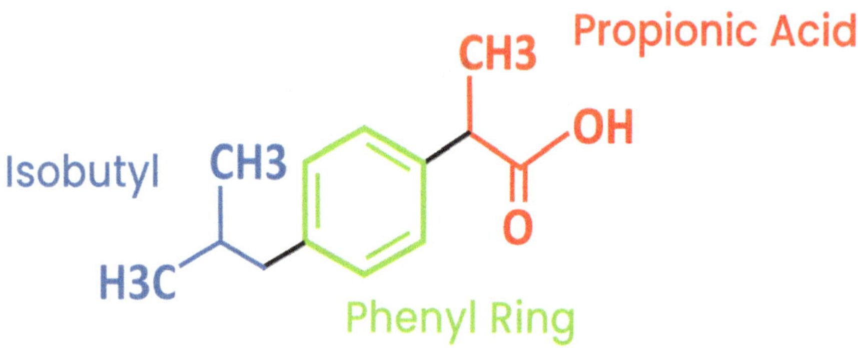

The chemical structure with the functional groups of ibuprofen highlighted is shown in **Fig. 2.1.** While its naming is straightforward, ibuprofen has several complex chemical variations, including 2-(4-isobutylphenyl) propanoic acid and 2-(p-isobutylphenyl) propionic acid —names that could make anyone's head spin![73,74]

To simplify matters, the International Union of Pure and Applied Chemistry (IUPAC), the global authority on chemical nomenclature, has designated ibuprofen an official IUPAC name.[75] The official name for ibuprofen is:

2-[4-(2-Methylpropyl)phenyl]propanoic acid

Despite its complex chemical identity, most people recognize it by its brand names, such as *Advil* and *Motrin* in the United States. Internationally, it is sold under various names and formulations.

Forms of Ibuprofen

Most people are familiar with ibuprofen as a small tablet or pill, but it comes in many forms to suit different needs, including:

- **Capsules**: Common for general pain relief.
- **Chewable tablets**: Preferred for young children or others who have trouble swallowing tablets.
- **Liquid suspensions** (dilute and concentrated): Preferred for young children or individuals needing precise dosing.
- **Topical gels or creams**: Targeted relief for muscle and joint pain without systemic side effects.
- **Sprays**: convenient for targeted pain relief, such as sports injuries.

This versatility makes ibuprofen a go-to option for managing pain and inflammation, whether it's for a headache, sore joints, or muscle pain. No matter the form, ibuprofen remains a trusted and widely used medication, offering relief in a way that fits everyone's needs.

The Invention of Ibuprofen

Ibuprofen was developed in the 1960s by chemist Dr. Stewart Adams at Boots Pure Drug Company in Nottingham, England.[76] Dr. Adams was a pharmacologist, and with the help of John Nicholson, an organic chemist, they researched a safer and more effective treatment for rheumatoid arthritis than existing options like aspirin and corticosteroids. After testing more than 600 compounds, they identified 2-(4-isobutylphenyl)propionic acid, later named ibuprofen, as the most promising candidate.

The first clinical trials were conducted in Edinburgh in the mid-1960s, demonstrating its anti-inflammatory effects. Ibuprofen was launched as a prescription drug in the UK in 1969 under the brand name *Brufen* and was primarily used to treat rheumatoid arthritis.[77]

Fig. 2.2. Timeline for ibuprofen's clinical approval

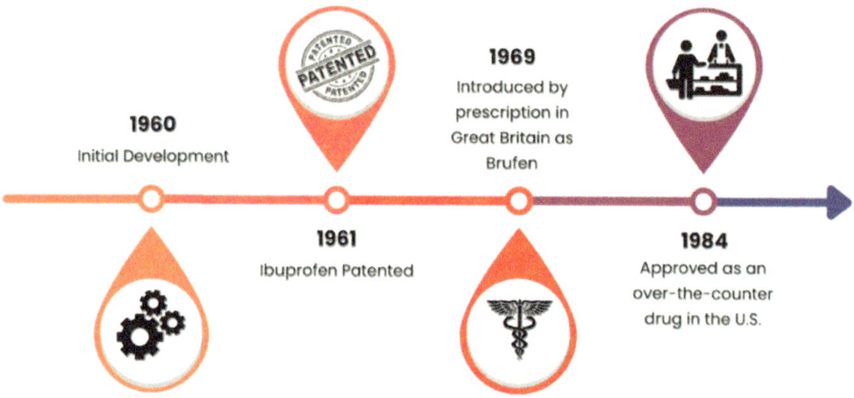

Thanks to its effectiveness in pain relief and lower risk of gastrointestinal (GI) side effects, ibuprofen's popularity grew rapidly and became available over-the-counter in 1983 in the UK and 1984 in the US (**Fig. 2.2**). Compared to other painkillers, such as aspirin and acetaminophen (the active ingredient in *Tylenol*), ibuprofen was associated with fewer stomach-related issues, including abdominal pain, nausea, diarrhea, and indigestion. Despite its risks, ibuprofen remains widely used because clinical trials confirmed that ibuprofen had one of the lowest incidences of GI side effects among these common medications.[78] Additionally, studies demonstrated that high doses of ibuprofen were effective for severe pain, while lower doses provided relief for mild to moderate pain.[77]

After extensive clinical trials confirmed its effectiveness and safety, ibuprofen was approved for over-the-counter (OTC) use in the United

States in 1984, making it accessible to millions just 15 years after its initial introduction.[77] Its widespread success even led the World Health Organization (WHO) to designate ibuprofen as an "Essential Medicine" in 1977, recognizing its reliability in reducing pain and inflammation.[79,80]

However, while ibuprofen and other NSAIDs provide significant benefits, they are not without risks. Long-term or improper use can increase the likelihood of cardiovascular issues, liver damage, and kidney impairment.[81] Therefore, understanding both the benefits and potential side effects of ibuprofen is essential for its safe and effective use, whether for occasional pain relief or chronic conditions.

Common Uses of Ibuprofen

Following these key regulatory milestones and its recognition as an essential medicine, ibuprofen is now a go-to remedy for various types of pain, including headaches, postoperative pain, dental pain, and injuries such as sprains or strains (**Fig. 2.3**). It is also widely used as a fever reducer, with research consistently confirming its effectiveness. This dual ability to alleviate pain and lower fever makes ibuprofen particularly useful for treating symptoms of illnesses like upper respiratory tract infections.[82,83] Additionally, ibuprofen's longer-lasting effects (6-8 hours) when treating a child's fever, compared to acetaminophen (4 hours), make it a preferred choice for overnight pain relief.[84]

For targeted relief, ibuprofen can be applied as a topical cream, which allows for a lower dose while still delivering effective pain reduction. Topical ibuprofen is also a safer alternative for individuals with GI issues or those taking medications that may not interact well with oral NSAIDs.[85] Studies have shown that topical NSAIDs, including ibuprofen creams, are highly effective for managing chronic musculoskeletal pain, particularly in conditions like osteoarthritis.[86] However, despite their proven benefits, topical ibuprofen remains available only by prescription, which can be frustrating for those seeking convenient, over-the-counter options. This is due to regulatory reasons: no manufacturer has successfully submitted and received approval for it by the FDA.

Fig. 2.3. Common uses of ibuprofen

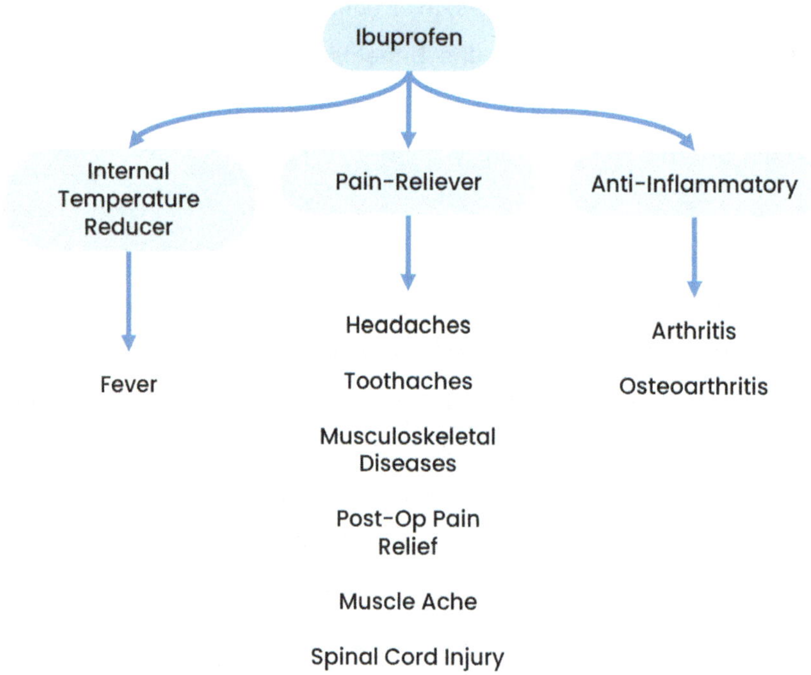

How Safe is Ibuprofen?

Ibuprofen has long been recognized as a safe and reliable option for pain relief. However, as research has expanded, even recommended doses of ibuprofen have been linked to potential adverse effects, including GI issues, cardiovascular problems, kidney damage, and liver complications.[81] Despite these risks, studies indicate that ibuprofen is still safer for the GI tract compared to many other pain relievers, such as acetaminophen (paracetamol) and aspirin.[87]

The most common reasons people use ibuprofen are shown in **Fig. 2.4**.

Fig. 2.4. Most common reasons people use ibuprofen

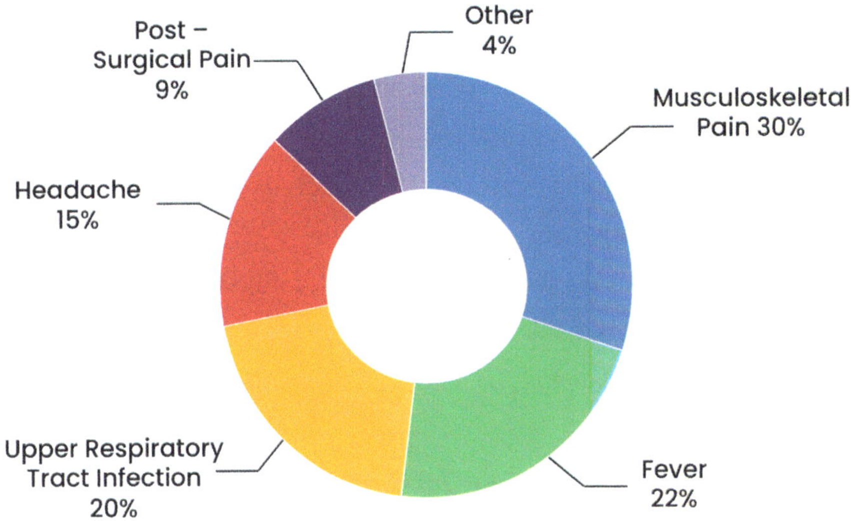

A large-scale study involving over 8,677 patients with acute pain found that ibuprofen was associated with fewer side effects than both aspirin and acetaminophen. For every 100 patients treated, four more experienced side effects with acetaminophen, and five more with aspirin compared to ibuprofen.[81] While these findings reaffirm ibuprofen's overall safety when used correctly, it is essential to recognize its potential risks. Even at standard over-the-counter dosages, ibuprofen has been linked to serious health conditions, including Stevens-Johnson Syndrome (SJS) and Toxic Epidermal Necrolysis (TEN)—both of which can be life-threatening.[88] These rare but severe reactions often occur in individuals with unknown medical predispositions, emphasizing the importance of awareness.

Moreover, misuse or overuse of ibuprofen can lead to severe complications, such as gastritis, GI perforation, acute kidney injury, chronic kidney disease, heart attacks, strokes, and liver damage. While ibuprofen is generally safe, excessive use could result in severe intestinal damage and even death (**Table 2.1**).[89]

These risks highlight the importance of public education on the proper use of ibuprofen and other NSAIDs. While some healthcare professionals have expressed concerns about the OTC availability of NSAIDs, most agree that they are safe when used as directed. However, understanding ibuprofen safety—both the benefits and potential risks—is crucial for safe and effective pain management. This knowledge helps reduce misuse and prevents people from inadvertently exceeding safe dosages or combining incompatible products that increase the risk of serious adverse effects like GI bleeding, kidney damage, or heart complications.[90]

Table 2.1. Factors Influencing Gastrointestinal (GI) Safety of Ibuprofen

Factor	Impact on GI Safety	Reference
Dose	OTC doses (≤1,200 mg/day) pose minimal risk; prescription doses (≥2,400 mg/day) increase ulcer/bleeding risk	91,92
Formulation	Fast-dissolving ibuprofen may cause more gastric damage than tablets	93
Duration	Short-term use (≤7 days) is safer; long-term use elevates the cumulative risk	92
Individual Susceptibility	History of GI disease or advanced age increases vulnerability	91

Bridging the Knowledge Gap

One of the biggest challenges with ibuprofen and OTC pain medications is that many people lack a clear understanding of which pain reliever to take, how much to take, when to take it, and what the potential risks are. This knowledge gap is widespread, as demonstrated by a study involving 140 middle school and 163 high school students. When asked basic questions about ibuprofen, naproxen, and acetaminophen, only 26% of the 303 students correctly identified their uses.[94] Even more concerning, fewer than 1 in 10 students (8%) knew the potential side effects or the risks of overdosing on these medications.

Additionally, only 21% of students correctly answered questions about safely combining OTC drugs.[94] Only 55% understood how to read medication labels, including maximum daily doses and identifying active ingredients across different products. Despite many students learning about OTC medications from parents or doctors, these findings highlight significant gaps in their understanding. However, it's worth noting that this study primarily involved white, male students, so the results may not fully reflect the knowledge levels of more diverse populations. Studies with more diverse populations consistently show varied results, underscoring the importance of inclusive research designs and educational practices.[95]

Another study involving 1,326 people who had taken ibuprofen in the past month found similar, concerning patterns.[26] Participants kept daily medication diaries for a week, and during that period:

- 55% took ibuprofen for three or fewer days, and 16% used it every day.

- Over one-third also used at least one other NSAID (such as aspirin or naproxen), often unaware that they were taking multiple NSAIDs simultaneously.

- 11% exceeded the recommended daily limit, and some even surpassed the single-dose limit.

A survey of runners further underscored this issue, with over 90% stating they wanted more information on the benefits and risks of NSAIDs.[96]

This widespread lack of awareness is a serious concern. It is important to involve pharmacists, schools, or public health campaigns to improve education about commonly used drugs. Every individual needs to understand how to use OTC medications safely, including:

- Proper dosages
- When and how often to take them
- Avoiding dangerous drug interactions

By addressing these knowledge gaps, we can help ensure the safer and more effective use of ibuprofen and other OTC medications.

How to Take Ibuprofen Safely

To ensure safe and effective use of ibuprofen, always take it as directed on the label or as advised by your healthcare provider. The appropriate dose varies based on considerations such as:

- Age and weight
- Reason for taking it (pain relief, fever reduction, inflammation)
- Type of ibuprofen (tablet, liquid, or topical)

Standard General Dosing Recommendations for Ibuprofen

Adults (ages 12 and older):

- **Typical dose**: 200–400 mg by mouth every 4 to 6 hours, as needed for pain or fever.
- **Maximum OTC dose**: 1,200 mg per day (usually 6 tablets of 200 mg).
- **Maximum prescription dose**: 3,200 mg per day. For conditions like arthritis, higher prescription doses (up to 3,200 mg/day) may be used, split into 3 or 4 doses.[97,98]

Children (under 12 years):

- Dosing is based on body weight, not age alone.
- Usual dose: 5–10 mg per kg (2.2 lbs) of body weight every 6 to 8 hours as needed.[99]
- Maximum daily dose: 40 mg per kg per day.[100]
- Do not use in children under 6 months of age unless directed by a healthcare provider.
- Example dosing by weight (using 100 mg/5 mL liquid formulation)[99,101]
    - 12–17 lbs (6–8 kg): 2.5 mL (50 mg) every 6–8 hours
    - 18–23 lbs (8–10.5 kg): 4 mL (80 mg) every 6–8 hours
    - 24–35 lbs (10.5–15.5 kg): 5 mL (100 mg) every 6–8 hours
    - 36–47 lbs (16–21 kg): 7.5 mL (150 mg) every 6–8 hours

- 48–59 lbs (21.5–26.5 kg): 10 mL (200 mg) every 6–8 hours
- 60–71 lbs (27–32 kg): 12.5 mL (250 mg) every 6–8 hours
- 72–95 lbs (32.5–43 kg): 15 mL (300 mg) every 6–8 hours
- Over 96 lbs (43.5 kg): 20 mL (400 mg) every 6–8 hours

Special Notes:

- For children, always use the dosing device provided with the medication for accuracy.
- Ibuprofen should be given with food or milk to reduce stomach upset.
- Do not exceed recommended doses or duration without medical advice.

For best results and to avoid stomach irritation, follow these guidelines:

- **Take ibuprofen with food:** Avoid taking it on an empty stomach. Instead, take it with or just after a meal, along with water.[102] This helps reduce the risk of gastric irritation and ulcers.
- **Avoid alcohol:** Combining ibuprofen with alcohol can increase the risk of stomach bleeding and liver damage.[51]
- **Know when to expect relief:** While ibuprofen starts relieving pain 20-30 minutes after oral intake, it can take more than four weeks to reduce inflammation fully when used for chronic conditions.[103,104]

By understanding how ibuprofen works and following these safety tips, you can maximize its benefits while minimizing potential risks.

Who Should Avoid Ibuprofen Without Medical Consultation?

While ibuprofen is generally safe for most people when used at low doses, certain individuals should avoid it unless advised otherwise by a healthcare professional (**Fig. 2.5**). These include people with:

- Asthma
- Crohn's disease
- Kidney or liver problems
- Lupus
- Peripheral arterial disease
- A history of stroke or stomach bleeding
- Moderate heart failure
- Uncontrolled high blood pressure
- A stomach ulcer
- Chickenpox or shingles
- Hypersensitivity to aspirin or other NSAIDs

Additionally, individuals who are pregnant, trying to conceive, or taking low-dose aspirin for heart health should consult their doctor before using ibuprofen.[105,106] You'll find a more in-depth discussion about why these and similar conditions raise the risk when using ibuprofen in later chapters.

After reading this information, you might feel a bit cautious about using ibuprofen. However, ibuprofen is highly effective for most people when used correctly and at the appropriate dose for short periods. The key is knowing how to use it safely, which we'll explore in the following chapters.

Fig. 2.5. Known conditions that could worsen ibuprofen's side effects

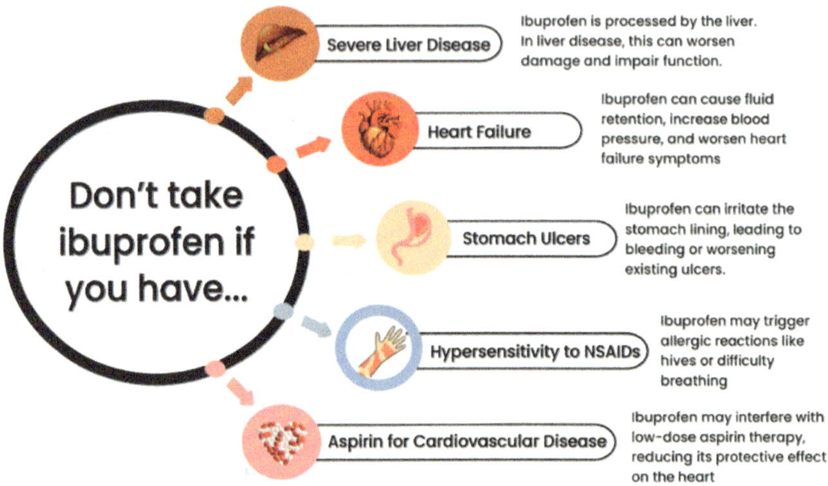

Why Age and Weight Matter

When you buy ibuprofen at a grocery or drugstore, the label typically recommends 200 mg every 4 hours for anyone over the age of 12. But does this one-size-fits-all dose work the same for everyone?

Consider this:

- Should a 5′2″, 105-pound woman take the same dose as a 6′4″, 210-pound man?
- Does body weight affect how much ibuprofen enters the bloodstream and tissues?

The answer is yes—weight matters. A lighter person taking 200 mg will have more ibuprofen per pound of body weight, meaning the medication's effects could be stronger compared to a heavier person taking the same dose.

Finding the Right Dose

- If you weigh 120 pounds or less, consider starting with 100 mg to see if it's effective before taking the full 200 mg. Some members of the Gomes lab use 100 mg ibuprofen tablets obtained from the children's section of pharmacies.

- For larger individuals, the standard 200 mg dose may be appropriate, but always follow the recommended maximum daily limit.

Understanding how age and weight impact ibuprofen's effects can help you use it more safely and effectively.

Beneficial Roles of Ibuprofen

At this point, you might be wondering: If ibuprofen carries risks, why is it so widely recommended? The answer lies in its proven benefits for managing fever, pain, inflammation, and various health conditions. It's also important to note that few if any medications are entirely risk-free. However, these risks can be mitigated with proper knowledge of its usage.

Ibuprofen and Fever

Fever is generally defined as a body temperature above 37°C (98.6°F), with 38°C (100.4°F) or higher considered significant. Ibuprofen is a widely used treatment for fever reduction in both adults and children, whether taken orally or intravenously.

How Effective is Ibuprofen for Fever?

In Adults:

A study tested intravenous ibuprofen in doses of 100 mg, 200 mg, and 400 mg on critically and non-critically ill patients.[107] Results showed that 400 mg was the most effective, reducing fever below 38.33°C (101°F) within 4 hours and keeping it lower for up to 24 hours.[107] The study confirmed ibuprofen's effectiveness for fever but was limited to short-term safety outcomes without assessing long-term risks. While short-term use is generally well tolerated, long-term use carries additional risks, such as GI complications that weren't evaluated in this particular fever study.[107]

In Children:

A separate study compared intravenous ibuprofen (10 mg/kg) and acetaminophen in children with fevers above 38.3°C (100.94°F).[108] Findings revealed that ibuprofen was more effective than acetaminophen, significantly reducing fever within 2 to 4 hours.[108]

When Ibuprofen May Not Work

While ibuprofen effectively lowers fevers, it doesn't prevent all types. For example, a study on children undergoing fiber-optic bronchoscopy (a lung examination) found no difference in fever prevention between ibuprofen syrup (10 mg/kg) and a placebo.[109]

Ibuprofen remains a powerful tool for fever management. However, its effectiveness depends on the condition being treated, individual factors, and medical conditions, making proper usage and medical guidance essential.

Ibuprofen and Pain Relief

Pain management is one of ibuprofen's most well-documented benefits, particularly in postoperative recovery and dental procedures. While opioids are often prescribed after surgery, they carry risks of addiction and side effects. Fortunately, NSAIDs like ibuprofen provide an effective and safer alternative.[110]

Managing Postoperative Pain

Postoperative pain affects about 80% of patients after surgery, with many experiencing moderate to severe discomfort.[110] Research has shown that ibuprofen is highly effective in reducing pain following various surgical procedures. It does this by inhibiting cyclooxygenase (COX) enzymes and reducing the production of prostaglandins, which is discussed in detail in the next chapter.

Study: Ibuprofen vs. Acetaminophen vs. Opioids

A double-blind study examined 105 patients recovering from carpal tunnel surgery, comparing 600 mg ibuprofen, 500 mg acetaminophen, and 5 mg oxycodone *(an opioid)* for pain relief.[111] The findings were significant: Ibuprofen and acetaminophen users reported the lowest pain levels.[111] Fifty percent of ibuprofen users felt well-managed with 10 pills, compared to 43.2% in the oxycodone group.[111] None of the ibuprofen users requested stronger medication.[111]

Study: Intravenous (IV) Ibuprofen for Surgery Pain Relief

A separate trial explored the effect of a single 800 mg IV dose of ibuprofen on 50 patients undergoing septorhinoplasty *(a nose and nasal septum correction surgery)*.[112] Results showed: Patients reported lower pain scores for 24 hours after surgery.[112]

Study: Ibuprofen Reducing Opioid Use

Another study analyzed pain management after radical cervical cancer surgery.[113] 60 female patients were divided into three groups:

1. Placebo
2. 400 mg IV ibuprofen
3. 800 mg IV ibuprofen *(every 6 hours for 48 hours)*

Findings:

- The 800 mg group used significantly less morphine (an opioid) for pain relief.[113]
- No significant side effects (renal toxicity, gastrointestinal bleeding, etc.) were observed.[113]

This suggests that higher doses of IV ibuprofen can effectively reduce opioid dependence after surgery, helping to minimize opioid-related risks. Reduced opioid use is preferred as it is associated with addiction, nausea, and sedation. Other studies support the use of ibuprofen instead of opioids for postoperative pain management.[114,115] Patients should always consult their healthcare provider before switching from opioids to ibuprofen or any other NSAID, as not all individuals are suitable candidates for ibuprofen use due to preexisting conditions, potential drug interactions, and other potential risks.

Ibuprofen for Dental Pain

Ibuprofen is also widely used for pain relief following dental procedures, such as root canals and tooth extractions, where discomfort can be severe.

Study: Ibuprofen vs. Opioids After Root Canal

A 2008 prospective, randomized, double-blind clinical trial involving 43 patients compared the effectiveness of 600 mg ibuprofen, a placebo, and the opioid combination pentazocine/naloxone for pain relief following root canal treatment. Patients took their assigned medication every 6 hours for 24 hours, and pain was assessed using a visual analog scale (VAS) at 0, 6, 12, 18, and 24 hours after treatment.[116] The Visual Analog Scale is a simple, reliable, and valid tool for measuring subjective symptom intensity by having patients indicate their experience along a continuous line, which is then quantified by measuring the distance from the scale's zero point to the patient's mark.

Results of the 2008 trial showed:

- Ibuprofen provided statistically greater pain relief at 6 and 12 hours, outperforming the placebo.[116]
- Ibuprofen was just as effective as the opioid medication.[116]
- No difference in effectiveness was noted between male and female participants.[116]

Study: Ibuprofen Liquid Gels for Tooth Extractions

In another randomized, double-blind study 200 mg and 400 mg ibuprofen liquid gels were compared against 1000 mg acetaminophen and a placebo for pain relief after impacted molar removal.[117] This study used the Visual Analog Scale to measure pain intensity.

Results found:

- Ibuprofen (200 mg and 400 mg) provided superior pain relief within 2 hours, outperforming both acetaminophen and the placebo.[117] Ibuprofen 400 mg achieved 1.7 times greater pain relief than acetaminophen.
- Even after 6 hours, ibuprofen users reported less pain compared to the placebo group.[117] Ibuprofen 400 mg provided 2.1 times greater overall pain relief than acetaminophen at 6 hours.

Ibuprofen is a highly effective and safer alternative to opioids for postoperative and dental pain relief. Studies consistently suggest that proper ibuprofen dosing reduces pain, lowers opioid use, and has minimal side effects.

Ibuprofen and Menstrual Pain

Menstrual pain, commonly experienced as cramping, is caused by the release of prostaglandins—bioactive compounds that trigger uterine contractions. NSAIDs, like ibuprofen help relieve this pain by blocking the enzyme responsible for prostaglandin production, effectively addressing the root cause of discomfort.

How Effective Is Ibuprofen for Menstrual Pain?

To evaluate NSAIDs' effectiveness in treating menstrual pain, researchers often conduct meta-analyses—studies that combine data from multiple previously published studies. This approach increases sample sizes, offering stronger, more reliable conclusions than individual studies alone.

One meta-analysis examined over 5,800 females, aged 15.8 to 32.2 years, and found that NSAIDs reduce menstrual pain by approximately 30% compared to a placebo.[118] A 30% reduction is considered a moderate effect and can mean the difference between being housebound and being able to go grocery shopping, work part-time, or engage in light exercise. While the meta-analysis includes many studies using different ibuprofen dosages, the most commonly used and studied dosage for menstrual pain relief is 400 mg taken three times daily during the days of pain.

The effectiveness of ibuprofen varies depending on the dosage. A recent randomized controlled trial compared 400 mg and 800 mg IV doses of ibuprofen in women with primary dysmenorrhea and found no significant difference in pain relief between these two dosages over the first hour, suggesting that higher doses do not necessarily provide additional benefit for most patients.[119] This supports the use of standard dosing (200–400 mg) as effective for most individuals. However, dosing protocols in meta-analyses can vary, and not all studies specify exact dosages, which is a limitation that should be acknowledged when interpreting pooled results.

Meta-analyses have shown that ibuprofen is not significantly more effective than other NSAIDs, such as aspirin or naproxen, for menstrual pain relief.[118]

These findings emphasize the importance of evidence-based medicine, enabling healthcare providers to make informed treatment recommendations based on robust data. Ibuprofen's availability, relative safety, and patient satisfaction help explain why it remains a go-to NSAID, even when its efficacy is similar to that of other options.

Ibuprofen for Headaches and Migraines

Ibuprofen has been widely studied for its effectiveness in treating migraines, offering relief for both pain and associated symptoms, such as nausea.

How Effective is Ibuprofen for Migraines?

A study involving 660 adults (aged 18 to 84) tested the impact of nonprescription ibuprofen in doses of 200 mg, 400 mg, or a placebo.[120] The results showed that both 200 mg and 400 mg doses significantly relieved migraine pain.[120] Even the lower 200 mg dose provided effective relief (41.7% of patients reported mild or no pain after 2 hours), emphasizing ibuprofen's potency.[120] The 400 mg dose resulted in 40.8% of patients reporting mild or no pain after 2 hours. Beyond pain relief, ibuprofen also reduces migraine-related symptoms, such as nausea.[120]

These findings highlight ibuprofen as a valuable, accessible option for migraine management, especially for individuals seeking a nonprescription solution.

Ibuprofen and Osteoarthritis Management

Osteoarthritis, the most common form of arthritis, primarily affects older adults, causing joint pain, stiffness, and reduced mobility.[121] Studies have shown that ibuprofen is an effective pain reliever for osteoarthritis, providing a 50–60% improvement in pain and function compared to placebo.[122] However, ibuprofen and other NSAIDs carry potential risks, including gastrointestinal and cardiovascular side effects, especially with long-term use or in higher doses. The use of ibuprofen for osteoarthritis should be carefully considered based on individual patient risk factors and in comparison with other available treatments.

How Effective is Ibuprofen for Osteoarthritis?

- A meta-analysis found that ibuprofen significantly reduced pain and improved joint stiffness in knee osteoarthritis patients. The effect size of ibuprofen on osteoarthritis was 0.44, which suggests a moderate reduction in pain.[123]

- Ibuprofen provides better pain relief than acetaminophen, which lacks anti-inflammatory properties.[123,124]

- However, ibuprofen increases the risk of GI and cardiovascular complications compared to other non-NSAID pain relievers, as discussed in other parts of this book.

Risks and Considerations

Risks

- Non-selective NSAIDs like ibuprofen (except for naproxen) may increase the risk of heart attacks.
- Ibuprofen can interfere with aspirin's heart-protective benefits, making it less ideal for some patients.[125]
- Medical organizations, including the Osteoarthritis Research Society International and the American Pain Society, often recommend acetaminophen as the first-line treatment for osteoarthritis in patients with higher GI or cardiovascular risks.[125] They also recommend the use of proton pump inhibitors for patients with higher GI risk.

Considerations

Ibuprofen inhibits COX enzymes, reducing prostaglandins that initiate and amplify inflammation and pain.[126] While this mechanism is the same for both types of arthritis, rheumatoid arthritis involves systemic autoimmune-driven inflammation, whereas osteoarthritis is localized, joint degeneration. Ibuprofen alleviates symptoms in both conditions but does not alter the disease progression of either rheumatoid arthritis or osteoarthritis. It provides rapid relief for pain, stiffness, and swelling. It is often used short-term while waiting for slower-acting disease-modifying antirheumatic drugs (DMARDs) to take effect.[127]

DMARDs (e.g., methotrexate) and biologics (e.g., TNF inhibitors) are the preferred first-line treatments for osteoarthritis. These target the immune system to slow joint damage and disease progression, but take 6-12 weeks to be fully effective.[128] While these drugs are better for long-term outcomes, some of these drugs carry risks such as immunosuppression.[129]

Hence, while ibuprofen is a valuable tool for immediate osteoarthritis symptom relief, for long-term disease control DMARDs and biologics are better. Its role is supportive rather than curative.

Ibuprofen is effective for osteoarthritis pain relief, though potential risks should still be considered. Treatment should be tailored to the patient's needs, balancing pain management with individual health risks.

Ibuprofen in Rheumatoid Arthritis Treatment

Rheumatoid arthritis (RA) is a chronic autoimmune disease where the immune system mistakenly attacks joint tissues, leading to inflammation, pain, and long-term joint damage. [130-134]

Role of Ibuprofen in RA Management

- Ibuprofen helps reduce inflammation and alleviate pain, but it does not treat the underlying immune dysfunction.[135,136]
- It is approved for temporary relief of acute pain associated with RA, making it useful for short-term symptom management while waiting for long-term treatments to take effect.[137-143]
- It is often combined with disease-modifying anti-rheumatic drugs (DMARDs), which target the root cause of RA.[137-143]

Considerations & Risks

- NSAIDs, including ibuprofen, are not a cure for RA—they only help manage symptoms.[137-143]

- About 1% of RA patients may experience serious GI complications, such as bleeding.[51]
- Prolonged use of ibuprofen increases the risk of cardiovascular and GI side effects, so it should be used cautiously, especially in high doses.[51,144]
- Long-term use of ibuprofen is associated with kidney damage, fluid retention, or hypertension.
- Some studies suggest that NSAIDs might increase blood levels and toxicity of some DMARDs, such as methotrexate.[145] However, the clinical significance of this interaction is still being investigated.

Ibuprofen is a helpful short-term pain reliever for RA flare-ups, but it should be used alongside DMARDs for long-term treatment. Patients should consult their doctor to weigh the benefits and risks of long-term NSAID use.

Ibuprofen in Cystic Fibrosis Treatment

Cystic fibrosis (CF) is a hereditary disease that mainly targets the respiratory and digestive systems, worsening over time. Chronic lung inflammation is a key driver of lung damage in CF, making inflammation control a crucial treatment goal.[146]

How Ibuprofen Helps

Ibuprofen has been studied for its anti-inflammatory effects in CF patients, aiming to reduce lung inflammation and slow disease progression.[146] A four-year, double-blind, placebo-controlled trial involving 85 CF patients with mild lung disease (ages 5-39) found that those taking ibuprofen orally twice daily for four years had a slower decline in lung function compared to the placebo group.[146] The ibuprofen dose was individually adjusted to achieve peak plasma concentrations of 50–100 μg/mL, a range shown to inhibit neutrophil migration and thus reduce inflammation.

Lung function tests confirmed that ibuprofen-treated patients experienced significantly less decline (39.7% less) in forced expiratory volume in one second (FEV1) than the control group, suggesting its potential to preserve lung health.[146]

Considerations & Future Research

Determining the right dose for different age groups is complex because metabolic rates, body composition, and organ function vary with age. However, dosage consistency is crucial, as ibuprofen levels need to be adjusted based on age to maintain similar plasma concentrations, which enhances clinical benefits and safety.[146] Further research is needed to determine long-term safety and effectiveness, particularly regarding side effects in CF patients.[146]

Ibuprofen shows promise as a treatment for slowing lung damage in cystic fibrosis patients. While more research is needed, these findings suggest it could be a valuable addition to CF management.

Can Ibuprofen Reduce Cancer Risk?

Chronic inflammation is a major factor in cancer development, as it weakens the immune system and creates an environment where cancer can thrive. Due to its anti-inflammatory properties, ibuprofen—along with other NSAIDs—has been studied for its potential role in reducing the risk of tumor formation. Research suggests that ibuprofen may help block certain cell signaling pathways that drive cancer growth.[147,148] However, its effectiveness depends on proper dosage, and more studies are needed to determine its long-term safety and impact.

One of the most intriguing discoveries about ibuprofen is its ability to trigger cancer cell death. Studies have shown that ibuprofen can induce programmed cell death in various cancer cells. For instance, research on human prostate cancer cells found that ibuprofen significantly reduced cancer cell survival.[149] Similarly, experiments on gastric cancer cells revealed that ibuprofen promoted cell death, potentially limiting the spread of cancer.[150]

A groundbreaking discovery also found that ibuprofen can trigger a unique form of programmed cell death called ferroptosis, which specifically targets tumor cells.[151] In animal studies, ibuprofen not only encouraged ferroptosis but also reduced the activity of genes that regulate this process.[151] While scientists are still unraveling the exact mechanisms, these findings suggest that ibuprofen could play a role in future cancer treatments. However, even though the research is promising, it is important to note that it is still in its early stages and not yet applicable in clinical cancer treatment.

Final Thoughts

Ibuprofen is widely recognized for its ability to reduce fever, relieve pain, and control inflammation, making it a versatile option for conditions such as arthritis, muscle aches, and post-surgical pain—and often serving as a safer alternative to opioids for short-term use. However, like any medication, ibuprofen carries risks, particularly for the heart and GI system. Long-term use or high doses can increase the risk of heart attack, stroke, stomach bleeding, and kidney or liver damage.

To minimize these risks, it is best to use the lowest effective dose for the shortest necessary duration—for example, a lower dose such as 200 mg to 400 mg may often suffice for mild pain or fever, and doses as low as 100 mg can sometimes be effective for headaches, especially in sensitive individuals. Responsible use also means following dosage guidelines, being aware of potential drug interactions (such as with alcohol or blood pressure medications), and consulting a healthcare professional if you have underlying health conditions or are taking other medications.

Studies suggest ibuprofen may have additional roles in medicine, including potential applications in cancer treatment or prevention. Some studies indicate that ibuprofen can inhibit cancer cell survival by blocking specific signaling pathways and inducing cell death. While these findings are promising, more research is needed to determine how ibuprofen might best fit into cancer treatment paradigms, whether as an adjunct to existing therapies—as a tool for symptom management, or as a preventive agent in at-risk populations.

The key to using ibuprofen safely is understanding when and how to take it, being mindful of its limitations, and staying informed about new developments in its use. With proper knowledge and caution, ibuprofen remains a powerful and accessible tool for pain and inflammation management.

Key Takeaways:

- Ibuprofen effectively reduces fever, pain, and inflammation, even at low doses (e.g., 200 mg for fever or pain).
- A 100 mg dose, often used for children, can also be effective for adults with mild headaches or pain.

- For joint pain, topical ibuprofen (gels or creams) is preferred over oral tablets to reduce systemic side effects.
- Ibuprofen works better than acetaminophen for osteoarthritis because of its anti-inflammatory benefits.
- As a safer alternative to opioids, ibuprofen can help with postoperative pain relief, but it should be used at the lowest effective dose to minimize GI risks.

Most Important Takeaway: *Use ibuprofen as needed, follow medical guidelines, and take the lowest effective dose. Always consider safer alternatives when appropriate, and consult a healthcare professional if you have questions about the best option for your situation.*

Chapter 3
How Ibuprofen Fights Pain and Inflammation

Most people know that ibuprofen relieves pain and inflammation, but few understand how it actually works inside the body. Upon ingestion, ibuprofen initiates a series of biological processes that work to reduce pain and swelling. By targeting key processes in the body, it not only blocks discomfort but also helps regulate the body's response to injury. In this chapter, we'll explore the science behind how ibuprofen works and why it's such a trusted remedy.

Ibuprofen's Mechanism of Action: Blocking Pain at the Source

To understand ibuprofen's effects, we first need to look at arachidonic acid, a fatty acid stored in cell membranes. This acid usually comes either from our food or from omega-6 fatty acids in the body. It plays a key role in triggering inflammation, pain, fever, and even blood clotting.

When cells are damaged or stressed, special enzymes called phospholipases break down cell membranes to release arachidonic acid. This sets off a chain reaction leading to the production of molecules that cause pain and swelling.

Once freed, cyclooxygenases (COX-1 and COX-2) and other specialized proteins convert arachidonic acid into a variety of biologically active molecules, including:

- **Prostaglandins** - Trigger inflammation, pain, and fever.[152]
- **Thromboxanes** - Involved in blood clotting and vasoconstriction.
- **Leukotrienes** - Involved in allergic reactions and inflammation, particularly in the lungs.
- **Lipoxins** - Reduce inflammation and promote healing.

Fig. 3.1. General overview of ibuprofen's effect on COX-1 and COX-2 enzymes.

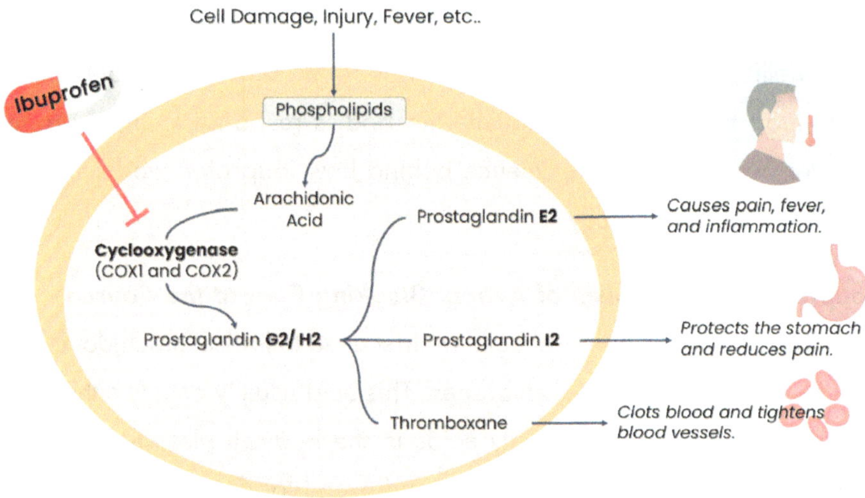

Ibuprofen works by blocking COX enzymes (COX-1 and COX-2), which are responsible for producing prostaglandins—chemical messengers that trigger pain, inflammation, and fever.[153-155] By binding to the enzyme's active site, ibuprofen prevents arachidonic acid from converting into prostaglandins, reducing swelling and discomfort.[156] This also limits vasodilation (blood vessel widening) and decreases immune cell activity in inflamed areas.[152] However, since ibuprofen's interaction with COX enzymes is reversible, its effects wear off as the drug is metabolized.

Importantly, the inhibition of COX-1 and COX-2 also helps explain why ibuprofen can cause side effects (such as stomach irritation, bleeding, and kidney problems), especially when used frequently or over long periods.

Why Do We Have Two COX Enzymes?

Since ibuprofen blocks both COX-1 and COX-2, it is classified as a non-selective COX inhibitor. While both enzymes contribute to inflammation,[157] they have distinct roles:

- **COX-1**: The "housekeeping" enzyme; it is always active in most tissues. It protects the stomach lining, supports blood clotting, and regulates kidney function.
- **COX-2**: Mostly inactive under normal conditions but becomes active during injury, infection, or inflammation. It is the main target of anti-inflammatory drugs since it directly contributes to pain and swelling.

Since COX-1 is essential for stomach protection, scientists avoid developing drugs that block it exclusively. Doing so could lead to ulcers and stomach bleeding, a common side effect of long-term NSAID use.

Ibuprofen and the Endocannabinoid System: A Surprising Link

One of ibuprofen's lesser-known effects is its interaction with the endocannabinoid system, a complex network that regulates pain, mood, appetite, and immune response.[156,158] Normally, COX-2 converts an endocannabinoid called 2-arachidonoylglycerol into compounds that influence pain and inflammation. However, ibuprofen selectively blocks this reaction, altering how the body processes pain.[159,160]

This discovery has sparked interest in developing ibuprofen-like drugs that specifically target the endocannabinoid system. Such medications could provide more precise pain relief with fewer side effects than traditional NSAIDs. However, ongoing research is needed to fully understand how ibuprofen interacts with COX-2 in real-world conditions.[156] **Table 3** shows a comparison of how COX-1 and COX-2 respond differently to fatty acids.

Table 3.1. Preferences of substrates for COX Enzymes

Cyclo-oxygenase	Preferences
COX-1	Exhibits a preference for oxygenating arachidonic acid.[161,162] This preference is the main reason why ibuprofen contributes to GI side effects (via reduced protective prostaglandins).
COX-2	Effectively catalyzes the oxygenation of various fatty acids, including arachidonic acid, eicosapentaenoic acid, and linoleic acid.[163,164] Facilitates the oxygenation of endocannabinoid substrates such as 2-arachidonoylglycerol and arachidonoylethanolamide.[165,166] COX-2's broader substrate range allows ibuprofen to simultaneously target inflammation (via arachidonic acid suppression) and amplify pain relief (via endocannabinoid retention).

Effects of Ibuprofen Use

Ibuprofen helps manage a range of symptoms by influencing various physiological processes in the body. Below are some of the key ways ibuprofen impacts these symptoms:

1. **Reducing Inflammation**
    - By limiting the recruitment of immune cells to the affected area, ibuprofen helps prevent excessive tissue damage (**Fig. 3.1**).[167]

2. **Relieving Pain**
    - Prostaglandins increase pain sensitivity. By inhibiting their production, ibuprofen helps reduce pain perception and reduces pain signals in the nervous system.[168]

3. **Lowering Fever**
    - Ibuprofen prevents prostaglandins from affecting the hypothalamus (the brain region that regulates body temperature), leading to reduced heat production and lower fever.[169] [170,171]

4. **Affecting Blood Clotting and Circulation**
    - Ibuprofen inhibits platelet aggregation (clumping), preventing blood from clotting.[172]
    - In certain situations, ibuprofen functions as a vasoconstrictor by inhibiting the vasodilating prostacyclin produced by COX-2.[126] Like other NSAIDs, it can decrease kidney blood flow, potentially affecting fluid balance and blood pressure.[173]

5. **Modulating Immune Response**
   - Ibuprofen can suppress certain immune cell activities, reducing inflammation, but also affecting how the immune system responds to injury or infection.[136,174,175]

6. **Interaction with the Endocannabinoid System**
   - Possible Cannabinoid Receptor Involvement: Some evidence suggests ibuprofen interacts with CB1 and CB2 cannabinoid receptors, which are involved in pain regulation and inflammation.[176]
   - Inhibits Fatty Acid Amide Hydrolase (FAAH): FAAH is an enzyme that breaks down anandamide, a key endocannabinoid. By inhibiting FAAH, ibuprofen may increase endocannabinoid levels, further helping with pain and inflammation.[177]
   - Inhibiting FAAH enhances pain relief by preventing the breakdown of endocannabinoids like anandamide (AEA), allowing these molecules to accumulate and activate cannabinoid receptors that modulate pain signaling.[178]

7. **Scavenges Free Radicals**
   - Ibuprofen can help neutralize harmful molecules like hydroxyl radicals and nitric oxide radicals, which contribute to tissue damage during inflammation.[179]

8. **Regulates Nitric Oxide (NO) Production**
   - While it doesn't directly block NO production, ibuprofen influences mRNA and protein levels related to nitric oxide synthesis, affecting NO production. NO induces

vasodilation, enhancing blood flow and regulating blood pressure. NO also inhibits platelet aggregation inflammation and maintains endothelial integrity.[136,180-182]

A Closer Look at Prostaglandins

Much of ibuprofen's effectiveness stems from its ability to block the production of prostaglandins—which are lipid molecules that play a central role in inflammation, as well as mediating pain and fever responses. For example, in conditions like osteoarthritis and rheumatoid arthritis, excessive prostaglandin production leads to persistent joint pain, swelling, and reduced mobility. By reducing prostaglandin levels, ibuprofen helps decrease inflammation, alleviate pain, and improve joint function, as demonstrated by significant improvements in symptom scores and physical functioning in clinical trials.[122,183]

If you're eager to dive into the finer details, keep reading! But if you're ready to move on, feel free to skip ahead to the next chapter, which focuses on ibuprofen's role in fighting cancer.

Prostaglandins: The Key Players in Pain and Inflammation

Prostaglandins and thromboxane A2, collectively known as prostanoids, are produced through a complex chain of enzymatic reactions involving phospholipases, COX enzymes, and specialized synthases. While both COX-1 and COX-2 contribute to prostanoid production, they serve distinct functions:

- COX-1: Maintains normal bodily processes, such as protecting the stomach lining and regulating blood clotting.
- COX-2: Is primarily activated in response to injury, infection, or inflammation, driving pain and swelling.

Since prostanoids are unstable and act locally, their effects are highly targeted—influencing only the area where they are produced.[184] This localized action explains why ibuprofen's anti-inflammatory effects are strongest at the site of pain or swelling.

Prostaglandin Biosynthesis and Function

Prostaglandins are powerful signaling molecules that play a central role in regulating inflammation, pain, and other physiological processes. Their synthesis begins with arachidonic acid, which undergoes a COX-catalyzed reaction to form an unstable intermediate called prostaglandin H2 (PGH2) (**Fig. 3.2**). From PGH2, the body produces five primary bioactive prostaglandins, each with distinct functions:

- **PGE2** – Major player in pain, fever, and inflammation.
- **PGF2α** – Involved in smooth muscle contraction (e.g., in labor and bronchial airways).
- **PGD2** – Plays a role in allergic reactions and sleep regulation.
- **PGI2** (prostacyclin) – Prevents blood clot formation and regulates blood vessel dilation.
- **Thromboxane A2** (TXA2) – Promotes platelet aggregation and blood vessel constriction.

Understanding how these molecules act in the body is key to appreciating their clinical significance. Once synthesized, each prostaglandin binds to its own set of specific G protein-coupled receptors (GPCRs) on the surface of target cells. This binding triggers a cascade of intracellular signals that ultimately shape how our bodies respond to injury or illness.

For example, when PGE2 binds to EP receptors on nerve endings, it lowers the threshold for pain signals, making us more sensitive to pain. In the brain, PGE2 can raise body temperature, leading to fever. In inflamed tissues, it promotes blood flow and attracts immune cells, fueling the redness and swelling typical of inflammation. This is why PGE2 is a major target for pain relievers like ibuprofen. By blocking its production, they can reduce pain, fever, and inflammation all at once.

Other prostaglandins are also critically important. For instance, excessive PGF2α can contribute to menstrual cramps, while overactive thromboxane A2 can increase the risk of blood clots after surgery.

By understanding the specific actions of each prostaglandin, researchers can design more targeted therapies for a wide range of conditions—from arthritis and allergies to post-surgical pain and even cancer.

Fig. 3.2. Diagram showing biological processes regulated by different prostaglandins created by COX-1 and COX-2 enzymes

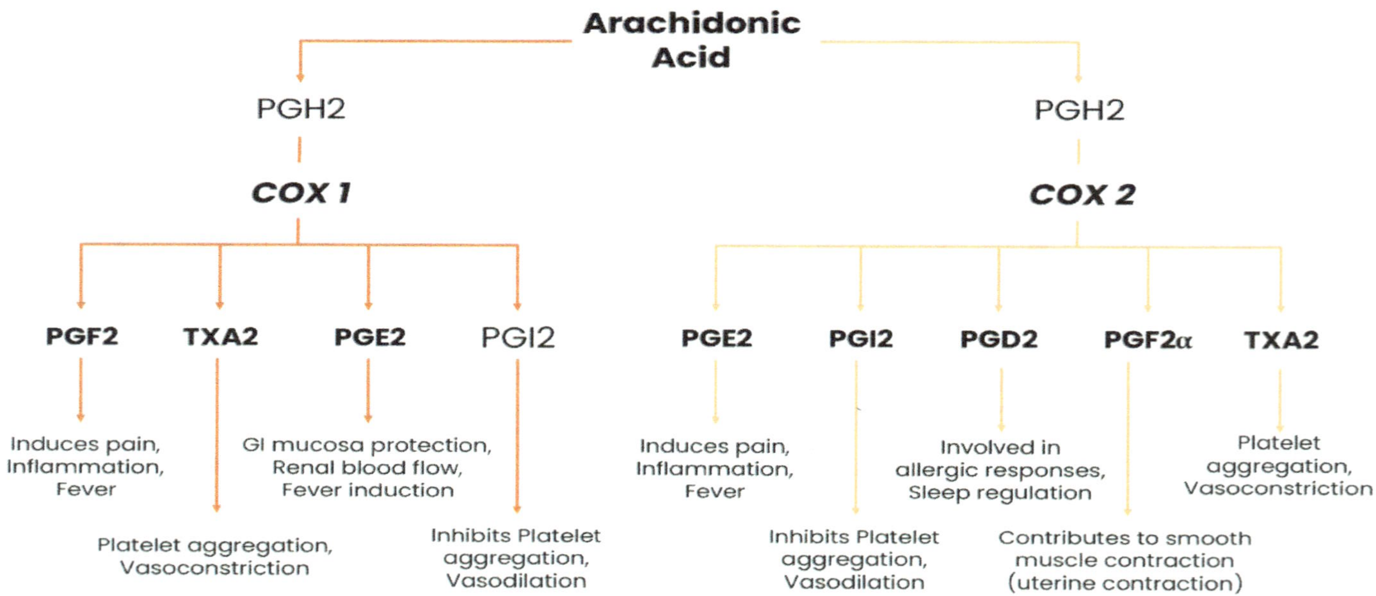

How Prostaglandins Activate Cellular Responses

Once prostaglandins bind to their respective GPCRs, they initiate different signaling pathways that regulate key cellular functions:

- **cAMP Production** – Some prostanoid receptors activate adenylyl cyclase, an enzyme that converts ATP into cyclic adenosine monophosphate (cAMP). Higher cAMP levels modulate gene expression, metabolism, and inflammation.
- **Calcium Signaling** – Other receptors influence phosphatidylinositol metabolism, increasing intracellular calcium levels. Phosphatidylinositol helps create messenger molecules (like inositol 1,4,5-trisphosphate (IP3)) that initiate the release of calcium from the sarcoplasmic reticulum. Calcium is essential for muscle contraction, neurotransmitter release, and immune responses.
- **Inflammatory Cascade** – Some pathways activate phospholipase C (which produces IP3) and Rho guanine nucleotide exchange factors, leading to cellular changes such as swelling, movement, and shape alterations. Rho guanine nucleotide exchange factors help turn on proteins that let the cell move or change in response to signals.

PGE2 and Inflammation

Prostaglandin E2 (PGE2) is the most abundant and influential prostaglandin in the inflammatory response. It plays a key role in causing:

- Redness (vasodilation)
- Swelling (increased vascular permeability)
- Pain (sensitization of nerve endings)

How PGE2 is Synthesized

PGE2 is produced from PGH2 by prostaglandin E synthases, including:

- Cytosolic PGE synthase (cPGES)
- Microsomal PGE synthase-1 (mPGES-1)

Studies show that blocking mPGES-1 significantly reduces inflammation in animal models, highlighting its role in inflammatory diseases.[185]

The Role of COX-2 in PGE2 Production

During inflammation, COX-2 is the primary enzyme responsible for PGE2 synthesis. By blocking COX-2 activity, ibuprofen prevents the conversion of arachidonic acid to PGH2, leading to a decrease in PGE2 levels at sites of inflammation. This reduction in PGE2 interrupts the cascade of events that normally amplify pain signals, such as increased vascular permeability (causing swelling), and recruitment of immune cells. This mechanism is fundamental to ibuprofen's effectiveness as a pain reliever and an anti-inflammatory.

Balancing Efficacy and Side Effects

While NSAIDs relieve inflammation, they can also cause GI issues by blocking COX-1, which helps protect the stomach lining. This has led to the development of selective COX-2 inhibitors, which:

- Provide anti-inflammatory benefits
- Reduce the risk of GI complications

However, some COX-2 inhibitors have been linked to cardiovascular risks, emphasizing the delicate balance between safety and efficacy in anti-inflammatory drug development.

PGI2 and Inflammation

Prostacyclin (PGI2) is a key player in cardiovascular health and inflammation regulation, helping to:

- Maintain blood vessel function
- Regulate blood flow
- Control inflammatory responses

How PGI2 is Produced

PGI2 is produced in a two-step process.

1. In the first step, COX enzymes break down arachidonic acid into an intermediate (PGH2)

2. Second, an enzyme called PGIS converts this intermediate molecule into PGI2.

While some PGI2 is produced by COX-1, COX-2 is the primary source of PGI_2 during instances of inflammation or injury. As mentioned earlier, COX-1 is always active and supports normal bodily functions, whereas COX-2 becomes more active during inflammation or tissue injury. Under such conditions, COX-2 more frequently works alongside PGIS, resulting in increased PGI2 production.

This production pathway links PGI2 to several important processes in the body, including the regulation of blood vessels, the immune response, and the formation of blood clots.

Factors That Influence PGI2 Production

Several physiological and pathological factors affect PGI2 levels:

Thrombin (Blood Clotting Signals)

- Boosts PGI2 production in endothelial cells
- Helps prevent excessive clotting, ensuring smooth blood flow

Oxidized LDL (Harmful Cholesterol)

- Increases COX-2 activity, triggering inflammation
- Contributes to atherosclerosis (plaque buildup in arteries)

Shear Stress (Blood Flow Against Vessel Walls)

- Regulates PGI2 levels in response to blood movement
- Healthy circulation increases COX-2 activity, promoting vascular health

Hypoxia (Low Oxygen Levels)

- Stimulates PGI2 production
- Helps adjust blood vessels to changing oxygen demands

Inflammatory Cytokines (TNF-α, IL-1β)

- Enhance PGI2 production
- Plays a role in immune responses and vascular inflammation

Balancing Inflammation and Cardiovascular Health

PGI2 can have both protective and harmful effects, depending on the context. It plays a beneficial role by:

- Reducing the risk of blood clots
- Supporting healthy blood vessel function
- Helping to regulate the immune system and inflammation

At the same time, PGI2 can also contribute to inflammation, especially during infections or injury, by enhancing the body's immune response. While this can be helpful in the short term, prolonged or excessive PGI2 activity may lead to chronic inflammation. For example, in conditions like rheumatoid arthritis, elevated PGI2 levels can worsen symptoms by increasing inflammatory signals and joint damage.[186]

Therefore, PGI2 has a dual role: it can support the body's defenses, but it may also contribute to disease when its activity becomes unbalanced.

Therapeutic Potential

Understanding PGI2's function opens avenues for new treatments targeting:

- Cardiovascular diseases (e.g., atherosclerosis, thrombosis)[187]
- Inflammatory disorders (e.g., arthritis, vascular inflammation) [187]
- Immune-related conditions[187]

Recent studies suggest that PGI2 therapy might help calm the immune system by boosting special cells (like T Cells) that prevent it from overreacting. This could open new ways of treating diseases where the immune system attacks the body by mistake, such as in autoimmune or inflammatory conditions.[188,189] These findings show that PGI2 is already useful in medicine and could play a bigger role in future treatments.

Key Takeaways:

- Ibuprofen works primarily by inhibiting the cyclooxygenase enzymes COX-1 and COX-2.

- Inhibition of COX-1 reduces the production of protective prostaglandins, which can lead to side effects such as stomach irritation, ulcers, and increased risk of bleeding, but does not significantly reduce pain, fever, or inflammation.

- The inhibition of COX-2 reduces the production of prostaglandins, particularly prostaglandin E2 (PGE2), the most critical component for promoting pain, swelling, fever, and inflammation. COX-2 inhibition does not affect the protective prostaglandins made by COX-1.

- Comprehensive insights into its mechanism of action reveal that it has multifaceted effects on various processes regarding inflammation and pain.

THE GOOD

Chapter 4
Ibuprofen and Cancer:
Does It Slow Cancer Growth?

Cancer remains one of the most pressing global health challenges, affecting millions each year.[190] While standard treatments like chemotherapy, immunotherapy, and surgery are widely used, researchers are exploring whether common drugs, like ibuprofen, could play a role in cancer prevention or treatment.

What is Cancer?

Normally, cell growth and death are carefully regulated, but cancer disturbs this balance. Cancer occurs when cells grow uncontrollably, forming tumors that can invade nearby tissues and spread to other parts of the body through metastasis. It is a very complex disease, shaped by genetic, epigenetic, and environmental factors that drive tumor growth, survival, and resistance to treatment.[191]

One of the biggest challenges in cancer research is that not all cancer cells are the same (tumor heterogeneity). They can vary not just from person to person, but even within the same tumor. This makes it hard to predict how the cancer will respond to treatment, making it more difficult to manage.[192]

Ibuprofen's Potential Role in Cancer Prevention

While ibuprofen is not an approved cancer treatment, studies suggest it may reduce the risk of developing certain cancers,[142-144] including:

Bladder Cancer: a case-control study (1,171 cases/1,418 controls) found that regular use of nonaspirin NSAIDs like ibuprofen was associated with a 40% reduced risk.[193]

Prostate Cancer: A 2005 meta-analysis of 91 studies reported a 39% risk reduction in prostate cancer with daily NSAID use (primarily aspirin/ibuprofen).[194] *In vitro* studies demonstrate ibuprofen's superior efficacy compared to other NSAIDs, inducing apoptosis in prostate cancer cells at clinically relevant concentrations.[149]

How Could Ibuprofen Help?

Ibuprofen belongs to the NSAID family, which inhibits COX enzymes, key players in both inflammation and cancer progression.[195]

COX-2 & Cancer: Many tumors overexpress COX-2, which contributes to tumor growth, blood vessel formation (angiogenesis), and metastasis.[195] By blocking COX-2, ibuprofen may reduce cancer-related inflammation, slow tumor growth, and limit the spread of cancer.[195]

Ibuprofen's potential anticancer effects extend beyond COX-2 inhibition, involving apoptosis induction and cell-cycle regulation through COX-independent pathways. Ibuprofen triggers apoptosis in prostate cancer cells (LNCaP, DU-145) by upregulating proapoptotic proteins via p38 MAPK signaling, independent of COX inhibition.[196]

In colon cancer models, ibuprofen induces apoptosis and G0/G1 cell-cycle arrest by downregulating cyclins A/B and elevating p27Kip-1.[196] In

PC3 cells, ibuprofen suppresses tumor migration and proliferation via PI3K/AKT/mTOR pathways and synergizes with radiotherapy by enhancing DNA damage response.[197] These multimodal mechanisms highlight ibuprofen's broader anticancer potential beyond COX-2 inhibition.

Future Research & Considerations

While these findings are promising, more studies are needed to determine the optimal dosage for cancer prevention, understand the long-term side effects, and identify which cancer types respond best. Currently, ibuprofen should only be used as directed for pain relief, and not as a cancer treatment. While ongoing research may uncover new therapeutic applications in the future, several challenges exist to translating the lab findings into clinical use. Long-term use of ibuprofen can lead to stomach problems such as ulcers and bleeding, and it may increase the risk of heart issues, especially for cancer patients undergoing treatments like chemotherapy or radiation. Additionally, genetic differences (e.g., CYP3A variants), and variations in the tumor environment can also make things more problematic.

Lung Cancer

Lung cancer is one of the deadliest cancers in the U.S., ranking as a leading cause of cancer-related deaths for both men and women (**Fig. 4.1**). Smoking remains the primary risk factor, responsible for about 80% of all lung cancer deaths.[198]

In fact, smokers are 15 to 30 times more likely to develop lung cancer than non-smokers.[199-201]

Fig. 4.1. Probability of developing bronchus and lung cancer in the US during 2017-2019

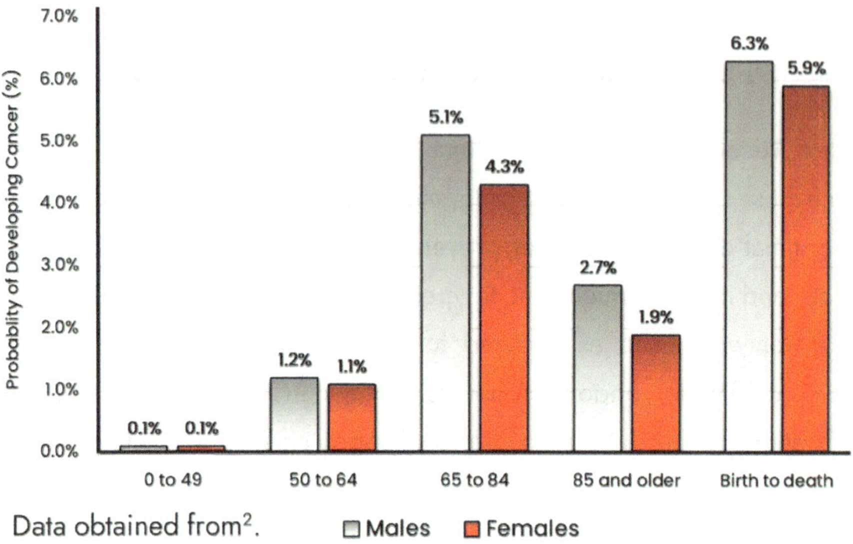

Data obtained from[2].

Recent research has explored new ways to reduce lung cancer risks and improve survival rates. A long-term study by Ohio State University followed over 10,000 participants, many of whom were current or former smokers over, 18 years. The study examined the effects of NSAID use and lifestyle factors on lung cancer outcomes and was adjusted for smoking intensity, duration, and demographics. Follow-up spanned 18 years, with mortality data linked to the National Death Index.

Surprisingly, researchers found that regular ibuprofen use (≥3 times/week) in 5,882 current/former smokers was linked to a 48% reduction in lung cancer mortality. However, other NSAIDs, like aspirin, and non-NSAIDs, like acetaminophen, did not show the same benefit.[202]

Ibuprofen may reduce lung cancer risk through COX-2 inhibition, suppressing pro-inflammatory prostaglandins linked to tumor angiogenesis, and downregulation of heat shock protein 70 (Hsp70), which induces apoptosis.[202,203] This latter COX-independent mechanism suggests ibuprofen's unique potential in lung cancer, distinct from other NSAIDs.[203]

Potential of NSAIDs in Lung Cancer Treatment

Research on lung cancer treatments has expanded beyond traditional therapies, exploring new drug combinations and delivery methods. Inflammation is known to be associated with lung cancer progression.[204]

One study in female ovariectomized mice, exposed to a tobacco carcinogen, investigated the effects of combining aspirin (25 mg/kg/day) or ibuprofen with anastrozole (25 mg/kg/day), a drug commonly used to treat breast cancer.[205] Eight weeks after carcinogen exposure, tumor count, size, and biomarkers were analyzed. The results showed that:

Parameter	**Aspirin + Anastrozole**	**Ibuprofen + Anastrozole**
Average number of tumors vs control	63% reduction ($P < 0.001$)	75% reduction ($P < 0.001$)
Tumor size reduction	41% reduction ($P < 0.001$)	Comparable effect
Macrophage infiltration	↓ 50%	↓ 45%

While ibuprofen with Anastrozole led to a 75% reduction in the average number of lung tumors, suggesting a powerful synergy between the two treatments, typical chemotherapy/ immunotherapy only achieves 20–50% response rates in advanced lung cancer.[206]

Supporting this study is a prospective NHANES III study that found a 48% reduced lung cancer mortality in smokers using ibuprofen regularly.[202]

These preclinical results suggest that NSAID combinations could enhance current regimens, particularly in high-risk subgroups like former smokers or patients with inflammatory comorbidities. While this promising combination could open the door to more effective lung cancer therapies involving NSAIDs, human trials are needed to validate efficacy and address risks like GI bleeding and cardiovascular diseases.

Several epidemiological studies also support the benefits of NSAIDs in reducing lung cancer risk. One study found that taking ibuprofen daily for at least two years was linked to a 68% decrease in lung cancer risk for both current and former smokers.[207] Additionally, a 2020 study revealed that ibuprofen could slow lung cancer progression by inhibiting certain inflammatory genes that help cancer cells grow and spread.[208]

Enhancing Ibuprofen's Effectiveness

What if ibuprofen could be even more effective in fighting cancer? Scientists in Turkey have been working on an innovative drug delivery system using Eudragit® RS 100, a material designed to precisely target lung cancer cells. This advanced method was shown to be 4 to 28 times more effective than regular ibuprofen in reaching cancerous cells.[209]

While these breakthroughs are still in the research phase, they offer hope that a widely available, affordable drug like ibuprofen could play a vital role in future lung cancer treatments.

Prostate Cancer and the Potential Role of Ibuprofen

Prostate cancer affects over 250,000 men in the U.S. each year and ranks among the most aggressive cancers.[200] However, research suggests that ibuprofen may help slow its progression. One study found that ibuprofen outperforms other NSAIDs, like aspirin, in reducing prostate cancer cell growth.[149] Additionally, Vitamin D3 supplementation has been shown to lower serum prostate-specific antigen (PSA) levels and reduce prostate volume.[210] Further studies indicate that combining ibuprofen with Vitamin D3 can significantly inhibit prostate cancer cell growth.[211] This may be due to its anti-proliferative and pro-apoptotic effects, particularly in aggressive prostate cancer forms.[212] Ibuprofen enhances the Vitamin D3 effect by suppressing the PI3K/AKT/mTOR pathways.[212]

Challenges in Translating Lab Findings to Clinical Use

While laboratory results are promising, applying them to real-world treatments presents challenges. The ibuprofen concentrations used in cell-based studies often exceed what is achievable through standard oral doses. The maximum clinically safe dosage of ibuprofen is 3200 mg/day, which may not consistently produce the same cellular effects seen in lab settings.[149] However, despite these limitations, ongoing research suggests that ibuprofen may still hold therapeutic potential in prostate cancer management. For example, new drug delivery methods (discussed in more detail in Chapter 16), such as ibuprofen-loaded nanoparticles, extended-release formulations, and combination delivery may help make ibuprofen a more practical option for cancer therapy in the future.[213]

How Ibuprofen Affects Prostate Cancer Cells

Ibuprofen's anti-cancer abilities appear to be multifaceted and occur through COX-2-dependent and independent pathways. Studies show that ibuprofen affects many pathways inside the cell[214]:

- At clinically relevant concentrations (0.5–1.5 mM), it reduces the ability of prostate cancer cells to divide and multiply.[149,215] It does this by shifting cancer cells into a resting phase, preventing their growth and replication.

- Suppresses tumor cell proliferation, potentially leading to cancer cell death.

One study on prostate adenocarcinoma cells found that ibuprofen treatment resulted in greater cancer suppression than aspirin or naproxen.[214] It should be emphasized that effective antitumor plasma concentrations (50–100 μg/mL) require individualized weight/age adjustments and pharmacokinetic monitoring due to the variable metabolism of ibuprofen and long-term safety risks of using ibuprofen at moderate to high doses.[216] Pharmacokinetic monitoring refers to how your body absorbs ibuprofen, moves it around, breaks it down, and gets rid of it.

Enhancing Ibuprofen's Effectiveness with Nanoparticles

Exciting new research explores whether ibuprofen nanoparticles could offer greater benefits with fewer side effects. Poly(lactic-co-glycolic acid) nanoparticles deliver ibuprofen directly into cancer cells, achieving significantly greater antiproliferative effects at equivalent doses compared to free ibuprofen.[217] Scientists found that these tiny ibuprofen particles protected DNA in white blood cells of prostate cancer patients, reducing genetic damage. In lung cancer patients, ibuprofen nanoparticles reduced DNA damage in white blood cells by 30–40% compared to bulk formulations.[218] This suggests that nanoparticle-based ibuprofen treatments could improve its potency while reducing potential harm.[219]

The PSA Mystery: Protection or Masking?

Prostate-specific antigen (PSA) is a protein in both normal and cancerous prostate cells and is used as a screening tool for prostate cancer, as elevated PSA levels can indicate prostate cancer. A study measuring PSA levels in 1,319 men over 40 years old found that regular NSAID use was associated with lower serum PSA levels.[220] By reducing PSA levels, ibuprofen could potentially be masking cancer risk during screening. However, researchers remain uncertain whether ibuprofen is truly reducing PSA levels or simply masking them. Further investigation is needed to determine its exact role in prostate cancer detection and progression. Until then, medical providers may need to consider NSAID use when interpreting PSA results, potentially requiring a 24-hour absence from NSAID use before testing.

Breast Cancer and the Role of NSAIDs

Breast cancer remains the most common cancer among women, accounting for about 1 in 3 of all new female cancers each year (over 300,000) in the U.S. Research on NSAIDs and their effect on breast cancer risk has produced mixed results.[221] Some studies suggest that prolonged NSAID use may lower breast cancer risk, particularly in postmenopausal women.

The Columbia University Study on NSAIDs and Breast Cancer Risk

A 2019 study from Columbia University and international collaborators examined whether NSAIDs could help women with a family history of breast cancer or those with elevated risks of breast cancer (such as those carrying BRCA1 or BRCA2 mutations).[222] These genes play a crucial role in DNA repair, and mutations can impair this function, making individuals more susceptible to tumor development.

The study included over 8,000 women aged 18 to 79 from seven centers across the U.S., Canada, and Australia. Many participants had close relatives (parents, siblings, or second-degree family members) diagnosed with breast cancer. Researchers collected detailed lifestyle, family history, and medication usage data, focusing on women who reported using aspirin, COX-2 inhibitors, ibuprofen, or other NSAIDs at least twice a week for a month or more before any breast cancer diagnosis. The goal was to assess whether these medications could reduce the risk of invasive breast cancer.[222]

Key Findings: Aspirin and COX-2 Inhibitors Show Strong Protective Effects

The results were striking:[222]

- Regular aspirin use was linked to a 37% reduction in breast cancer risk.
- COX-2 inhibitors, another class of anti-inflammatory drugs, showed even stronger protective effects, with 71% reductions in cancer risk.
- These associations held steady across different factors, including family history, genetic risk, hormone receptor status, and age.
- Ibuprofen and acetaminophen showed no significant impact on breast cancer risk.

Why Didn't Ibuprofen Show a Protective Effect?

The lack of risk reduction for ibuprofen may be due to how these drugs work:

- Ibuprofen is a nonspecific COX inhibitor, meaning it blocks both COX-1 and COX-2 enzymes. However, it may not inhibit COX-2 as effectively as other NSAIDs, which could limit its potential anti-cancer benefits. COX-2 drives tumor progression via prostaglandin E2 (PGE2)-mediated angiogenesis, apoptosis inhibition, and metastasis.[223] COX-2 is overexpressed in 40–50% of breast cancers, correlating with poor prognosis.[224]

- Although COX-1 helps with early tumorigenesis (e.g., colorectal polyp formation) it is less directly involved in advanced cancer pathways.[145]
- Differences in drug usage patterns could also play a role. Aspirin is often preferred over ibuprofen due to its well-known cardiovascular benefits, leading to more frequent and consistent use, potentially influencing the observed protective effects.

Conflicting Evidence on NSAIDs and Breast Cancer Risk

While some studies suggest that NSAID use may lower breast cancer risk, other research has failed to confirm the same protective effects. One study found that regular NSAID use, defined as more than once a week, did not significantly reduce overall breast cancer risk. However, a study found that long-term ibuprofen use elevated overall breast cancer risk by 51%.[225,226] Similarly, daily aspirin use showed no notable association with a reduced risk of breast cancer.[225] However, the California Teachers study found increased ER/PR-negative breast cancer risk (81%) with long-term aspirin use.[225]

However, when researchers analyzed the data by breast cancer subtypes, some intriguing patterns emerged:[225]

- Long-term daily aspirin use (five years or more) appeared to lower the risk of estrogen receptor (ER)-positive and progesterone receptor (PR)-positive breast cancer, but the reduction was not statistically significant.

- Surprisingly, long-term aspirin use was linked to a significantly higher risk of ER/PR-negative breast cancer, which is a more aggressive form of the disease.
- Ibuprofen use was associated with an increased overall risk of breast cancer.
- Long-term daily ibuprofen users faced an even higher risk of advanced, non-localized tumors, nearly doubling their risk compared to non-users.

The Complex Role of NSAIDs in Breast Cancer Development

These findings suggest that the effects of NSAIDs on breast cancer risk may depend on the specific drug, the amount used, and the cancer subtype. If these associations are proven to be causal, aspirin might help prevent some ER/PR-positive breast cancer cases, but could also increase the risk of ER/PR-negative cases. Similarly, long-term ibuprofen use may contribute to a higher number of breast cancer cases, particularly those diagnosed at advanced stages.[225]

For aspirin, higher cumulative doses (e.g., >8,600 mg) showed stronger protective effects, suggesting dose-dependent mechanisms.[227] Despite these and other findings, it remains unclear whether NSAIDs directly influence breast cancer risk. It is important to note that many of these studies are observational, which can generate hypotheses; however, they cannot definitively prove causation. Further randomized trials or mechanistic studies are needed to confirm these results and gain a deeper understanding of NSAIDs' role in breast cancer development.

This chapter underscores the complexity of balancing risks and benefits when using common medications like aspirin and ibuprofen. The lack of statistical significance in several studies may be due to insufficient power or heterogeneity in aspirin and ibuprofen dosing across populations. It is recommended that future clinical studies be done on larger group sizes if possible.

Bladder Cancer

Bladder cancer affects tens of thousands of men and women annually, but emerging research suggests ibuprofen may have a surprising role in reducing risk. A study by the National Cancer Institute found that regular ibuprofen use (more than twice a week), along with other non-aspirin NSAIDs, was linked to about a 40% reduction in bladder cancer risk, but only for nonsmokers. Interestingly, this protective effect was not observed in former or current smokers.[228] Cigarette smoke contains β-naphthylamine and tobacco-specific nitrosamines, both direct bladder carcinogens that may overwhelm ibuprofen's anti-inflammatory effects.[229] Smoking is also known to induce cytochrome P450 enzymes, which could speed up ibuprofen clearance and reduce its bioavailability.[193]

Limitations and Unanswered Questions

While these findings are promising, the study had several limitations:

- It did not account for specific ibuprofen doses.
- Ibuprofen was grouped with other non-aspirin NSAIDs, making it unclear if the effect was due to ibuprofen alone.
- Data was based on self-reported questionnaires, which can sometimes be inaccurate.

- It did not account for occupational carcinogens (e.g., aromatic amines in dyes/rubber industries) and arsenic in drinking water – both established bladder cancer risks.[230]
- Lifestyle factors, such as the use of antioxidants that may affect the results, were not considered.

Despite these challenges, the research raises the possibility that ibuprofen could offer some protective benefits for bladder cancer.

Ibuprofen's Potential in Bladder Cancer Treatment

Beyond risk reduction, some studies suggest ibuprofen may enhance the effectiveness of bladder cancer treatments. Researchers at Bond University in Australia found that ibuprofen improved the effectiveness of Mitomycin C, a common bladder cancer treatment, while reducing its side effects.[231]

- Mitomycin C is known to cause discomfort, including frequent and painful urination.
- In mouse studies, ibuprofen reduced these side effects, making treatment more tolerable.
- The study also found that ibuprofen boosted Mitomycin C's ability to kill bladder cancer cells.

However, determining the optimal ibuprofen dosage remains a challenge. Researchers determine human-equivalent drug doses from animal studies primarily through allometric scaling, which accounts for metabolic differences by normalizing doses to body surface area rather than body weight alone.[232] However, in the experiments, ibuprofen was provided in drinking water, making human dosage calculations unclear, as humans don't ingest ibuprofen every time they drink water.

The Need for Further Research

Currently, there is not enough evidence to confirm that ibuprofen lowers the risk of bladder cancer or improves treatment outcomes in humans. While early findings are intriguing, more comprehensive studies are needed to determine whether ibuprofen could play a beneficial role in bladder cancer prevention or therapy.

Colorectal Cancer

Colorectal cancer, also known as colon cancer, originates in the mucosa, the innermost layer of the colon. This layer contains specialized cells responsible for producing mucus and other fluids. When these cells undergo mutations, they can form polyps (adenomas), which may develop into cancer over time.[233] While the rates of colorectal cancer for people over 50 have been decreasing, they have increased for those below 50.[234] As such, in 2021, the United States Preventive Services Task Force updated its guidelines to recommend that colorectal cancer screening begin at age 45, rather than the previous starting age of 50.[235]

Recent research suggests that ibuprofen may play a role in reducing the progression of colorectal cancer and preventing its recurrence (**Fig. 4.2**). Prospective data linked regular ibuprofen use to a 48% lower advanced adenoma risk and 19% lower colorectal cancer risk, supporting its chemopreventive potential.[236] This compares favorably to colonoscopy, which reduces colorectal cancer mortality by 40-50%.

Studies show ibuprofen acts by breaking apart the enzyme group WNK1/GSK3β/SRPK1, which colorectal cancer cells need to activate RAC1B. This effect specifically harms cancer cells that depend on RAC1B for survival, without relying on ibuprofen's usual anti-inflammatory mechanisms.[237]

While targeted therapies achieve 8-12 month survival gains in metastatic disease, ibuprofen's benefit is primarily preventive with milder (but chronic) side effects, compared to chemotherapy's toxicity.[238,239]

Ibuprofen and Adenoma Recurrence

A prospective study conducted by the University of Pennsylvania investigated the effects of ibuprofen and aspirin on colorectal adenoma recurrence.[236] Researchers classified 13 years of self-reported patient data into three groups based on their ibuprofen intake:

- Fewer than 4 pills per month
- 4 to 30 pills per month
- More than 30 pills per month

The study found that taking more than 30 ibuprofen pills per month reduced the risk of advanced adenomas by 24% and the risk of new adenomas by 52%. However, while ibuprofen helped slow the severity of adenomas, it did not significantly impact their overall recurrence.[236]

When looking at colorectal cancer itself, the study found that patients taking more than 30 ibuprofen pills per month had a 19% lower risk of developing cancer. This suggests that ibuprofen may help slow the progression of adenomas and reduce the chances of them becoming cancerous.[236] However, while the study adjusted for smoking and family history, it lacked data on NSAID dosage consistency or concurrent medications.

Ibuprofen and Post-Surgery Cancer Recurrence

Another study, conducted by the University of Copenhagen, examined whether taking ibuprofen shortly after colorectal cancer surgery could reduce the risk of recurrence. Researchers analyzed 2,308 colorectal cancer surgery cases, with 702 patients receiving a daily dose of ibuprofen (800 mg or four pills) for at least two days within the first week post-surgery.[195]

Fig. 4.2. Potential anti-cancer effects of ibuprofen

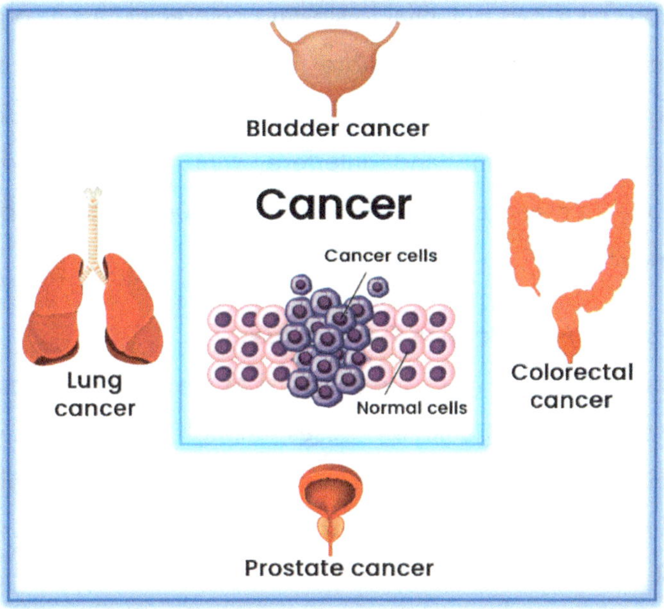

Their findings revealed that ibuprofen use reduced the risk of cancer recurrence within five years by 17%. Researchers believe this effect is linked to ibuprofen's ability to inhibit COX-2, an enzyme that is often overexpressed in colorectal cancer. By blocking COX-2, ibuprofen reduces inflammation and suppresses tumor growth.[195]

The Genetic Influence of Ibuprofen on Colorectal Cancer Cells

Beyond its anti-inflammatory effects, ibuprofen may also impact the genetic mechanisms of colorectal cancer. Some colorectal cancer cells carry a mutation in the B-Raf proto-oncogene, which leads to the overproduction of a tumor-associated protein that promotes cancer growth.[237] Ibuprofen disrupts this process by preventing the instructions (mRNA) needed to produce this tumor-promoting protein from being properly processed. Without these instructions, the protein cannot be made, slowing tumor growth.[237]

While ibuprofen shows potential in slowing colorectal cancer progression and reducing recurrence risk, more research is needed to determine optimal dosages and long-term effects. Its ability to reduce inflammation, suppress tumor growth, and interfere with cancer-related genetic processes makes it an exciting area of study in colorectal cancer prevention and treatment.

How Ibuprofen May Reduce Cancer Risk

Regular ibuprofen use shows the potential to lower cancer incidence by targeting early carcinogenic processes, though the evidence remains observational and preclinical.[194] Daily intake of NSAIDs, primarily aspirin, produced risk reductions of 39% in breast cancer and 73% for esophageal cancers. Researchers continue to explore how this widely used drug may influence cancer development at a biochemical level. While the exact mechanisms are not yet fully understood, several key pathways have been identified. Since cancer is a complex group of diseases with varying characteristics, the effects of ibuprofen can differ depending on the type of cancer. However, one of the most intriguing findings is ibuprofen's potential role in reducing cancer cell stemness.

Diminishing Cancer Cell Stemness

Cancer stemness refers to a cancer cell's ability to behave like a stem cell—dividing rapidly, forming new tumors, and resisting treatment. The more stem-like a cancer cell is, the more aggressive and treatment-resistant it becomes. Ibuprofen may help weaken cancer by reducing this stemness, making tumors less likely to grow, spread, or resist treatment.

At the molecular level, ibuprofen interferes with genes and proteins that support cancer stem cells. One of its key targets is a gene called Intercellular Adhesion Molecule 3 (ICAM3), which is linked to the aggressive behavior of cancer cells. By blocking ICAM3, ibuprofen makes it harder for cancer cells to retain their stem-like properties, potentially slowing tumor progression.[208]

Beyond gene interference, ibuprofen also affects how DNA is packaged inside cancer cells. Cancer cells rely on certain enzymes, histone deacetylases, and lysine demethylases, to activate genes that promote stemness. These enzymes modify histones, the proteins that act as spools for DNA, controlling gene activation. Unlike other NSAIDs, ibuprofen simultaneously suppresses histone deacetylases and lysine demethylases, amplifying its anti-stemness effects in cancers.[208] By disrupting these enzymes, ibuprofen prevents cancer cells from turning on harmful genes, thereby reducing their ability to grow and spread.[208]

While ibuprofen is widely known as a pain reliever, emerging research suggests it may also serve as a powerful tool to weaken cancer cells. By reducing cancer stemness, interfering with key genes, and altering histone modifications and DNA packaging, ibuprofen could potentially slow tumor growth, prevent cancer spread, and enhance treatment effectiveness. Histone modifications control how tightly DNA is packed, which turns genes on or off. In cancer, abnormal histone changes can switch on cancer-causing genes (oncogenes) or turn off genes that protect against cancer (tumor suppressors).

However, these findings presented are based on human cell lines and xenograft models; clinical trials are needed to fully understand its role and determine the best ways to harness its potential in cancer prevention and treatment.

Targeting Cellular Stress Responses

One possible way ibuprofen may fight cancer is by interfering with HSP70, a protein that cancer cells often overproduce to survive stressful conditions, including chemotherapy. In 2014, researchers from the University of Tokushima, Japan, found that ibuprofen reduces HSP70 levels in human lung cancer cells. This is significant because HSP70 helps cancer cells resist stress across multiple cancer types, including damage from chemotherapy drugs like cisplatin. Elevated HSP70 correlates with poor prognosis in breast, lung, endometrial, cervical cancers, and acute myeloid leukemia.[240] By lowering HSP70, ibuprofen enhances processes that lead to cancer cell death, effectively supporting chemotherapy in its anti-cancer role.[203]

Overcoming Chemoresistance

Chemoresistance, the ability of cancer cells to resist the effects of chemotherapy, remains one of the biggest challenges in cancer treatment. A 2020 preclinical study revealed that ibuprofen, when combined with cisplatin, may help weaken chemoresistant cancer cells by targeting a specific protein[241]:

- EF-hand domain-containing protein D2 (EFhd2) is a key player in non-small cell lung cancer and is linked to increased chemoresistance.

- Higher levels of EFhd2 make cancer cells less responsive to chemotherapy and are associated with lower survival rates.

- Ibuprofen suppresses EFhd2, via proteasomal and lysosomal degradation (COX-independent), making chemotherapy treatments like cisplatin more effective.

Interestingly, this effect is independent of ibuprofen's usual anti-inflammatory role as a COX inhibitor. This suggests that ibuprofen has anti-cancer benefits beyond its well-known ability to reduce inflammation, potentially offering a new pathway to enhance cancer treatment.[241] However, while these results highlight ibuprofen's ability to reduce cancer stemness and chemoresistance in preclinical settings, clinical relevance remains unconfirmed.

Future Directions

While ibuprofen shows promising anti-cancer effects, several challenges must be addressed before it can be widely used in cancer treatment:

Determining Safe & Effective Doses

- Many studies have focused on high-dose, long-term ibuprofen use, which can cause GI issues, cardiovascular risks, and kidney damage.

- Preliminary evidence suggests that ibuprofen doses in the range of 200–400 mg taken orally every 4 to 6 hours, with a maximum daily limit of 1200 mg, are considered generally safe for short-term use in adults.[126]

- For cancer prevention, one study found that 300 mg of ibuprofen daily was the lowest effective dose in certain cancer prevention trials.[242]

- Future research must identify safe yet effective doses that minimize risks while maximizing therapeutic benefits.

Expanding Research to Other Cancer Types

- Current studies highlight ibuprofen's impact on lung, bladder, and prostate cancers, but its effects on pancreatic, kidney, and other less-studied cancers remain unknown.
- Investigating its potential against a wider range of cancers could unlock new treatment possibilities. Ibuprofen's anti-cancer potential seems to stem from its dual role in dampening inflammation-driven pathways and enhancing immune-mediated tumor clearance.

Clinical Trials & Combination Therapies

- A low-dose phase II trial for chemotherapy-related cognitive impairment was completed in 2023. Cancer patients (breast, colorectal, others) receiving chemotherapy were randomized to ibuprofen (200 mg twice daily) or placebo for 6 weeks. The results showed that low-dose ibuprofen reduced the cognitive side effects of chemotherapy by improving processing speed and visual memory compared to placebo. No GI bleeding or serious adverse events linked to ibuprofen were observed in the 87 patients used in this study.[243]
- While preclinical and epidemiological data are promising, more clinical trials are needed to confirm ibuprofen's anti-cancer effects in real-world treatment settings.
- Given its COX-independent mechanisms, ibuprofen could complement existing cancer therapies by targeting pathways that other drugs do not.

Table 4.1: Types of Cancer and Interactions with Ibuprofen

Type of Cancer	Overall Conclusion
Bladder	Ibuprofen seems to be beneficial in reducing the risk of bladder cancer by 40% in nonsmokers. However, more studies are needed to confirm the dosage of ibuprofen, as well as how much lower the bladder cancer risks are with ibuprofen.
Breast	Ibuprofen's effects on breast cancer are inconclusive. Some studies found a reduced risk of breast cancer after extended use of ibuprofen, while others did not.
Lung	Ibuprofen seems to be beneficial in reducing the risk of lung cancer. Lung cancer might be reduced by up to 44% through ibuprofen intake. However, the studies do not report on doses and duration of therapies, so more studies are required.
Prostate	Ibuprofen seems to be beneficial in reducing the risk of prostate cancer with a maximum clinically acceptable dosage of 3200 mg/day. It effectively increases mitosis and decreases metastasis in prostate cancer.
Colorectal	Ibuprofen seems to be beneficial in reducing the recurrence risk of colorectal cancer. Recurrence of colorectal cancer may be reduced by 19% with 800 mg/day of ibuprofen intake after resection.

By addressing these challenges, ibuprofen could move closer to becoming a practical tool in cancer treatment. Whether used alone or in combination with chemotherapy, its ability to target cellular stress, reduce chemoresistance, and work through COX-independent pathways makes it a promising candidate for future cancer therapies. Another challenge would be addressing the GI bleeding, kidney damage, or cardiovascular issues associated with long-term NSAID use.

Key Takeaways:

- There is currently no clear scientific consensus on ibuprofen's role in cancer prevention or treatment.
- Although several observational and preclinical studies suggest that regular ibuprofen use may lower the risk of certain cancers—such as prostate, colorectal cancer, and lung cancer—these findings remain inconclusive and should be interpreted with caution.
- Ibuprofen is not approved for the prevention or treatment of any type of cancer and should not be used as a substitute for medically recommended therapies.

Chapter 5
Ibuprofen and Brain Health:
More Than Just a Painkiller?

What if ibuprofen could offer more than just pain relief? What if it had a hidden capability, one that could help safeguard brain health? In recent years, scientists have explored whether this common pain reliever might play a role in reducing the risk of neurological disorders like Alzheimer's, Parkinson's, and epilepsy. Emerging research suggests that ibuprofen may influence brain aging and disease risk through multiple pathways, though the evidence remains mixed and context-dependent. In this chapter, we'll examine the science behind ibuprofen's unexpected connection to brain health, uncovering what we know, what remains uncertain, and what the future may hold.

Beyond Pain Relief: Ibuprofen and the Brain

For the past decade, researchers have been intrigued by ibuprofen's potential effects on brain function. In one study, researchers used a brain-aging measurement tool called BrainAGE that uses MRI scans to estimate how old your brain "looks" compared to your actual age. They found that, in humans, a single 200 mg dose made the brain appear 1.18 years younger on specific brain scans.[244] This effect is likely linked to ibuprofen's anti-inflammatory properties. However, increasing the dosage doesn't necessarily amplify the benefits; researchers found that a 600 mg dose offered no additional brain-aging effects. [244]

Despite these intriguing findings, ibuprofen is not currently approved for improving brain function or preventing neurological diseases. Nevertheless, these results highlight the drug's potential, sparking further scientific investigation into its ability to protect against brain disorders.

The Key to Brain Health

Your brain is the command center of your body, influencing everything from cognition to emotions, behavior, and more. According to the World Health Organization, maintaining optimal brain health enhances mental and psychological well-being while supporting everyday functioning.[245] However, keeping your brain in peak condition isn't always straightforward. Many factors—such as genetics, age, environment, and overall health, affect brain function and resilience.

Neurological disorders, which impact the brain and nervous system, are often associated with aging. However, they are far more common than many people realize and can affect individuals at any stage of life. In fact, nearly one billion people worldwide suffer from neurological conditions such as Alzheimer's, Parkinson's, or epilepsy.[246] Given the rising prevalence of these disorders, researchers are working tirelessly to uncover new ways to prevent and treat them.

Could Anti-Inflammatory Drugs Like Ibuprofen Help?

Since brain diseases can be challenging to treat, scientists are exploring alternative ways to protect brain health. One promising area of research focuses on anti-inflammatory drugs, such as NSAIDs like ibuprofen. These medications are being studied as potential therapies for neurological disorders due to their ability to reduce inflammation—a key factor in several brain diseases, including Alzheimer's and multiple sclerosis.[247,248] While research is still in its early stages, the possibility that ibuprofen and similar drugs could help safeguard brain function is an exciting avenue for future medical advancements.

How NSAIDs, Like Ibuprofen, May Protect the Brain

Ibuprofen's ability to cross the blood-brain barrier—a protective shield that prevents harmful substances from reaching the brain—makes it an intriguing candidate for treating neurological diseases, like Parkinson's, Alzheimer's, and epilepsy (**Fig. 5.1**).[249-251] Scientists are particularly interested in its anti-inflammatory properties, which may help reduce brain inflammation, a common factor in brain diseases.

Ibuprofen and Epilepsy

Epilepsy is a widespread neurological disorder characterized by abnormal brain activity, leading to seizures, behavioral changes, and even unconsciousness. While some cases of epilepsy are genetic, the condition can also develop after a stroke, brain injury, or infection.[252,253] Most patients manage their symptoms with anti-seizure medications, while others may require surgery or alternative treatments such as nerve stimulation.[254]

Fig. 5.1. Potential beneficial effects of ibuprofen on the brain

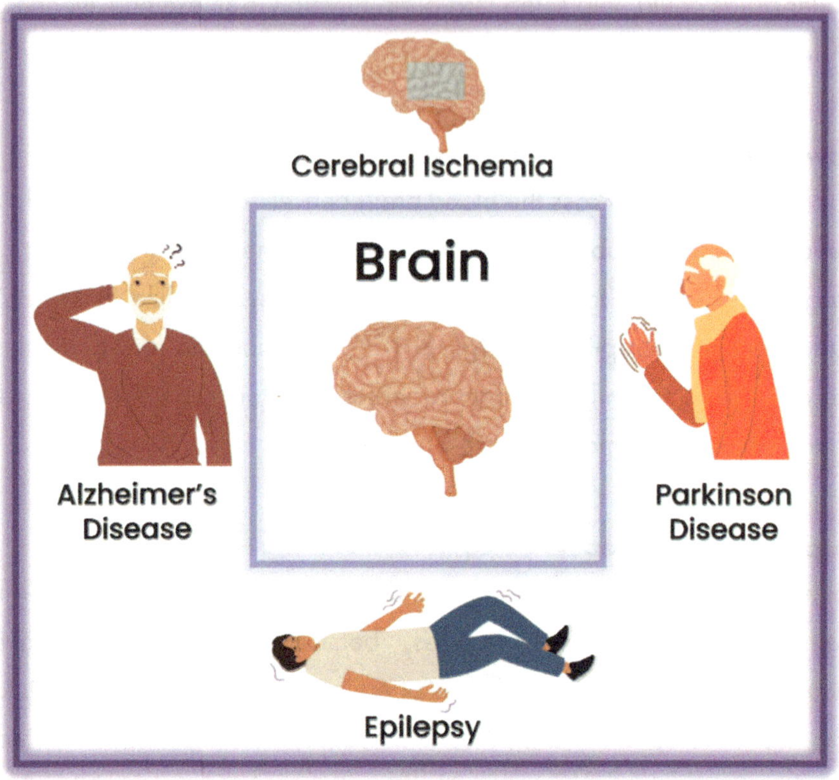

Interestingly, recent research suggests that ibuprofen could play a role in managing epilepsy. Scientists are investigating whether its anti-inflammatory effects could help reduce the severity and frequency of seizures. A key study conducted in 2020 provided promising results, indicating that ibuprofen might help suppress seizure activity in animal models, as discussed below.[247]

Scientific Findings: Ibuprofen's Effect on Seizures

A 2020 study by Durankus et al. examined the impact of ibuprofen on seizure activity in animal models.[247] Researchers induced seizures in rats using pentylenetetrazole (PTZ), a chemical known to trigger convulsions. The animals were then given ibuprofen to assess its potential effects. The results indicated that ibuprofen significantly reduced seizure severity, suggesting a possible therapeutic benefit.

The study divided 48 male rats into two experimental groups:

- **Electroencephalogram (EEG) Group** – Monitored seizure activity through brain wave recordings.
- **Behavioral Test Group** – Determined seizure severity and response to treatment.

Each group was further split into four subgroups (n = 6 per group):

1. **Control Group** – No treatment.
2. **Saline Group** – Received a placebo (saline injection).
3. **Low-Dose Ibuprofen Group** – Treated with 200 mg/kg ibuprofen.
4. **High-Dose Ibuprofen Group** – Treated with 400 mg/kg ibuprofen.

EEG Findings: Reduced Seizure Activity

EEG recordings tracked seizure-related brain spikes, a key indicator of seizure intensity. The results showed statistically significant differences:

- Control Group (No PTZ) – 0% spike activity (no seizures).
- Saline Group – 74.5% spike activity (most severe seizures).

- 200 mg/kg Ibuprofen Group – 55.9% spike activity (moderate improvement).
- 400 mg/kg Ibuprofen Group – 45.1% spike activity (greatest reduction in seizure severity).

These findings suggest that higher doses of ibuprofen were more effective in lowering seizure-related brain activity.[247] As previously noted, animal studies should be viewed with caution as they don't always translate to humans. The levels of ibuprofen used in these studies may seem extremely high (200 and 400 mg/kg), but rats have a significantly higher metabolism than humans. These concentrations would correspond to 1,945 mg in a 60kg human. Two other studies using lower amounts of ibuprofen (35mg/kg, which corresponds to a dose of 340 mg in a 60 kg human) showed reduced frequency, latency, and duration of seizures.[255,256]

PTZ-induced epilepsy in mice involves inflammatory pathways, together with its direct seizure-inducing effects. Inflammatory-related epilepsy is distinct from other epilepsy types due to its direct link to immune system activation and neuroinflammation. Since most anti-seizure medications work by stabilizing neuronal activity, whereas ibuprofen primarily targets inflammation, ibuprofen may be complementary to current anti-seizure medicines.

Behavioral Findings: Delayed Seizure Onset and Reduced Severity
Seizure severity was assessed using the Racine Convulsion Scale (RCS), where 0 = no convulsions and 6 = lethal seizures.[247] The results indicated:

- Saline Group had the highest seizure severity.[247]

- Ibuprofen-treated groups (200 mg/kg and 400 mg/kg) had significantly lower RCS scores.[247]
- Rats receiving ibuprofen experienced a delay in the onset of myoclonic jerks (early seizure indicators), suggesting that the drug helped slow seizure progression.[247]

Anti-Inflammatory Effects: Lower Prostaglandin Levels

The study also measured prostaglandin F2 alpha (PGF2α), an inflammatory molecule that rises during seizures.

- Rats treated with 400 mg/kg ibuprofen showed statistically significantly lower PGF2α levels compared to the saline group. The 400 mg/kg ibuprofen showed significantly stronger efficacy than 200 mg/kg in lowering seizure severity.
- This suggests that ibuprofen's anti-inflammatory action played a crucial role in reducing seizure severity. These reductions were not due to random variation as the p-value was < 0.001.[247]
- These preclinical findings highlight ibuprofen's potential to mitigate seizure-associated inflammation, though human relevance remains unconfirmed.

Takeaways

These studies provide compelling evidence that ibuprofen may help reduce seizure severity, delay seizure onset, and lower inflammation in an epilepsy model.[247] However, further clinical trials in humans are needed to determine its safety, optimal dosage, and long-term effects as a potential epilepsy treatment. If future studies confirm similar effects, ibuprofen or drugs with similar anti-inflammatory properties could one day be explored as adjunct therapies for epilepsy.

How Does Ibuprofen Help with Seizures?

Ibuprofen may help manage seizures by reducing brain inflammation. It works by blocking COX enzymes, which produce inflammatory chemicals like PGF2α. Since brain inflammation can be a trigger for seizures, lowering these inflammatory molecules may help prevent or lessen seizure severity. However, the effectiveness of ibuprofen appears to be dose-dependent, and more research is needed to determine its optimal dosage and mechanism in epilepsy treatment.[247]

Ibuprofen and Astrocyte Regulation

Preclinical studies demonstrate that astrocyte activation reduces seizures in rodent models.[257] Astrocytes are specialized brain cells that are essential for maintaining the health and function of the central nervous system through their roles in structural support, metabolic regulation, synaptic maintenance, immune modulation, and response to injury. A study focused on a type of brain cells called astrocytes, by Peng et al., suggests that ibuprofen may have anti-epileptic potential.[255] Under normal conditions, the body maintains a balance of astrocytes through autophagy, a process that clears out damaged cells. However, in epilepsy, astrocyte proliferation increases, contributing to abnormal brain activity.[258]

In their experiment, researchers studied 60 male rats and found that ibuprofen reduced the growth of astrocytes, and appeared to protect against seizures. The study suggests that when too many astrocytes grow, they disrupt potassium and glutamate levels in the brain, which can lead to seizures. By preventing this overgrowth, ibuprofen may help maintain healthier brain activity and reduce the risk of seizures.[255]

Ibuprofen and Neuronal Excitability

Seizures occur when neurons become overly excited, leading to uncontrolled electrical activity. Liu et al. investigated whether ibuprofen could reduce this neuronal over-excitation in rats exposed to pentylenetetrazole (PTZ), a seizure-inducing chemical.[256]

Their key findings included:

- **Reduced neuronal damage** – Ibuprofen-treated rats had statistically less brain cell damage compared to untreated rats.[256]
- **Lower frequency of action potentials** – Rats that received ibuprofen showed fewer electrical discharges, indicating less seizure activity.[256]
- **Inhibition of COX pathways** – Since ibuprofen blocks COX enzymes, which are linked to inflammation, the study suggests that inflammatory pathways play a key role in seizure generation.[256]
- **Inhibition of Ion Channels** - Ibuprofen appears to block certain calcium channels and protect brain cells from damage, meaning it likely works through both anti-inflammatory effects and direct support of brain health.[256]

These results highlight ibuprofen's potential neuroprotective role in epilepsy, though further studies on humans are needed.

Does Ibuprofen Prevent Febrile Seizures?

Unlike epilepsy, febrile seizures occur in young children during high fevers and may involve different mechanisms. Researchers conducted a clinical trial comparing ibuprofen and acetaminophen to assess their ability to prevent recurrent febrile seizures.[259]

Trial Details: 231 children (aged 4 months to 4 years) were given either:

- Ibuprofen (10 mg/kg)
- Acetaminophen (15 mg/kg)
- Placebo
- Doses were administered up to 4 times daily if fever exceeded 38°C.

Results:

- 23% of children experienced recurrent febrile seizures, regardless of treatment.[259]
- Neither ibuprofen nor acetaminophen was effective in preventing febrile seizures.[259]

Takeaways

- Ibuprofen may help manage epileptic seizures by reducing inflammation, astrocyte overgrowth, and neuronal excitability.
- Its effectiveness appears dose-dependent, but more research is needed in humans.
- While ibuprofen did not prevent febrile seizures in this study, further research is needed to understand whether its effects differ across seizure types.

Ibuprofen and Alzheimer's

Alzheimer's disease is one of the most common neurodegenerative conditions, leading to memory loss, confusion, and cognitive decline. While there is currently no cure, researchers have been investigating whether NSAIDs, like ibuprofen, could help delay its onset or slow its progression. The idea is that by reducing inflammation in the brain, these drugs might protect neurons and prevent the buildup of toxic proteins like β-amyloid, which are key contributors to Alzheimer's disease.[260]

Some observational studies have suggested that consistent, long-term use of NSAIDs may be associated with a lower risk of developing Alzheimer's when used before symptoms appear. However, observational studies show correlation, not causation, and clinical trials have not consistently shown a clear benefit with NSAID use.[261] Additionally, once Alzheimer's has fully developed, NSAIDs, including ibuprofen, appear to be less effective.[262] As the disease progresses, the brain undergoes significant changes, including neuron degeneration, β-amyloid aggregation, and the formation of neurofibrillary tangles that contribute to inflammation.[263]

Early Research and Observational Studies

One of the earliest studies in this field examined people who had been using NSAIDs for two or more years. Findings suggested that these individuals had a lower risk of developing Alzheimer's, compared to those who did not take NSAIDs.[264] The longer someone used NSAIDs, the lower their risk appeared to be. These results sparked further research into whether starting NSAID use earlier in life could delay or even prevent Alzheimer's disease.

Evidence from Animal Models

Animal studies have provided additional insights into ibuprofen's potential role in Alzheimer's prevention. For example, a study by Van Dam et al. found that ibuprofen reduced β-amyloid plaques in mice genetically modified to develop Alzheimer's-like symptoms.[265] These ibuprofen-treated mice performed better in memory tests, such as the Morris water maze, compared to placebo-treated mice. While these findings are promising, mice do not completely replicate human pathology, so translating these findings to humans remains a challenge.

Large-Scale Epidemiological Findings

A major meta-analysis by Zhang et al. pooled data from 16 cohort studies involving over 236,000 participants to clarify the relationship between NSAIDs and Alzheimer's risk. The results showed that individuals who had used NSAIDs were nearly 20% less likely to develop Alzheimer's compared to non-users. This protective effect was observed across different types of NSAIDs, but was not seen with aspirin or acetaminophen, suggesting that the anti-inflammatory properties of traditional NSAIDs may be key.[266]

However, like all meta-analyses, this study combined data from research with different methodologies, participant populations, and NSAID dosages, which can introduce variability and limit how strong the conclusions can be. Further subgroup analysis revealed that the protective effect was strongest in prospective cohort studies, which track participants over time, and in studies conducted in Europe, where Alzheimer's risk dropped by about 28%. In contrast, retrospective studies, which rely on past medical records, showed weaker or no significant associations, highlighting how study design can affect the reliability and interpretation of results.[266]

Limitations and Considerations

Although these results are encouraging, they are not without their drawbacks. Observational studies cannot establish a direct cause-and-effect relationship, and factors such as healthier lifestyles among NSAID users may have contributed to the reduced Alzheimer's risk. Additionally, the duration and dosage of NSAID use varied widely between studies, making it difficult to determine the optimal regimen for potential benefits.[266]

The Complexities of Clinical Trials

Building on earlier research that suggested NSAID use might lower the risk of Alzheimer's disease, Jack Rivers-Auty and colleagues looked more closely at this connection using data from the Alzheimer's Disease Neuroimaging Initiative (ADNI). They used statistical models to compare how different NSAIDs affected both the chances of having Alzheimer's and how quickly thinking and memory skills declined, aiming to better understand why past studies have shown mixed results [267]

The researchers confirmed earlier findings that NSAID use was associated with lower Alzheimer's prevalence. These results supported that NSAIDs may reduce the risk of developing Alzheimer's disease, particularly when taken over long periods. However, when researchers looked at the progression of cognitive decline in patients already diagnosed with mild cognitive impairment or Alzheimer's disease, the results were less encouraging. The study found that commonly used NSAIDs did not significantly slow cognitive decline, as measured by widely accepted metrics like the Mini-Mental State Examination (MMSE) and Alzheimer's Disease Assessment Scale (ADAS). This finding aligns with earlier clinical trials that failed to demonstrate NSAID efficacy in treating established Alzheimer's disease.[267]

Limitations and Considerations

Rivers-Auty et al. found that one specific NSAID, diclofenac, was linked to slower memory and thinking decline in people with Alzheimer's, while ibuprofen and other NSAIDs were not. They suggest this difference might be because diclofenac blocks a particular inflammation pathway in the brain, called the NLRP3 (NOD-, LRR-, and pyrin domain-containing protein 3) inflammasome, which ibuprofen and naproxen do not effectively target.[267]

Interestingly, paracetamol (also known as acetaminophen), which does not reduce inflammation, was also linked to a lower risk of Alzheimer's, similar to NSAIDs. The authors suggest this may not be because the drug itself helps, but because people who regularly take medications for pain might also have other healthy habits that lower their risk. These findings highlight the importance of separating the effects of the drug from the effects of people's overall behavior when studying ways to prevent Alzheimer's.[267]

The researchers proposed several reasons for the disconnect between observational studies and clinical trials:

1. **Timing of NSAID Use:** Rivers-Auty and colleagues suggested that NSAIDs might be effective only if taken long before symptoms of Alzheimer's disease develop. Observational studies, which follow healthy people over many years, show a possible lower risk of Alzheimer's in long-term NSAID users. However, these studies can be biased, since healthier people are more likely to use medications regularly and report their habits accurately. In contrast, clinical trials usually test interventions over a relatively shorter period (6–12 months), in individuals who are already showing early signs of Alzheimer's, when brain damage is already underway. This timing mismatch could explain why clinical trials have failed to replicate the protective effects seen in epidemiological studies.

2. **Population Differences:** Observational studies capture real-world NSAID use in diverse populations. This may include individuals who

regularly take pain relievers like NSAIDs or paracetamol, and who might also engage in other health-conscious behaviors that contribute to reduced Alzheimer's risk, such as exercising, eating a balanced diet, or managing cardiovascular health. In contrast, clinical trials often involve narrowly defined groups. These confounding factors make it challenging to draw definitive conclusions from observational studies alone.

Major studies like the Rotterdam and Cardiovascular Health studies controlled for diet, exercise, smoking, cardiovascular health, and socioeconomic factors. NSAID use remained associated with a 24–37% lower Alzheimer's risk after these adjustments.[268,269]

3. **Drug Selection:** Researchers found that diclofenac showed promise in slowing cognitive decline in their analysis, warranting further investigation into whether specific NSAIDs might have unique properties that benefit Alzheimer's patients. [267]

Together, these two studies provide a nuanced understanding of the relationship between NSAIDs and Alzheimer's disease. Zhang et al. found an association between long-term NSAID use and reduced Alzheimer's risk, while Rivers-Auty et al. showed that this potential benefit does not appear to extend to slowing disease progression in patients already diagnosed. These findings suggest that, if NSAIDs have any effect, it may be limited to the early stages of the disease, emphasizing the importance of further research into timing and prevention strategies.

While challenges remain, these studies highlight a potential area for further investigation in addressing Alzheimer's disease. Current evidence on NSAIDs is inconclusive, and it remains unclear whether they offer any real protective effect. Moving forward, future research should focus on well-designed, randomized controlled trials to determine whether NSAIDs provide measurable benefits, identify which types might be most effective, and clarify the best timing and duration for use.

Ibuprofen and Neuroprotection

i. Ibuprofen and Cerebral Ischemia

Cerebral ischemia, commonly known as an ischemic stroke, occurs when blood flow to the brain is blocked or reduced. If left untreated, it can lead to cerebral infarction—permanent brain damage from oxygen deprivation—potentially leading to severe disability or even death.[270] Given the serious consequences of strokes, researchers continue to explore potential treatments to minimize damage and improve long-term recovery.

One key mechanism behind stroke-related brain damage is glutamate-induced excitotoxicity, a process where excessive activation of glutamate receptors leads to neuronal injury or death. This occurs when the neurotransmitter glutamate accumulates in the synapse—the communication junction between neurons—instead of being cleared away due to impaired clearance. The resulting overstimulation damages brain cells and worsens stroke outcomes.

To counteract this effect, scientists have investigated the neuroprotective potential of ibuprofen, a common anti-inflammatory drug. Research by Iwata et al. examined how ibuprofen might shield neurons from excitotoxic damage.[271] Using cultured brain cells in a laboratory setting, they simulated stroke-like conditions to assess ibuprofen's protective effects. Their findings suggest that ibuprofen may help reduce neuronal injury by mitigating inflammation and excessive excitation.

While these findings point to a possible way that ibuprofen could protect brain cells, it's still unclear whether this effect is replicated in humans. So far, no human studies have confirmed that the laboratory results apply in real-life medical settings. More research in animals and humans is needed to determine if ibuprofen could be truly useful as a stroke treatment.

For Medical Experts and Others Interested:

Mixed cortical cultures (a combination of different cell types such as neurons and glial cells) and near-pure neuronal cultures were obtained from fetal mice at 13 to 15 days of gestation. These cell cultures were then exposed to 12.5 µmol/L N-methyl-D-aspartate (NMDA) or 50 µmol/L kainate to induce excitotoxic injury, and neuronal cell death was quantified to establish a baseline for comparison.[271] Researchers subsequently applied ibuprofen at concentrations of 25, 50, and 100 µg/mL.

They found:

1. NMDA-induced neuronal death (74.5 ± 3.8%) was significantly reduced by ibuprofen:
    - 25 µg/mL ibuprofen: neuronal death reduced to 56.1 ± 4.0%
    - 50 µg/mL ibuprofen: neuronal death reduced to 38.7 ± 2.8%
    - 100 µg/mL ibuprofen: neuronal death reduced to 12.3 ± 1.4%
2. Kainate-induced neuronal death (36.1% ± 3.5%) was reduced to 20.0 ± 3.1% with 100 µg/mL ibuprofen in mixed cultures.

Researchers discovered that ibuprofen significantly increased cell survival, with higher doses offering even greater neuroprotection. Hence, ibuprofen protects neurons from NMDA or kainate-induced glutamatergic excitotoxic neuronal cell death after ischemia.[271] Ibuprofen does this primarily through mechanisms beyond just COX inhibition, including by inhibiting microglial NADPH oxidase, reducing oxidative stress in these cells.[179]

Ibuprofen and Parkinson's Disease

Parkinson's disease is a progressive neurological disorder that affects movement, often causing tremors, stiffness, and difficulty with coordination. In the United States alone, approximately one million people live with Parkinson's, with 90,000 new cases diagnosed each year.[272] Notable figures like actor Michael J. Fox, boxing legend Muhammad Ali, and singer Linda Ronstadt have all been affected by this condition.

Although the exact cause of Parkinson's disease is still unknown, scientists believe that long-term brain inflammation and damage from oxidative stress play a major role in how the disease develops. This has led researchers to explore whether anti-inflammatory drugs like ibuprofen might help protect the brain. Animal studies suggest ibuprofen may reduce harmful brain inflammation, but human trials have not confirmed this.[273] Some population studies show a possible link between ibuprofen use and a reduced risk of Parkinson's, though more research is needed to understand if the drug is truly protective.[250]

From Animal Models to Human Studies

Early evidence of ibuprofen's neuroprotective effects comes from animal studies. Research using mouse models has shown that ibuprofen can reduce the loss of dopaminergic neurons and suppress neuroinflammation.[274] For example, a study by Zaminelli et al. found that ibuprofen's antioxidant properties helped improve motor function and reduce oxidative damage in mice.[272] While promising, these findings are still preclinical, meaning human studies are needed to confirm these effects.

Epidemiological Evidence: Insights from Human Studies

A major review by Badawoud et al. analyzed multiple studies to determine whether NSAIDs could lower Parkinson's risk.[275] Their meta-analysis, which combined data from numerous observational studies, found a 27% reduction in Parkinson's risk among ibuprofen users compared to non-users.[275] Researchers believe ibuprofen's protective effects stem from its ability to inhibit COX-1 and COX-2, which are responsible for producing inflammatory chemicals in the brain. By blocking COX-2, ibuprofen reduces the synthesis of pro-inflammatory prostaglandins in the brain, thereby reducing inflammation and its associated effects.

Interestingly, the study also looked at aspirin and other NSAIDs, but only ibuprofen showed a significant protective effect. This suggests that ibuprofen may have a unique mechanism that makes it particularly beneficial for Parkinson's prevention. However, more research is needed to fully understand how it works and whether it could be used as a treatment for high-risk individuals.[275]

Adding to this, a long-term study by Chen et al. examined data from two large U.S. cohorts: the Health Professionals Follow-up Study and the Nurses' Health Study.[276] These studies tracked over 140,000 participants for decades to investigate the link between NSAIDs and Parkinson's. Among 415 newly diagnosed cases, researchers found that regular ibuprofen users had a 45% lower risk of developing Parkinson's compared to non-users.[276]

Chen's team proposed that ibuprofen's benefits may go beyond simple inflammation control. In preclinical models, ibuprofen has been shown to scavenge free radicals and inhibit NF-κB activation, a protein complex involved in inflammation.[276] These mechanisms could help reduce oxidative stress and chronic inflammation, both of which are strongly linked to Parkinson's. However, the study also highlighted a dose-response trend, meaning the protective effects were stronger with prolonged, consistent use.[276]

That said, long-term ibuprofen use carries risks, including GI bleeding, kidney/liver toxicity, and cardiovascular issues. Therefore, while ibuprofen shows promise, individuals considering it for Parkinson's prevention should do so under medical supervision.[276] Future research is needed to confirm ibuprofen's neuroprotective role via PPARγ activation or inflammasome inhibition, pathways suggested in preclinical models.[250] Research is also needed to identify subgroups most likely to benefit from ibuprofen use, such as individuals with early biomarkers of neuroinflammation or genetic susceptibility.

Genetic and Lifestyle Factors

In 2020, researchers explored how NSAIDs might benefit individuals with a genetic mutation linked to Parkinson's, known as Leucine-rich repeat kinase 2 (LRRK2).[277] The study divided participants into two groups:

- 259 individuals who had Parkinson's symptoms
- 318 individuals who carried the mutation but had not yet developed symptoms

Researchers found that participants who carry a gene linked to Parkinson's disease (called LRRK2) but don't have any symptoms were more likely to regularly use anti-inflammatory drugs like NSAIDs (31.8%) compared to those who did develop Parkinson's (10.9%).[277] This suggests that people who regularly take NSAIDs might be less likely to get Parkinson's, with the data showing their risk could be about two-thirds lower.[277]

One possible reason for this is that the LRRK2 gene is highly expressed in immune cells and plays a role in inflammatory pathways. Long-term inflammation is thought to play a role in brain damage that leads to Parkinson's. Since NSAIDs help reduce inflammation, they might also help protect the brain in people who carry this gene.

However, the researchers stress that this doesn't prove that NSAIDs prevent Parkinson's. More long-term studies are needed to confirm whether these drugs actually help reduce the risk and to figure out how they might work.

Chronic Pain and Parkinson's

Chronic pain and Parkinson's disease are strongly linked through shared neuroinflammatory and neurodegenerative mechanisms, with pain affecting 40–85% of Parkinson's disease patients.[278] Parkinson's disease damages brain regions like the basal ganglia and frontal cortex, which process pain signals. Neuroinflammation, marked by the activation of microglia and the release of pro-inflammatory cytokines, plays a central role in both conditions and contributes to the loss of dopaminergic neurons seen in Parkinson's disease. This ongoing inflammation not only worsens neurodegeneration but also disrupts pain processing pathways in the brain.[279,280]

A 2013 study by Lin et al. investigated the link between chronic pain, Parkinson's risk, and ibuprofen use. Using data from two large-scale health surveys in Taiwan, China, researchers found that individuals who experienced moderate to severe pain were more likely to develop Parkinson's.[281] However, ibuprofen use appeared to reduce this risk, suggesting that pain could be an early warning sign of the disease and that ibuprofen may offer protective benefits.

Conclusions

Ibuprofen's ability to inhibit COX enzymes reduces the production of inflammatory mediators, like prostaglandins, offering potential neuroprotection against various neurological disorders.[247] Research suggests that ibuprofen may slow Alzheimer's progression by reducing neuroinflammation and amyloid-beta deposition, though results remain inconsistent between animal models and human trials.[282] In cerebral ischemia, findings are mixed, with some studies indicating neuroprotection, while others highlight the need for further investigation into the factors influencing its effectiveness. Studies on Parkinson's disease suggest a possible reduction in disease risk with NSAID use, though long-term clinical validation is required.[250] Overall, ibuprofen has shown promise in mitigating neurological disease progression, impacting brain function through multiple mechanisms, including oxidative stress reduction, modulation of cellular signaling pathways, and indirect effects on neurotransmitter systems.[179,283,284]

Future Directions

The existing research highlights ibuprofen's potential as both a preventive and therapeutic agent for neurological disorders. However, translating these findings into clinical applications requires further exploration, particularly in determining optimal dosages and long-term effects in human populations. While many promising results stem from preclinical studies, validation of ibuprofen's neuroprotective benefits requires well-designed, large-scale clinical trials. Future research should prioritize Phase III randomized controlled trials to carefully measure the effectiveness and safety of treatments in a wide range of patients.

In epilepsy, ibuprofen has demonstrated potential in reducing seizure severity through COX pathway modulation, while in Alzheimer's, it has been linked to delayed cognitive decline in animal studies. For ischemic stroke, it may help reduce neuronal death, and in Parkinson's, it appears to mitigate chronic neuroinflammation and protect dopaminergic neurons.

Future research should focus on refining treatment strategies, evaluating long-term safety, and understanding how ibuprofen interacts with genetic and environmental factors. For example, the effectiveness of NSAIDs, like ibuprofen, in Alzheimer's disease may depend on an individual's APOE genotype, with some studies suggesting benefits primarily seen in APOEε4 carriers.[268] Personalized approaches could involve tailoring ibuprofen dosage or combining it with other targeted therapies based on an individual's genetic profile and environmental exposures. With continued investigation, ibuprofen could play a meaningful role in neuroprotection, offering new hope for individuals affected by debilitating neurological conditions.

Table 5.1. Summary of the effects of ibuprofen on neurological diseases.

Neurological Disease	Effects of Ibuprofen as a Treatment	Overall, is it effective in mice/humans?
Epilepsy	• Decreased PGF2α • Decreased spike occurrence • Decreased astrocytes • Increased autophagy	Yes, in animal studies/Need for human clinical trials to confirm efficacy and safety; mechanisms of action in human epileptic tissue remain unclear.
Alzheimer's	• Decreased pathology-related behavior	Yes, in animal studies/Epidemiological studies suggest long-term use lowers risk and delays onset.[267] Need for more early-stage intervention and prevention studies in at-risk populations
Cerebral Ischemia	• Decreased neuronal cell death • Decreased CA1 (hippocampal memory) neuron injury	Yes, in animal studies/Limited human data; need for translational studies to determine optimal dosing, timing, and patient selection for neuroprotection after stroke.

Parkinson's	• Decreased dopamine turnover • Decreased neuroinflammation • Reverse negative effects of dopaminergic neuron degeneration (motor impairment) • Decrease risk for those with LRRK2 gene (associated with Parkinson's)	Yes, in animal studies/Epidemiological studies show reduced risk of Parkinson's disease with regular ibuprofen use, especially in LRRK2 variant carriers.[250,275] Need for dose-response relationships and optimal dosing regimens and impact of genetic variants (e.g., LRRK2) on response to ibuprofen

Key Takeaways:

- **Ibuprofen's Potential in Brain Health**: Ibuprofen, known for its anti-inflammatory effects, shows promise in treating neurological diseases like Alzheimer's, Parkinson's, epilepsy, and stroke.

- **Reduces Seizure Activity in Epilepsy**: Studies suggest ibuprofen may help lower the frequency and severity of seizures by reducing brain inflammation and lowering the levels of molecules that trigger seizures, such as prostaglandin F2 alpha.

- **Alzheimer's Disease**: Ibuprofen might slow Alzheimer's progression if taken early, although its benefits lessen in later stages of the disease. It has demonstrated some protective effects in animal models by reducing the buildup of harmful β-amyloid proteins.

- **Neuroprotection in Stroke**: Ibuprofen has the potential to protect neurons from damage after ischemic strokes by reducing inflammation and excitotoxicity.
- **Parkinson's Disease**: Ibuprofen has been found to reduce inflammation and slow down the loss of dopamine-producing neurons in the brain, which are key to the progression of Parkinson's disease.
- **Further Research Needed**: While animal studies are promising, challenges remain in applying these results to human populations, particularly concerning dosing and long-term safety. More human studies are needed to confirm ibuprofen's effectiveness in treating neurological conditions.

Chapter 6
Little Patients, Big Relief: Ibuprofen for Children

When a child has a fever, ear infection, or discomfort after vaccination, parents and caregivers often seek safe and effective ways to ease their pain. Ibuprofen, one of the most commonly used NSAIDs for children, helps reduce fever and relieve common aches. In some cases, it is also used to manage inflammation in conditions like juvenile idiopathic arthritis and dental pain, though these applications are less frequent.[285] It is used for these conditions because its anti-inflammatory action helps reduce swelling and tissue inflammation, while its analgesic effect addresses pain.

While ibuprofen is generally safe for children, their bodies process medications differently from adults. This makes it crucial to follow proper dosage recommendations, consider age and weight guidelines, and be aware of potential risks. This chapter explores the role of ibuprofen in pediatric care, providing practical guidance for parents, caregivers, and healthcare providers.

How Should Ibuprofen Be Used?

Ibuprofen is considered safe for children over six months old. However, the FDA has not approved its use for infants younger than six months due to limited safety data. Acetaminophen is the preferred alternative for infants between three and six months old, as it has been more extensively studied in this age group.

To accommodate different ages and preferences, ibuprofen is available in multiple formulations (**Fig. 6.1**).

Regardless of the form used, following the correct ibuprofen dosage is essential for both safety and effectiveness. When choosing the right ibuprofen formulation for children, age and developmental stage are important considerations. The recommended oral dose for children is 5-10 mg per kilogram every 6-8 hours as needed, with a maximum daily limit of 40 mg per kilogram.

Fig. 6.1. Common forms of ibuprofen used by children

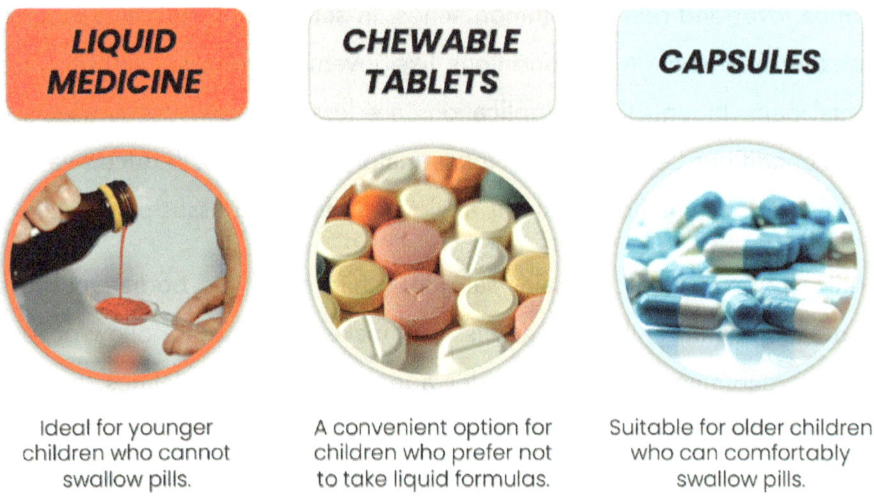

Ibuprofen can sometimes irritate the stomach lining because it blocks the production of prostaglandins that help protect the stomach from its own acid. This irritation can lead to symptoms like indigestion, nausea, or even ulcers, especially with higher doses or prolonged use. Taking ibuprofen with food or milk helps buffer the stomach lining and reduces the risk of these side effects, making it a safer option for children who may be more sensitive to stomach upset. Additionally, it should not be used for more than three days to treat fever or pain unless directed by a healthcare provider. For specific dosing charts, refer to the appendix.

While dosing may seem straightforward, medication errors are a leading cause of hospital visits among children. Measuring liquid ibuprofen accurately is especially critical, as even small miscalculations can lead to underdosing (reducing effectiveness) or overdosing (increasing the risk of side effects).

The most accurate way to measure liquid ibuprofen is with a medication syringe. If one is not included with your ibuprofen, pharmacies offer syringes for precise dosing. Avoid using household teaspoons or tablespoons, as they are not designed for accuracy and can result in incorrect measurements. A 2010 study found that people using teaspoons received 8.4% less medication than intended, while those using tablespoons received 11.6% more. Though these differences may seem minor, repeated overuse, especially near the maximum dose, can increase the risk of side effects.[286] Despite these risks, 34.5% of people still use household spoons to measure liquid medicine.[287]

Consult a doctor if fever persists for more than 24 hours in a child under 2 years, or if the child seems unusually drowsy, irritable, or "acts very sick." Other important warning signs include difficulty breathing, persistent vomiting, severe pain, rash, dehydration, or a seizure.[288]

By carefully following dosing guidelines, using the correct tools, and understanding when and how to use ibuprofen, parents and caregivers can ensure ibuprofen remains a safe and effective way to relieve children's pain, fever, and inflammation.

Safety Precautions and Side Effects

While ibuprofen is generally safe, some precautions are necessary, especially for children with asthma or underlying medical conditions. Though some studies have suggested a potential link between ibuprofen and asthma, a review of 24 studies found no strong evidence supporting this connection. However, ibuprofen may worsen asthma symptoms in some children, so it should be used with caution under medical guidance.[289]

Most ibuprofen side effects are mild, including stomach pain, vomiting, mild abdominal discomfort, or skin rashes. However, prolonged use or high doses can lead to more serious complications, such as kidney issues (especially in dehydrated children), GI bleeding, and in rare cases, hypersensitivity reactions like hives, wheezing, or anaphylaxis (a life-threatening allergic reaction).[285,290]

Common Mistakes When Giving Ibuprofen to Children

Medication errors are surprisingly common. A 2014 study found that 26.42 per 10,000 people annually experience medication-related errors, with pain relievers like ibuprofen among the most misused medications. It is estimated that more than 25% of children given ibuprofen receive the wrong dose.[291,292]

Some of the most frequent mistakes include incorrect dosing using an oral syringe, dropper, or dosing cup; giving an extra dose by accident; and administering doses too frequently.[291,292] Ibuprofen should only be given every 6 to 8 hours and never more than four times in 24 hours.

Moreover, a common error is increasing the dose or shortening the time between doses because a child's fever isn't dropping quickly enough. Some caregivers also alternate between ibuprofen and acetaminophen or even give both medications simultaneously without proper guidance. Though this may seem like an effective way to control fever, it can increase the risk of serious side effects, including GI bleeding and liver damage. [291,292]

Best Practices to Prevent Ibuprofen Misuse

Use the correct dosing tool: Use the oral syringe, dropper, or dosing cup that comes with the medicine. Never use kitchen spoons, which are not accurate.

Dose by weight, not just age: Use your child's current weight to determine the right dose.[293] If you are unsure, ask your doctor or pharmacist for guidance.

Double-check the concentration: Before giving a dose, confirm whether you have infant drops or children's suspension, and use the correct amount for your child's weight and the product's strength.

Write down the time and amount of every medication given: This prevents accidentally giving an extra dose or giving doses too close together.

Review all instructions and ingredients on the bottle: Check all medicines your child is taking to ensure you are not giving more than one product containing ibuprofen.

Consult your doctor: If you are considering alternating ibuprofen with another medicine (like acetaminophen), or if your child is under six months old, has other medical conditions, or is taking other medications, always check with your healthcare provider first.

Know when to seek help: If you think your child has received too much ibuprofen, call the poison control center (1-800-222-1222 in the U.S.) or seek emergency care immediately. Signs of overdose include nausea, vomiting, fatigue, abdominal pain, or more severe symptoms.

Common Questions Parents Have About Ibuprofen

Can You Breastfeed While Taking Ibuprofen?

Ibuprofen is generally considered safe for breastfeeding mothers. It is present in breast milk in only minimal amounts, has a short half-life, and is well tolerated at doses higher than those found in milk. Considering this, ibuprofen is often the preferred pain reliever for nursing mothers.[294]

Are There Any Foods That Should Be Avoided When Giving Ibuprofen?

While research on ibuprofen's interactions with food is limited, studies on other medications suggest that certain foods may interfere with its effectiveness. Here are a few that warrant particular attention:

- **Grapefruit & Grapefruit Juice:** These are known to affect drug metabolism and could increase ibuprofen levels in the bloodstream.[295]

- **High-Fat Foods:** Fatty meals may delay the drug's onset of action, meaning it could take longer to work.[296]

- **Carbonated Soft Drinks:** Some contain phosphoric acid, which might affect how the body absorbs ibuprofen.[296]

Ibuprofen vs. Acetaminophen: Which Is Better For Children?

Both ibuprofen and acetaminophen are widely used to manage pain and fever in children, but they have key differences:

- **Efficacy:** Ibuprofen lasts longer (6-8 hours) than acetaminophen (4-6 hours) and is more effective for inflammation-related pain. Multiple studies and meta-analyses show that both drugs provide similar relief for moderate to severe pain, but ibuprofen is more effective at reducing fever, especially within the first 6 hours after dosing.[297,298]

- **Safety:** Acetaminophen is the preferred choice for children who are dehydrated or have kidney issues, as it poses less risk to kidney function. Ibuprofen can reduce blood flow to the kidneys, making it particularly risky for dehydrated children, such as those experiencing vomiting, diarrhea, or excessive sweating. One study found that more than half of dehydrated children who received ibuprofen developed some degree of kidney impairment, with drug exposure doubling the risk of acute kidney injury compared to those who did not receive ibuprofen.[299]

- **Research summary:** A review of studies up to 2010 found that ibuprofen was more effective than acetaminophen for treating pain and fever in both children and adults, with similar safety profiles.[300]

When deciding whether to use ibuprofen or acetaminophen, consider your child's symptoms. Both medications are effective for reducing fever and pain, but ibuprofen also reduces inflammation, which can be helpful for conditions like sprains or sore throats. Studies show that ibuprofen is often more effective at lowering fever and easing pain in the first 24 hours, with a similar safety profile to acetaminophen when used as directed.[301]

However, acetaminophen may be preferred if your child has kidney problems, is dehydrated, or has a history of stomach issues, as ibuprofen can worsen these conditions. If you're unsure whether ibuprofen or acetaminophen is best for your child's condition, consult your healthcare provider.

Should You Alternate Ibuprofen and Acetaminophen?

A 2024 review analyzing 31 trials with 5,009 children found that alternating ibuprofen and acetaminophen in the first six hours did not increase side effects compared to using either drug alone.[302] However, the long-term effects of alternating these medications are not well studied.[303]

Many major health organizations, including the American Academy of Pediatrics, advise parents to stick to a single medication rather than alternating.[304,305] That said, some doctors and parents still use alternating doses, and studies show that less experienced doctors are more likely to recommend this approach.[306,307] This may be due to gaps in awareness or understanding of current guidelines.

However, some doctors who recommend alternating medications may do so because studies indicate these drugs work through different mechanisms and are processed by different organs. Acetaminophen is processed through the liver, and ibuprofen through the kidneys. It is also possible that they do so because studies found that alternating acetaminophen (10 to 15 mg/kg per dose) with ibuprofen (5-10mg/kg) every 4 hours was more effective at lowering fever in children than using either continuously.[308,309]

Are Medical Practitioners Using Best Practices?

Guidelines from major organizations like the FDA, the British National Formulary, the World Health Organization (WHO), and the American Academy of Pediatrics generally align on key recommendations for ibuprofen use in children. However, studies show that some doctors do not always follow these best practices. For example, a survey of pediatricians in Italy found that some continue to alternate ibuprofen and acetaminophen (with 9% alternating and 7.1% combining the two drugs), despite official guidelines advising against it. Others even use these medications preventively before vaccinations, which is not recommended.[310] This behavior is not unique to Italy; similar patterns have been reported in other countries, with both parents and healthcare professionals sometimes alternating these medications for pain or fever management in children.[311] Using ibuprofen or acetaminophen before vaccinations is discouraged because studies suggest these medicines may blunt the immune response to vaccines, potentially reducing vaccine effectiveness.[312]

Is Your Child at Risk for an Allergic Reaction To Ibuprofen?

Ibuprofen is one of the most common triggers for drug hypersensitivity reactions in children. Recent research (2017-2024) has helped develop a risk-stratification tool to identify children who are at low risk of reacting to ibuprofen.[290]

- Lower Risk: Children with no history of angioedema (rapid swelling of deeper skin layers) or anaphylaxis (severe allergic reaction) are less likely to experience an adverse reaction. Severe allergic reactions include trouble breathing, severe drowsiness, dizziness, fainting, skin turning pale or blue, or swelling of lips, face, mouth, throat, or tongue.

- Higher Risk: Children aged 10 or older who have previously experienced angioedema or anaphylaxis may be at greater risk of a reaction to ibuprofen.
- If your child has a history of allergic reactions, consult a doctor before giving them ibuprofen.

If your child takes ibuprofen and develops any of the above symptoms-especially trouble breathing, swelling of the face or throat, or sudden severe symptoms-stop giving ibuprofen immediately and seek emergency medical help (**call 911**).

How to Ensure Safe Use of Ibuprofen

Healthcare professionals play a crucial role in educating families about proper ibuprofen use. However, as a parent or caregiver, it's important to take an active role in ensuring you're using ibuprofen safely and correctly:

- Ask your doctor about the correct dose based on your child's weight, the maximum single dose, the total daily limit, and the time interval between doses.
- Ask your doctor to consider your child's age, organ function, or special health conditions which can make standard doses unsafe.[313]
- If buying over-the-counter ibuprofen, consult a pharmacist to confirm the appropriate dose for your child's age and weight.
- Follow the dosing instructions exactly and avoid guessing or adjusting the dose on your own.

By taking these precautions, you can safely and effectively use ibuprofen to relieve your child's discomfort while minimizing the risk of medication errors.

Key Takeaways:

- Ibuprofen is an effective treatment for fever, pain, and inflammation in children when used correctly.
- Side effects are rare but possible; caregivers should be aware of potential risks, particularly with misuse or overuse.
- To ensure safety, always follow weight and age-appropriate dosing, avoid excessive use, and monitor the child's response to the medication.
- Be aware of specific risks, such as potential side effects and overdose, and consider any underlying medical conditions your child may have, such as kidney problems or dehydration, which may make ibuprofen unsafe.
- Always use the oral syringe or dosing cup that comes with the medicine for accurate measurement—never use household spoons—to prevent dosing errors.
- If you are unsure about the correct dose, the appropriate formulation, or whether ibuprofen is safe for your child, consult your healthcare provider before administering the medication.

Chapter 7
Ibuprofen During COVID-19: Impact on Patient Outcomes and Public Perception

The COVID-19 pandemic, caused by the SARS-CoV-2 virus, profoundly impacted lives worldwide, sparking widespread concern about how to manage symptoms effectively. Among the many questions that arose was whether common medications, such as ibuprofen, could influence the severity of the disease. Early in the pandemic, conflicting reports fueled uncertainty: some suggested ibuprofen might worsen COVID-19 symptoms, while others claimed it had no impact or could even be beneficial.

Given how commonly ibuprofen is used, millions likely took it before or during a COVID-19 infection—often without knowing they were sick, since many cases were asymptomatic. This raises a crucial question: does ibuprofen help, harm, or have no effect on COVID-19 symptoms? By mid-2020, the scientific consensus was that ibuprofen does not worsen COVID-19. This was important, as understanding its potential impact could shape public health guidance and influence the choices of those managing the illness.

Why the Initial Confusion?

In March 2020, French health authorities issued a warning that ibuprofen might increase the risk of severe or fatal COVID-19 symptoms. Their concern stemmed from the idea that ibuprofen could boost the production of a receptor called angiotensin-converting enzyme 2 (ACE2). ACE2 proteins are found on the surface of human cells and serve as the entry point for the SARS-CoV-2 virus. The virus's spike proteins latch onto these receptors, allowing it to invade cells and multiply.[314]

The warning was based on a study involving rats, which suggested that ibuprofen could increase the number of ACE2 receptors **(Fig. 7.1)**.[315] Further research on both human and rat cells supported these findings, indicating that ibuprofen might indeed upregulate ACE2 expression[315]. This led to fears that taking ibuprofen during a COVID-19 infection could create more pathways for the virus to enter cells and spread.

Fig. 7.1. Infection of Human Cells With The SARS-CoV-2 Virus That Causes COVID-19

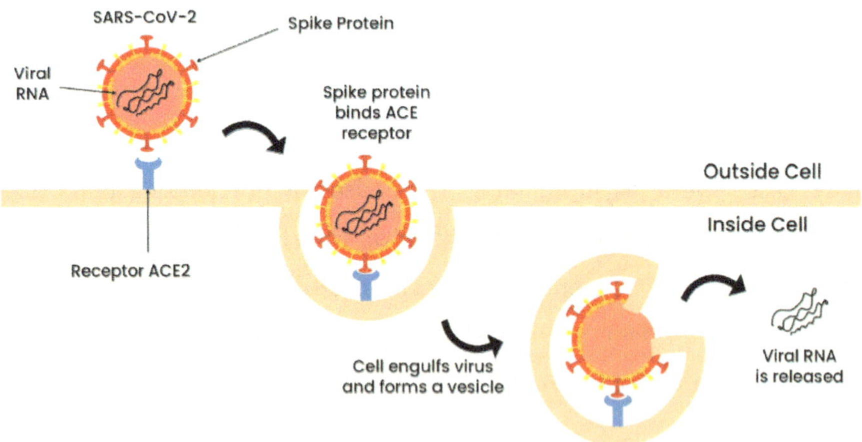

While early studies suggested ibuprofen might increase the number of ACE2 receptors, potentially making it easier for the SARS-CoV-2 virus to enter cells, further research revealed a more complex picture. The same study found that ibuprofen also activated mechanisms that reduced the virus's ability to invade cells.

To understand this, imagine cells have "doors" (ACE2 receptors) that the virus uses to enter. Ibuprofen may increase the number of doors, but it also installs stronger locks, making it harder for the virus to get inside. This happens because ibuprofen interferes with two key enzymes, ADAM17 and TMPRSS2, which the virus relies on to open these "doors." As a result, while there may be more entry points, the virus has a harder time using them. [315]

What Do the Studies Say?

Several studies have examined whether ibuprofen use affects the severity of COVID-19 symptoms. The overall evidence suggests that ibuprofen does not significantly impact COVID-19 outcomes, but there are important considerations regarding study size, design, and potential biases.

Shamir Medical Center Study (Israel, 403 patients):

This retrospective study analyzed data from 403 COVID-19 patients, evenly split between men and women, with an average age of 45 years.[316] The week before their diagnosis with COVID-19, 22% used ibuprofen and 32% used paracetamol for symptom relief.

Comparing outcomes:

- Ibuprofen users: 3.4% (3 patients) passed away, and 10.3% (9 patients) required respiratory support.

- Non-ibuprofen users: 2.8% (9 patients) passed away, and 11% (35 patients) required respiratory support.[317]

The differences in mortality and need for respiratory support were minor and not statistically significant, suggesting ibuprofen did not worsen clinical outcomes compared to paracetamol or no antipyretic use.

Limitation: This study's small sample size (403 patients) means its findings should be interpreted with caution, especially compared to larger studies.

Denmark Nationwide Study (4,002 patients):
This larger study analyzed data for 4,000 COVID-19 patients, 6.6% (264 patients) of whom had filled an ibuprofen prescription before their diagnosis.

After adjusting for age, sex, and comorbidities, there was no significant association between ibuprofen use and severe COVID-19 outcomes (defined as severe respiratory syndrome, ICU admission, or death).[317]

Strength: Larger sample size and adjustment for key confounders make these findings more robust.

Other Large-Scale Evidence:
A 2023 study analyzed 1.7 million participants with chronic pain conditions who regularly used ibuprofen. It found no increased risk of COVID-19 infection, hospitalization, or severe outcomes compared to users of other pain relievers.[318]

A study across 255 healthcare facilities in England, Scotland, and Wales found no significant differences in in-hospital mortality, need for ventilation, oxygen requirements, or acute kidney injury between NSAID users and non-users.[319]

Limitations and Final Thoughts

Some concerns have been raised about the methodology of these studies. Many relied on patient recall, which can introduce bias, and some had relatively small sample sizes (fewer than 1000 patients) of ibuprofen users, making it harder to generalize findings. Patient recall can distort research findings by introducing systematic errors in how participants remember and report past events or exposures, while small sample sizes weaken research reliability by limiting the detection of true effects and increasing error rates.[320,321] However, despite these limitations, the majority of evidence suggests that ibuprofen does not increase the severity of COVID-19 symptoms.

In summary, early fears about ibuprofen's role in COVID-19 outcomes were unfounded. Multiple studies show no strong clinical or scientific evidence that ibuprofen is harmful for those with COVID-19. Given its widespread use for pain and fever relief, this is reassuring news. So, if you contract COVID-19, you can safely take ibuprofen to manage fever and discomfort without unnecessary fear. This chapter underscores the importance of making health decisions based on high-quality, up-to-date scientific evidence rather than early reports or speculation.

Key Takeaways:

- **Ibuprofen and COVID-19 Concerns**: Early in the pandemic, there was significant anxiety about the use of ibuprofen in COVID-19 cases.[322] However, the majority of studies suggest no significant worsening of symptoms.

- It is important to note that much of the available research is observational and subject to limitations such as recall bias, small sample sizes, and lack of data on asymptomatic carriers.

- **Limited Role in Symptom Management**: While ibuprofen is effective for managing pain and fever in COVID-19, there is no scientific evidence that it provides additional benefits, such as reducing the length of COVID-19 symptoms. Ongoing research is actively exploring ibuprofen's role in inflammation regulation during COVID-19, which could clarify its potential benefits or risks beyond symptom relief.[323]

THE BAD

Chapter 8 **Ibuprofen and the Heart:** A Silent Threat?

For many people, reaching for an ibuprofen pill is second nature. It's a trusted remedy for headaches, muscle aches, and everyday discomfort. But what if this familiar pill carried an unexpected risk—one that could silently harm your heart?

In recent years, mounting research has uncovered a troubling side to ibuprofen and similar pain relievers, linking them to increased cardiovascular risks.[324] Could something so widely used be endangering your heart without you even realizing it?

Does Ibuprofen Increase the Risk of Heart Disease?

Research suggests that some NSAIDs, including ibuprofen, may increase the risk of heart problems (**Fig. 8.1**). A review of multiple studies found that ibuprofen and other drugs that block COX-2, an enzyme involved in inflammation, can raise blood pressure and even double the risk of congestive heart failure.[325-327]

In brief, when COX-2 is blocked, prostacyclin levels drop, but thromboxane (which promotes clotting) is not affected. This imbalance can make blood clots more likely, raising the risk of heart attack and stroke.[328]

COX-2 inhibitors can cause the body to retain salt and water, leading to increased blood pressure.[328]

Fig. 8.1. Ibuprofen associated with increased risk of cardiovascular diseases and overall mortality

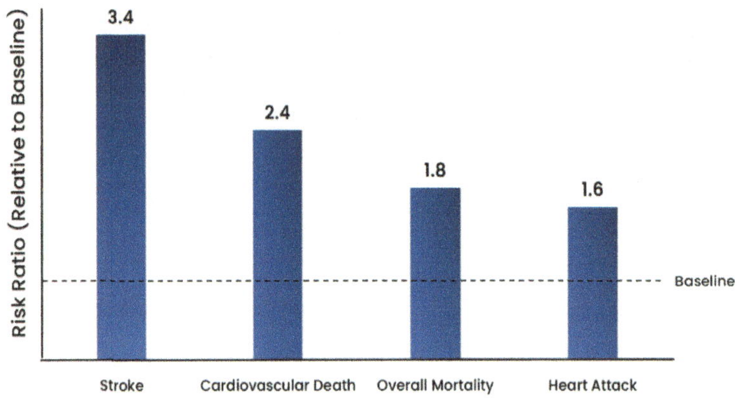

Looking specifically at ibuprofen, high doses have been linked to a significantly increased risk of major coronary events.[137] In a meta-analysis of 31 clinical trials involving over 116,000 patients,[329] ibuprofen was associated with:

- A 3.4 times higher risk of stroke[329]
- A 2.4 times higher risk of cardiovascular death[329]
- A 1.8 times higher risk of death from any cause[329]
- A 1.6 times higher risk of heart attack[329]

Among the seven NSAIDs studied (ibuprofen, naproxen, diclofenac, celecoxib, etoricoxib, rofecoxib, and lumiracoxib), ibuprofen posed the highest stroke risk.[329] However, it's important to note that these findings are based on high-dose usage. The risks for those who take ibuprofen occasionally or in lower doses are likely much lower.

It should also be noted that different NSAIDs have varying cardiovascular risks. For example, naproxen does not appear to significantly increase the risk of blood clot formation in arteries, a process called atherothrombosis, which can lead to heart attacks.[330]

What Does the FDA Say About NSAIDs and Heart Risks?

Concerns about NSAIDs and heart health are not new. The FDA has warned about the cardiovascular risks of non-aspirin NSAIDs, including ibuprofen, for years.

In 2005, public attention was drawn to these risks following the controversy surrounding Vioxx, a once-popular NSAID that was linked to a sharp increase in heart attacks. The drug, which specifically targeted COX-2, was estimated to have caused 140,000 heart attacks before being pulled from the market in 2004.[331]

A year later, the FDA issued its first official warning about NSAIDs and heart risks. Then, in 2015, after further research confirmed the dangers, the FDA strengthened its warning, emphasizing the increased risk of heart attacks and strokes even with short-term NSAID use.[332]

COX-2 inhibitors like Vioxx were developed to reduce pain and inflammation without causing stomach problems associated with traditional NSAIDs that inhibit both COX-1 and COX-2. However, blocking COX-2 reduces the production of prostacyclin, a molecule that normally helps keep blood vessels dilated and prevents platelets from clumping together. When prostacyclin levels drop but thromboxane (which promotes clotting) remains unchanged (because it is produced via COX-1), the risk of blood clot formation, high blood pressure, and other cardiovascular problems increases.[328,333,334] The Vioxx case highlighted the importance of understanding the different roles of COX-1 and COX-2 and the potential for serious cardiovascular side effects when selectively inhibiting COX-2.

What This Means for You

If you occasionally take ibuprofen for a headache or sore muscles, there's no need to panic for most users. The greatest risks appear to be linked to high doses and long-term use. However, if you rely on NSAIDs frequently or have pre-existing cardiovascular conditions, it is worth discussing alternative pain management options with your doctor.

Pain relief is important, but so is your heart health. Knowing the risks can help you make informed decisions about what's best for your body.

The FDA now requires that prescription labels for NSAIDs reflect important updates regarding cardiovascular risks:

1. Heart Attack and Stroke Risks Begin Early

- The risk of heart attack or stroke can start within the first few weeks of NSAID use, and prolonged use further increases this risk.[335]

2. Dose-Dependent Risk

- Higher doses of NSAIDs (more than 1200 mg/day) are linked to a greater risk of cardiovascular complications.

3. NSAID-Specific Risks Remain Unclear

- While it was previously believed that all NSAIDs carried the same cardiovascular risks, new data suggest that risk levels may vary between different NSAIDs. However, there is not enough conclusive evidence to declare any specific NSAID as definitively safer or riskier than others.

4. Risks Apply to Everyone, Not Just Those with Heart Disease

- The FDA warns that NSAIDs increase the risk of heart attack and stroke for all users, regardless of pre-existing heart conditions. However, individuals with heart disease or cardiovascular risk factors face an even higher baseline risk, which NSAIDs can further exacerbate.

5. Post-Heart Attack Risks

- Taking NSAIDs after a heart attack is associated with an increased likelihood of death within the following year compared to those who do not take them.

6. Higher Risk of Heart Failure

- NSAID use has been linked to an increased risk of heart failure, particularly in individuals who are already at risk.

These warnings are supported by extensive research showing that NSAID use is associated with increased cardiovascular disease risks. While NSAIDs like ibuprofen are effective for pain relief, frequent or high-dose use may come with serious heart-related consequences.

Some studies suggest that naproxen may be a safer alternative for individuals concerned about cardiovascular risks. In a 2011 study, naproxen was not linked to statistically significant increases in myocardial infarction, stroke, or cardiovascular death compared to placebo.[329] However, the potential dangers are likely to depend on dosage, duration, and individual health factors. Consulting a healthcare provider before choosing any pain relief option remains essential.

How Does Ibuprofen Contribute to Cardiovascular Disease?

The precise mechanism behind ibuprofen's impact on heart health is still under investigation, but research indicates that it affects key enzymes critical to heart and blood vessel function.

Ibuprofen works by inhibiting the COX-1 and COX-2 enzymes, which are essential for regulating blood vessel dilation, blood pressure, and platelet clumping factors that directly influence cardiovascular health.[114,336,337]

- COX-1 enzyme inhibition leads to increased thromboxane production, which promotes platelet aggregation (clumping) and blood vessel constriction.[336] This can increase the likelihood of blood clot formation and hypertension.

- COX-2 inhibition disrupts the balance between prostacyclin (PGI2, a vasodilator and platelet inhibitor produced by COX-2 in blood vessels) and thromboxane A2 (TXA2, a vasoconstrictor and platelet aggregator produced by COX-1 in platelets). By selectively blocking COX-2, prostacyclin levels drop, while thromboxane remains unaffected. This imbalance promotes vasoconstriction, platelet clumping, and thrombus formation, increasing the risk of heart attacks and strokes.[336,337]

Additionally, recent research, including studies from our own lab (the Gomes Lab), has revealed that ibuprofen, along with other NSAIDs such as naproxen, meclofenamate sodium, and diclofenac, can also lead to increased levels of reactive oxygen species (ROS) in heart cells.[338,339] Elevated ROS levels can cause oxidative stress, which is a known contributor to cardiovascular diseases such as hypertension, atherosclerosis, and heart failure.

Takeaway

While ibuprofen remains a widely used pain reliever, its potential cardiovascular risks should not be ignored, especially for individuals who take it frequently or at high doses. Understanding these risks and discussing safer alternatives with a healthcare provider can help minimize potential harm while ensuring effective pain management.

What is ROS?

Reactive Oxygen Species (ROS) are natural byproducts of oxygen metabolism within cells. At low concentrations, they play an essential role in cell signaling and maintaining homeostasis. However, when ROS levels become excessive, they can cause severe cellular damage by harming lipids, proteins, and DNA, ultimately disrupting normal cellular function.[340]

NSAIDs can increase ROS production mainly by disrupting mitochondrial function, depleting antioxidants like glutathione, and affecting enzymes such as NADPH oxidase. This overproduction of ROS contributes to the tissue damage and side effects sometimes seen with NSAID use.

Research shows that NSAIDs significantly increase ROS levels in various cell types, mainly by disrupting mitochondrial function, depleting antioxidants like glutathione, and affecting enzymes such as NADPH oxidase. This overproduction of ROS contributes to the tissue damage and side effects sometimes seen with NSAID use. However, this effect is particularly pronounced in cardiac cells, potentially leading to an elevated risk of cardiovascular disease.[338]

How Do Ibuprofen and Other NSAIDs Increase ROS?

Studies, including research from our lab, suggest that ibuprofen and other NSAIDs increase ROS levels in the heart by disrupting mitochondrial function (**Fig. 8.2**;[338,339,] unpublished results). Mitochondria, often called the powerhouses of the cell, generate energy (ATP) through a series of protein complexes (Complexes I to IV).

Certain NSAIDs interfere with this process:

- Naproxen and diclofenac affect Complex III, impairing energy production.[338,339]
- Meclofenamate sodium inhibits both Complex I and III, reducing mitochondrial efficiency.[338,339]
- Ibuprofen (unpublished results from our lab) appears to inhibit Complexes I and III, contributing to elevated ROS levels in cardiac cells.

When mitochondrial complexes are disrupted, ROS can accumulate, leading to oxidative stress, a condition where excess ROS overwhelms the body's natural antioxidant defenses.[341] While our cells have built-in antioxidants (such as vitamin E) to neutralize ROS, persistent oxidative stress can damage key cellular structures, increasing the risk of cardiovascular disease.

Fig. 8.2. Ibuprofen inhibits mitochondrial complexes increasing oxidative stress inside the heart

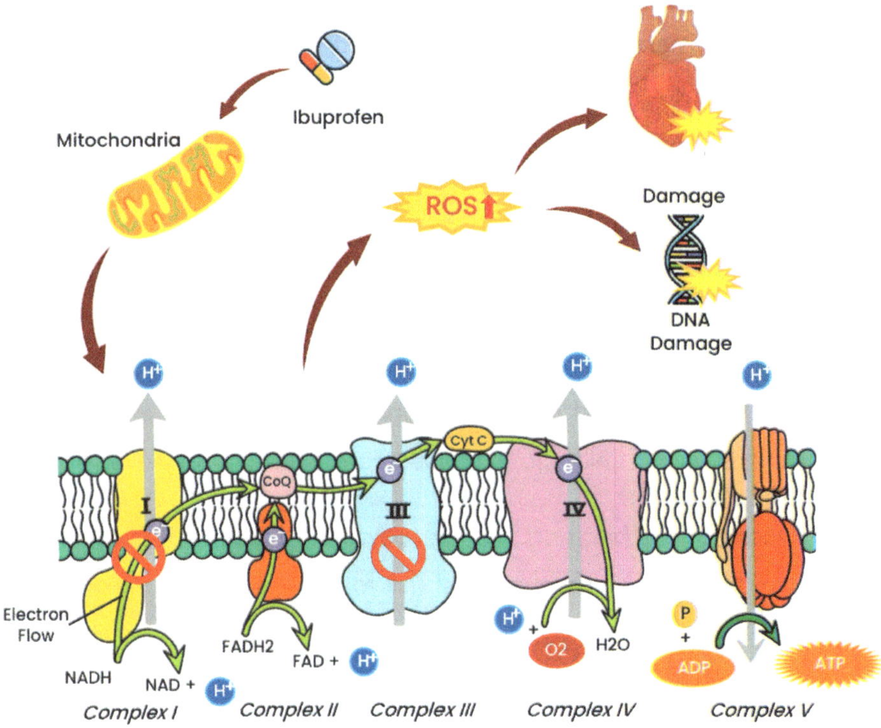

The Role of NSAIDs in Heart Function and Fibrosis

As noted in the previous section, NSAIDs induce ROS. Studies show that excessive ROS disrupts vascular integrity, promotes inflammatory plaque development, and degrades endothelial function, causing cardiovascular pathology.[342-344] ROS also reduces nitric oxide (NO) bioavailability, which impairs vasodilation and promotes vasoconstriction.[345]

Long-term exposure to NSAIDs, particularly diclofenac, has been shown to disrupt calcium balance in the heart, negatively impacting both diastolic and systolic function.[325] Additionally, ibuprofen has been linked to upregulation of the mitogen-activated protein kinase (MAPK) pathway in cardiac fibroblasts, which are responsible for producing collagen and maintaining heart tissue.[346] Overactivation of this pathway leads to excessive collagen production, contributing to fibrosis.

Cardiac fibrosis is a condition where scar-like tissue builds up in the heart, impairing its ability to contract and pump blood efficiently. Over time, this can lead to heart dysfunction and increased cardiovascular risks.[325]

Takeaway

NSAIDs like ibuprofen are effective for short-term pain relief, but emerging research highlights potential concerns about cardiovascular safety with prolonged or high-dose use. Studies suggest that chronic NSAID use may contribute to oxidative stress, mitochondrial dysfunction, and cardiac fibrosis—mechanisms linked to increased cardiovascular risk over time.

- **Occasional Use** (e.g., a few days for acute pain or fever) at standard doses poses minimal risk for most healthy individuals.
- **Chronic or High-Dose Use** (e.g., daily use for weeks/months) is associated with greater risks, particularly for those with pre-existing heart conditions, hypertension, or kidney disease.

For individuals requiring long-term pain management, especially those at risk for heart disease, discussing alternative strategies (e.g., physical therapy, acetaminophen, or non-pharmacologic options) with a healthcare provider is advisable.

Ibuprofen's Other Potential Mechanisms

While the exact impact of ibuprofen on cardiac dysfunction remains unclear, it may affect several biological pathways beyond ROS production. Emerging evidence suggests that ibuprofen-induced oxidative stress can directly impair proteasome function, creating a toxic cycle of protein misfolding and cellular damage.

Role of the Proteasome in Cardiac Health

The proteasome is a cellular complex responsible for breaking down damaged or misfolded proteins, ensuring proper cellular function. However, when cells experience mitochondrial damage and increased ROS, proteasome activity often declines, leading to a buildup of non-functional proteins that can harm cardiac cells.[347]

While earlier studies linked proteasome inhibition to drugs like diclofenac (an NSAID), recent research demonstrates that ibuprofen also disrupts proteasome function and mitochondrial health.[348]

Alterations in the mitochondrial electron transport chain by diclofenac have been linked to reduced proteasome activity due to ROS-induced oxidation of the proteasome subunits, ultimately increasing cardiac cell death.[338,349] In mouse hearts, at physiological human doses, increased ROS and caused by mitochondrial dysfunction.[348]

Why This Matters

Proteasome dysfunction decreases the heart's ability to remove damaged proteins, accelerating cardiac cell death and fibrosis. This mechanism may explain why long-term ibuprofen users exhibit higher rates of heart failure, particularly in older adults with pre-existing protein homeostasis deficits.[350,351]

Ibuprofen and Platelet Aggregation

Ibuprofen inhibits COX enzymes, which play a key role in producing prostaglandins and thromboxanes. By blocking COX-1, ibuprofen reduces thromboxane A2 (TXA2) levels. TXA2 is a molecule that promotes platelet aggregation and vasoconstriction. However, its antiplatelet effects differ significantly from aspirin's, with critical implications for cardiovascular risk and bleeding.

Key Mechanisms and Comparisons

Reversible vs. Irreversible Inhibition:

- Ibuprofen binds reversibly to COX-1, causing temporary suppression of TXA2. Platelet function normalizes within 24 hours after discontinuation, as new platelets enter circulation.
- Aspirin irreversibly acetylates and inhibits COX-1, blocking TXA2 production for the lifespan of platelets (8–9 days). This sustained inhibition contributes to its cardiovascular protective effects.[352]

Clinical Implications:

- While short-term ibuprofen use may temporarily reduce clotting ability, it does not provide long-term cardiovascular protection like low-dose aspirin.[352]
- In healthy individuals, even high-dose ibuprofen (600 mg every 8 hours for 7 days) only temporarily impairs platelet aggregation, with function returning to normal within 24 hours.[353]

Patients taking anticoagulants or those with conditions affecting bleeding risk should consult their healthcare provider before using ibuprofen or any NSAID to avoid potential complications.

Ibuprofen for Acute Pericarditis

Acute pericarditis is inflammation of the pericardium, the thin membrane surrounding the heart, often causing chest pain. Ibuprofen is commonly used to treat this condition due to its anti-inflammatory and pain-relieving properties.[354]

A 2024 Danish nationwide cohort study of 12,381 patients (median age of 51 years and 29% female) with acute pericarditis found that ibuprofen use for acute pericarditis did not increase cardiovascular risks (as measured by ischemic stroke, congestive heart failure, myocardial infarction, or cardiovascular death).[355] However, the study relied on prescription data, making it unclear how long and at what dosage patients actually used ibuprofen.

Can Ibuprofen Trigger Heart Rhythm Issues?

Emerging evidence from preclinical studies suggests ibuprofen may influence cardiac electrical activity, interfering with the electrical impulses that regulate heartbeat, but human data remains limited.

One study on over 1000 patients between 40 to 89 years with atrial fibrillation in the United Kingdom found that current use of NSAIDs was associated with a 44% increased risk of chronic atrial fibrillation.[356] This risk rises to 80% in users with a treatment duration of more than one year (long-term users), and may be related to short-term effects on kidney function and fluid balance, which can trigger arrhythmias.

A study on guinea pigs investigated ibuprofen's effects on cardiac electrical activity using both live animals (*in vivo*) and isolated heart tissues (*in vitro*).[357]

Study Overview:

- Researchers measured the heart rhythms of guinea pigs before and after administering ibuprofen at varying doses (10-30 μM).[357] These doses are lower than typical human therapeutic levels.

- Guinea pigs are used as they have similar ion channel properties as human hearts.
- Electrocardiograms (ECGs) were used to track electrical signals in the heart.[357]
- In separate experiments, researchers removed the hearts, isolated papillary muscles, and stimulated them with electrodes to assess electrical activity.[357]

By analyzing heart action potentials, researchers aimed to determine whether ibuprofen disrupts normal heart function.[357] They found that ibuprofen caused prolonged QRS duration, shortened action potential duration and effective refractory period, and increased susceptibility to ventricular fibrillation *in vitro*.

In a human case study involving a 13-year-old girl, heart palpitations occurred after standard oral ibuprofen dosing (three doses of 400mg).[358] The girl had no structural heart disease or prior arrhythmia history, and her symptoms resolved upon discontinuation.

While the full implications for human heart health are still being explored, this research suggests that ibuprofen may have unexpected effects on cardiac electrical activity, warranting further study. While OTC doses in healthy individuals likely pose minimal risk, caution is warranted in those with cardiovascular comorbidities. Patients with preexisting heart disease or electrolyte imbalances (e.g., hyperkalemia) may face higher risks due to compounded electrophysiological instability.

Takeaways

Proteasome Function in Cardiac Health

- The proteasome function is critical for degrading damaged or misfolded proteins in cardiac cells. Reduced proteasome activity causes accumulation of toxic protein aggregates and increased risk of cardiomyocyte death and heart failure.

- Chronic ibuprofen use (equivalent to 500 mg/day in humans) causes sex-specific proteasome dysfunction: Female mice show 10x more protein changes than males, including increased immunoproteasome activity and impaired mitochondrial function. Male mice showed fewer protein changes, but still caused proteasome and mitochondrial dysfunction.

- These changes may exacerbate cardiovascular risks by impairing protein quality control and energy production.

Antiplatelet Effects: Ibuprofen vs. Aspirin

- Ibuprofen's effect on platelet aggregation is temporary and weaker than aspirin's, meaning it does not provide long-term cardiovascular protection.

- Aspirin is used to prevent blood clots, whereas ibuprofen does not provide this benefit, making it a less protective choice for heart patients.

- Ibuprofen is effective for acute pericarditis, but more research is needed to determine its long-term safety in heart patients.

- Emerging studies suggest ibuprofen may impact heart rhythms, highlighting the need for further investigation into its potential cardiovascular effects.

Patients with preexisting heart conditions should consult a healthcare provider before prolonged ibuprofen use, especially if they are at risk for heart disease, clotting disorders, or arrhythmias.

Main Findings

Ibuprofen administration led to significant changes in the electrocardiograms (ECGs) of guinea pigs. The QRS complex representing the heart's electrical impulse conduction was prolonged, indicating slowed electrical activity. Simultaneously, the QT interval, a key component of heartbeat rhythm, was shortened. While heart rate variability remained largely unchanged, some guinea pigs exhibited premature beats and, in certain cases, ventricular fibrillation, a severe and potentially fatal arrhythmia, at doses as low as 5 or 10 mg/kg.[357] The guinea pig ECG model is useful because studies show that it is a robust tool for predicting human cardiac responses to new drugs, particularly for identifying proarrhythmic risks and evaluating the cardiac safety of candidate compounds.[359]

At the cellular level, ibuprofen has been shown to slow fast-response action potentials, which are crucial for coordinating heart contractions. This effect is likely due to ibuprofen's interaction with fast sodium ion (Na^+) channels, which play a vital role in maintaining a steady heartbeat. Disruption of these sodium channels can lead to conduction abnormalities, increasing the risk of arrhythmias-especially in individuals with pre-existing heart conditions, where the heart's electrical system is already more vulnerable.[360] By interfering with these channels, ibuprofen may increase the heart's susceptibility to irregular rhythms and potentially life-threatening arrhythmias.[357]

Additionally, ibuprofen altered slow-response and spontaneous action potentials, impacting the consistency of cardiac cell contractions. In studies with guinea pig hearts, lower doses caused mild irregularities that could be reversed. However, at higher doses, two out of eight guinea pig hearts ceased beating entirely, and heart rate declined in 75% of experiments, indicating a severe, dose-dependent impact.[357]

The study concluded that ibuprofen can significantly affect the heart's electrical activity, increasing the risk of arrhythmias, particularly at high doses.[357] While these effects may not pose a major risk for healthy individuals, those with pre-existing heart conditions should exercise caution and consult a healthcare provider before taking ibuprofen—especially for long-term or high-dose use—to mitigate potential cardiovascular risks.

In humans, there have been rare case reports of arrhythmias and palpitations following ibuprofen use, including atrial fibrillation and broad complex tachycardia, particularly in overdose situations or in those with other risk factors.[358] However, large-scale clinical studies confirming a direct, consistent impact of ibuprofen on heart rhythms in the general population are lacking, and further research is needed to fully understand the risk in humans.[357]

NSAIDs for Osteoarthritis Patients

While NSAIDs are effective for managing osteoarthritis symptoms, their safety profile in patients with underlying cardiovascular issues remains a concern. For individuals with osteoarthritis who rely on NSAIDs like ibuprofen for pain relief, a major study has highlighted key differences in how these medications may affect heart health, particularly for those at higher cardiovascular risk.

The Therapeutic Arthritis Research and Gastrointestinal Trial evaluated the safety of lumiracoxib, a selective COX-2 inhibitor (lumiracoxib) designed to reduce inflammation while minimizing GI side effects. Unlike traditional NSAIDs like ibuprofen, which inhibit both COX-1 and COX-2 enzymes, lumiracoxib specifically targets COX-2, a key player in the inflammatory process.[361]

It is important to note that lumiracoxib has since been withdrawn from many markets due to concerns about liver toxicity. However, its inclusion in these studies remains relevant for understanding the comparative cardiovascular risks of different NSAIDs in osteoarthritis management.

The TARGET trial enrolled over 18,000 patients aged 50 and older with primary osteoarthritis.[361] Patients were randomized into three groups:

- Lumiracoxib 400 mg once daily
- Naproxen 500 mg twice daily
- Ibuprofen 800 mg three times daily

Each group included both high- and low-risk cardiovascular patients. High-risk patients were those with conditions like diabetes or at least one cardiovascular risk factor, including hypertension, high total cholesterol, or low levels of high-density lipoprotein cholesterol. The trial lasted 52 weeks, with regular monitoring. The primary goal was to assess their impact on cardiovascular health, particularly concerning heart attack and stroke risk among high-risk osteoarthritis patients.[361]

Study Findings

The results showed that the risk of heart attack and stroke varied between the different treatments, especially for those with high cardiovascular risk:[361]

- **Ibuprofen and Aspirin**: High-risk patients taking both ibuprofen and aspirin had a heart attack and stroke rate eight times higher than those taking lumiracoxib and 1.5 times higher than those taking naproxen.

- **Naproxen**: For high-risk patients without aspirin, naproxen appeared safer, showing a lower cardiovascular risk than ibuprofen.

- **Low-Risk Patients**: For patients with low cardiovascular risk, no significant differences were observed between lumiracoxib, ibuprofen, or naproxen.

The researchers also looked into the risk of developing congestive heart failure in patients taking ibuprofen. They found that congestive heart failure developed in 1.28% of patients on ibuprofen, compared to just 0.14% of those on lumiracoxib—a nearly ninefold difference. In contrast, the rate of congestive heart failure among patients taking naproxen was similar to that seen with lumiracoxib.[361] To put these findings in perspective, for every 1,000 patients treated, about 13 developed congestive heart failure on ibuprofen versus just 1 to 2 on lumiracoxib over a year.

What This Means for Osteoarthritis Patients

If you have osteoarthritis and a higher risk of cardiovascular disease, choosing the right NSAID is crucial. Research suggests that naproxen may be a safer option than ibuprofen, particularly if you're also taking aspirin. While NSAIDs can effectively relieve pain, it's important to discuss their potential heart risks with your doctor—especially if you're using higher doses or combining them with heart medications.

Ibuprofen and Blood Pressure Medications

Taking ibuprofen alongside blood pressure medications can have clinically significant effects on blood pressure control, especially for those with hypertension. While the original 1987 study remains frequently cited and foundational, more recent research has confirmed its key findings and provided additional context for today's clinical practice.[362,363] The 1987 randomized, placebo-controlled trial examined 45 patients with essential hypertension, all on at least two antihypertensive medications. During the three-week intervention, patients received ibuprofen at 400 mg every 8 hours (totaling 1200 mg/day—a moderate strength dose), acetaminophen at 1 g every 8 hours, or placebo. The researchers aimed to determine whether ibuprofen interferes with blood pressure control.[362]

Participants were divided into three groups, each receiving either ibuprofen, acetaminophen, or a placebo every eight hours for three weeks. Throughout the study, researchers closely monitored their blood pressure, heart rate, and other vital signs to assess the impact of these medications.[362]

The study was conducted over nine weeks and consisted of three phases:

- **Phase I (4 weeks):** Patients were checked for their baseline blood pressure while on their regular medications. Only those with diastolic pressure (the pressure when the heart relaxes) between 90 and 114 mmHg were eligible for the study.

- **Phase II (3 weeks):** Patients were randomly assigned to take ibuprofen (two 200 mg tablets), acetaminophen (two 500 mg tablets), or a placebo.

- **Phase III (2 weeks):** This was a "washout" phase, where all participants took the placebo to see if the effects of ibuprofen wore off after stopping the medication.

Study Findings

In the ibuprofen group, the mean increase from baseline after 3 weeks was:

The study revealed that patients taking ibuprofen experienced an increase in systolic blood pressure (the pressure during heart contractions) and mean arterial pressure (the average blood pressure throughout the heartbeat cycle) during Phase 2 of the trial.

- Supine diastolic blood pressure: +6.4 mm Hg
- Supine mean arterial pressure: +6.6 mm Hg
- Sitting mean arterial pressure: +5.8 mm Hg
- Supine systolic blood pressure: +7.1 mm Hg compared to a decrease of 4.5 mm Hg in the placebo group.

In contrast, acetaminophen and placebo did not cause significant changes in blood pressure. However, once the ibuprofen group entered Phase 3 and stopped taking the drug, their blood pressure returned to baseline levels.[362]

Clinical Implications and Relevance Today

These results are still relevant, as more recent studies, such as the 2017 PRECISION-ABPM trial, have confirmed that ibuprofen can raise blood pressure in patients with osteoarthritis or cardiovascular risk factors.[363] In this study, ibuprofen (600–800 mg three times daily) increased mean 24-hour systolic blood pressure by 3.7 mm Hg over four months, and 23% of patients with normal baseline blood pressure developed hypertension while on ibuprofen. Naproxen and celecoxib had smaller or negligible effects.

Mechanism of Action: Ibuprofen and other NSAIDs can blunt the effects of antihypertensive drugs, particularly those that rely on vasodilation (such as ACE inhibitors, ARBs, and some beta-blockers).[362] This is thought to occur because NSAIDs inhibit prostaglandin synthesis, reducing the vasodilatory effect that helps keep blood pressure in check.

Even modest increases in blood pressure (5–7 mm Hg) are clinically meaningful, especially in patients at risk for cardiovascular events. Persistent elevation can increase the risk of stroke, heart attack, and heart failure. These findings align with previous research showing that long-term ibuprofen use can interfere with antihypertensive drugs, though short-term or occasional use typically does not have the same impact.[364]

A Closer Look at the Risks

Beyond its effects on blood pressure, ibuprofen has also been linked to more serious cardiovascular risks, including cardiac arrest. A major study from Denmark has highlighted a concerning link between certain NSAIDs and an increased risk of out-of-hospital cardiac arrest. Using data from the Danish nationwide health registries, researchers investigated how NSAID use in the days before a cardiac event might contribute to this serious risk.[365]

The study followed a case-time-control model, where each participant served as their own control.[365] Researchers compared two periods:

1. A "case period"—when the participant had used NSAIDs in the 30 days before cardiac arrest.

2. A "control period"—when the same participant had not used NSAIDs in the 30 days before the event.

To further validate the findings, the study also included a separate control group from the general population.[365]

The researchers analyzed data from nearly 29,000 individuals (all aged over 10) who suffered cardiac arrest between 2001 and 2010. They examined both non-selective NSAIDs (such as ibuprofen, naproxen, and diclofenac), and COX-2 inhibitors (including rofecoxib and celecoxib).[365]

Key Findings

Cardiac Risk: A Danish nationwide study (2001–2010) of 28,947 cardiac arrest patients found ibuprofen use increased cardiac arrest risk by 31% within 30 days of use.[365] One limitation of the study was that it only included prescription NSAIDs, meaning over-the-counter ibuprofen use was not accounted for. As a result, the actual exposure to ibuprofen in the general population may have been underestimated, and further studies including OTC NSAID use are needed to clarify the true real-world risk levels.[365]

Short-Term Use: Even short-term use of ibuprofen—even for brief periods (≤30 days)—was associated with a higher likelihood of cardiac arrest compared to those who did not take the drug.[365] This underscores an important reminder: Even widely used medications like NSAIDs carry potential risks. While acetaminophen carries well-known liver risks at high doses, it remains safer than NSAIDs for patients with cardiovascular or kidney conditions when used appropriately. For individuals with cardiovascular concerns, exploring alternative pain relief options and consulting a healthcare provider before regular NSAID use could be crucial for heart health.[365]

A summary of ibuprofen's effects on the heart is illustrated in **Fig. 8.3**.

Conclusion

Fig. 8.3. Ibuprofen's effect on the heart

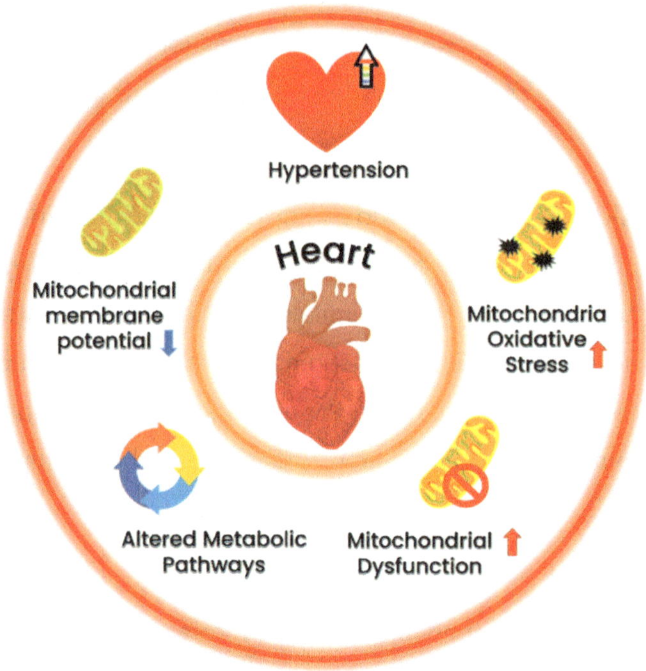

While medications like ibuprofen are common and accessible, their potential impact on heart health highlights the importance of making informed choices. Understanding these risks empowers us to balance pain relief with long-term well-being. By making small but thoughtful adjustments in how we manage our health, we can prioritize both comfort and cardiovascular safety—paving the way for a stronger, healthier future. For individuals with cardiovascular risks, consulting a healthcare provider before regular NSAID use is crucial.

Key Takeaways:

- Common pain relievers, like ibuprofen, can significantly increase cardiovascular risks—especially with long-term (daily use for more than 30 days) or high-dose use (doses above 1,200 mg per day).
- NSAIDs can counteract blood pressure medications, potentially raising blood pressure in hypertensive patients. As such, patients on blood pressure medications should consult their healthcare provider before using NSAIDs regularly.
- Ibuprofen at moderate prescription doses can significantly raise blood pressure in patients on antihypertensive therapy, with effects seen within weeks.
- Acetaminophen does not appear to have the same effect and may be a safer alternative for pain relief in hypertensive patients.
- By inhibiting COX enzymes, NSAIDs impact not only inflammation but also essential, protective vascular functions.
- Those with peripheral artery disease, hypertension, or existing heart conditions face greater risks when using NSAIDs (**Fig. 8.4**).

Fig. 8.4. Pre-existing conditions that increase the risk of heart related side effects from ibuprofen

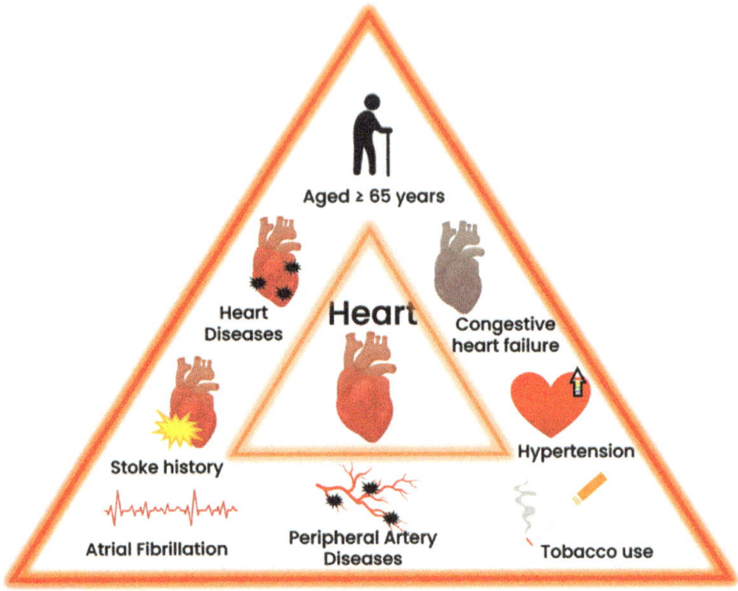

- When possible, take NSAIDs at the lowest effective dose, and as infrequently as needed, to reduce potential risks. Occasionally, short-term use of ibuprofen is less likely to cause cardiovascular problems.
- Understanding these risks helps individuals make safer, more informed choices about pain management and heart health.

Chapter 9
Ibuprofen and the Liver:
A Balancing Act

Understanding Liver Diseases

The liver is one of the body's most essential organs, responsible for processing nutrients, filtering toxins, and producing bile to aid digestion. Despite its remarkable ability to regenerate, liver diseases remain a major global health issue, contributing to nearly two million deaths each year.[366] These diseases can arise from a range of factors, including viral infections, excessive alcohol consumption, exposure to harmful substances, autoimmune conditions, and genetics.[367]

Some of the most common liver diseases include[368]:

→ **Fatty Liver Disease (NAFLD/NASH):** An accumulation of fat in the liver, often linked to obesity, diabetes, and metabolic syndrome. It can progress to inflammation and scarring (NASH), potentially leading to cirrhosis.

→ **Cirrhosis:** A condition where long-term damage causes severe scarring, impairing the liver's ability to function. Common causes include chronic alcohol use and viral hepatitis.

→ **Hepatitis (A, B, C):** Viral infections that inflame the liver. Hepatitis B and C can become chronic, increasing the risk of cirrhosis and liver cancer.

→ **Inherited Conditions:**

- *Hemochromatosis:* Excessive iron buildup, leading to liver damage.

- *Wilson's Disease:* Copper accumulation causes liver and neurological damage.

→ **Liver Cancer:** Often a complication of chronic liver diseases, liver cancer poses a severe health risk if not detected early.

Recognizing Symptoms of Liver Disease

Early detection of liver disease is challenging, as symptoms are often subtle or easily mistaken for other conditions. However, some of the more noticeable and common signs to be aware of include: [368,369]

- Persistent fatigue and weakness.
- Abdominal discomfort or pain, especially in the upper right side.
- Jaundice (yellowing of the skin and eyes), signaling impaired liver function.
- Noticeable bloating in the abdominal area (ascites) or legs, due to fluid buildup.
- Unexplained weight loss and loss of appetite.
- Easy bruising or bleeding due to reduced production of clotting factors.

Recognizing the symptoms of liver disease is crucial for early detection and timely treatment, which can help prevent irreversible damage. Cirrhosis, for example, ranks as the 11th leading cause of death worldwide, highlighting the urgent need for awareness and proactive management of liver health.[366,367]

Drug-Induced Liver Injury (DILI) and Hepatotoxicity

Hepatotoxicity refers to liver damage caused by drugs, chemicals, or other harmful agents. In many cases, this condition is reversible once the offending substance is discontinued.[370] However, because hepatotoxicity is often asymptomatic or mimics other liver diseases, diagnosing it can be challenging. Still, it is one of the leading causes of acute liver failure (ALF) in the United States.

Doctors typically identify hepatotoxicity by measuring levels of specific liver enzymes, known as aminotransferases, in the blood. Elevated enzyme levels can signal liver damage, prompting further investigation.[371]

Although drug-induced liver disease is relatively rare, widely used medications like ibuprofen contribute to several cases each year in the United States.[372] In Iceland, drug-induced liver disease occurs in approximately 19 cases per 100,000 people annually, while ibuprofen-induced liver injury is estimated to affect fewer than 1 in 100,000 users.[373]

Most recent studies suggest that most individuals will not experience liver problems from typical ibuprofen use and that ibuprofen-induced liver damage is much less frequent than with other drugs like acetaminophen. However, recent research also highlights the importance of caution when using ibuprofen, especially with high doses, prolonged use, or in individuals with existing liver conditions. Currently, there is no credible evidence from recent studies to suggest that ibuprofen has protective effects on the liver. Knowing how vital the liver is, the dangers of liver disease, and how common medications like ibuprofen can impact liver health highlights the importance of informed healthcare decisions. Continued research and education remain key to minimizing risks and ensuring the safe use of this widely available drug. Patients with liver disease should consult a doctor before using ibuprofen, particularly for prolonged periods.

What Do We Know?

In developed countries, NSAIDs are responsible for approximately 3-10% of all drug-induced liver injuries. The specific NSAIDs responsible for these cases vary by region, reflecting differences in prescribing habits, drug availability, and regulatory environments.

Regional Data and Sources

- In Spain, analysis of the Spanish DILI Registry-a nationwide, multicenter database dedicated to tracking drug-induced liver injury-found that ibuprofen was the most frequent cause of NSAID-related liver injury, accounting for 29% of cases.[374] This registry-based finding provides a high level of credibility and reflects data collected from multiple hospitals across the country.

- In India, a single-center study reported that ibuprofen was the second most common NSAID associated with liver injury (25%) between 1997 and 2008.[375] However, because this data is from one hospital, it may not represent India as a whole and should be interpreted with caution.

Environmental and regulatory factors, such as the maximum allowable OTC dosage per pill, likely influence these regional differences. For example, the maximum allowable over-the-counter ibuprofen dosage per pill varies by country. In the United States, the limit is 200 mg per pill, while in Spain, it can be as high as 400 mg.[376] These regional differences in dosage and accessibility may impact the reported rates of adverse effects.

Access to higher-dose formulations, such as those available in Spain, may increase the risk of liver injury by resulting in higher systemic drug exposure, especially if patients take multiple doses per day without medical supervision. Additionally, individuals with preexisting liver conditions are more vulnerable to the harmful effects of ibuprofen. Patients with rheumatic disorders, such as rheumatoid arthritis and systemic lupus erythematosus, as well as those with existing liver diseases, face a higher risk of ibuprofen-induced liver toxicity.[372] Furthermore, in patients with cirrhosis, NSAID use has been linked to an increased risk of renal failure, although ibuprofen specifically has not been singled out in this context.[377]

While ibuprofen is generally considered to have a favorable safety profile, its contribution to NSAID-induced liver injury varies by region. As research continues to evolve, both individuals and healthcare professionals need to consider these factors when using or recommending ibuprofen, particularly for those with underlying health conditions.

Does Ibuprofen Harm Healthy Livers?

For most individuals with a healthy liver, ibuprofen is considered safe when taken at recommended doses. However, research suggests that ibuprofen may have unintended effects on liver function (**Fig. 9.1**).

Studies in mice indicate that ibuprofen can influence liver enzymes and metabolic processes more profoundly than previously understood.[25] Research from the Gomes Lab found that ibuprofen may impair mitochondrial function—the cell's energy powerhouse—while also increasing reactive oxygen species, which can contribute to oxidative stress. Additionally, it was shown to impair proteasome function, a critical system responsible for breaking down and removing damaged or unnecessary proteins in cells.[25]

Fig. 9.1. Ibuprofen's effect on liver

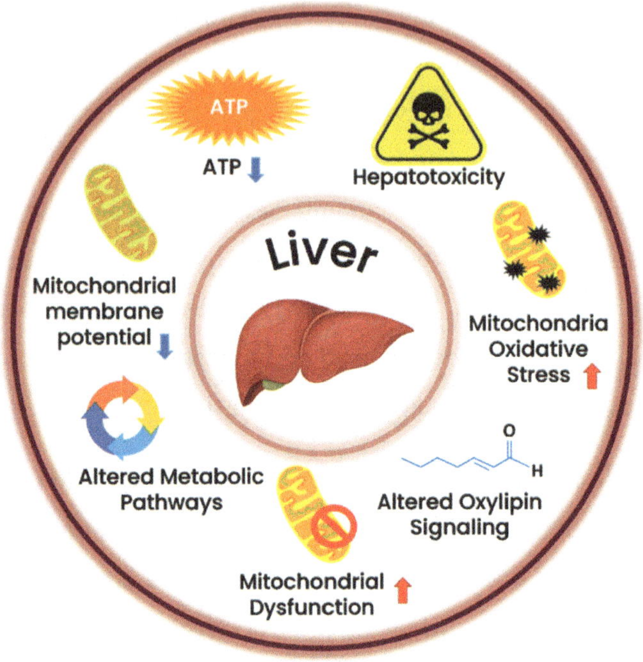

While these findings raise important questions, further research is needed to determine the full extent of ibuprofen's impact on liver health in humans.

However, these findings should be interpreted with caution, as results from animal studies do not always translate directly to humans. While most individuals with healthy livers can tolerate ibuprofen, several case studies have shown that a single overdose can lead to acute liver injury.[378] In extreme cases where individuals consumed 20,000 mg, 60,000 mg, or

9,600 mg of ibuprofen, liver transplantation was required.[379,380] These doses far exceed the recommended daily limit of 1,200 to 3,200 mg.

Severe liver damage from ibuprofen at recommended doses is exceptionally rare in individuals with healthy livers. In fact, ibuprofen-induced liver injury occurs in only about one per 100,000 patients.[379] Case studies suggest that when liver injury does occur in otherwise healthy individuals, it is often idiosyncratic, meaning it results from unique individual factors rather than a predictable dose-dependent reaction.[372]

This underscores the importance of using ibuprofen as directed and considering individual risk factors, such as preexisting conditions or interactions with other medications. While the overall risk remains low, continued research is crucial to understanding the mechanisms behind these rare cases and ensuring the safest possible use of this widely available drug.

Impact of Oxylipins and COX Inhibition

One crucial aspect of ibuprofen's mechanism involves oxylipins, signaling molecules that regulate essential bodily functions, such as gene expression and ion channel activity. Oxylipins, including prostaglandins and thromboxanes, are produced by COX enzymes in the arachidonic acid pathway.[381,382] Disruptions in the P450 pathway, caused by ibuprofen, may increase liver enzyme activity, contributing to hepatotoxicity, particularly in individuals with pre-existing liver conditions.[383,384]

Since ibuprofen inhibits COX enzymes, researchers expected it to lower prostaglandin levels in the liver.[381] A 2021 study confirmed this effect in both male and female mice.[381] However, the study also revealed sex-based differences in oxylipin alterations, with distinct changes observed in male mice compared to females. This finding highlights the potential need for personalized medication approaches based on sex.

Beyond COX inhibition, ibuprofen also influences the cytochrome P450 (CYP450) pathway, which involves soluble epoxide hydrolase (sEH) and microsomal epoxide hydrolase (mEH)—two enzymes crucial for metabolizing epoxy fatty acids (EpFAs). These fatty acids have anti-inflammatory properties, and inhibiting sEH can enhance their effects.[385,386] However, the same study found that ibuprofen treatment increased both sEH and mEH activity in the liver.[381] Since elevated sEH levels have been associated with high blood pressure, this suggests a possible link between ibuprofen use and cardiovascular risks.

Sex-Based Differences in Ibuprofen's Effects

While research in human subjects is still lacking, studies in mice suggest that ibuprofen affects liver processes differently in males and females. These studies reveal that ibuprofen can alter liver metabolism and protein pathways differently in males and females. For example, ibuprofen reduced glycolysis-related enzymes (which help generate energy) in male mice but not in females. This reduction can lead to decreased ATP levels and increased oxidative stress in the liver. In contrast, female mice did not show these same changes, suggesting a protective or different metabolic response.[25]

However, while these findings are significant, there is a clear gap in human research. The implications of these sex-based differences in animal models cannot be directly applied to humans without further validation. Human studies are needed to determine whether similar metabolic and enzymatic changes occur, and if so, how they might influence ibuprofen's safety and efficacy in men and women.

Implications for Liver Function and Drug Metabolism

In males, impaired glycolysis and increased oxidative stress could make the liver more susceptible to injury during prolonged or high-dose ibuprofen use, while in females, the absence of these changes suggests a different risk profile, possibly due to variations in drug-metabolizing enzymes and hormone levels.

Additionally, ibuprofen was shown to affect other liver pathways, such as proteasome function and cytochrome P450 enzyme activity, in a sex-specific manner. For instance, cytochrome P450 activity, which is involved in breaking down drugs, was increased in female mice but decreased in males. This could influence how long ibuprofen and other medications remain active in the body, potentially affecting drug interactions and side effects.

Human Studies and Clinical Relevance

Limited human studies suggest that ibuprofen's analgesic effects may also differ by sex. For example, some research showed that ibuprofen is less effective at reducing pain in women than in men, and this difference does not appear to be due to pharmacokinetics alone.[387,388] These findings highlight the need for more human-based research to clarify the underlying mechanisms and to determine whether dosing recommendations should be adjusted based on sex.

Ibuprofen and Alcohol: A Dangerous Combination

Ibuprofen is generally safe when used as directed, but combining it with excessive alcohol can pose serious health risks. The CDC defines moderate drinking as up to two drinks per day for men and one for women.[389,390] However, when ibuprofen is taken alongside alcohol, it can increase oxidative stress in the liver, making it more vulnerable to damage.

A synergistic effect occurs when ibuprofen and alcohol are consumed together, meaning their combined impact is greater than their individual effects. This heightened oxidative stress leads to the production of harmful chemicals that can severely damage liver cells.[391] A recent study on liver cells confirmed this, showing that exposure to both ibuprofen and alcohol caused significantly more damage than either substance alone.[392]

The combination of alcohol and ibuprofen poses increased risks for several specific groups, particularly those with preexisting liver conditions, adults over 65, long-term ibuprofen users (more than 30 days of daily use), heavy drinkers (those consuming more than three alcoholic beverages each day), and those with kidney disease.

To minimize liver toxicity:

- Avoid ibuprofen if you've been drinking heavily. Even occasional drinkers should be cautious about taking ibuprofen too close to alcohol consumption.

- Monitor symptoms. Liver damage from ibuprofen may be overlooked in individuals who regularly consume alcohol.

- Seek alternatives. If a friend or loved one needs pain relief after drinking, encourage hydration and rest instead of ibuprofen. If medical care is needed, consult a healthcare professional for safer alternatives.

By understanding these risks and using ibuprofen responsibly, we can help prevent avoidable liver damage while ensuring safe and effective pain management.

Case Study: Stevens-Johnson Syndrome (SJS)

Stevens-Johnson syndrome (SJS) is a rare, severe, and potentially life-threatening disorder of the skin and mucous membranes, most often triggered by adverse reactions to medications or, less commonly, infections. SJS typically begins with flu-like symptoms such as fever, sore throat, fatigue, and burning eyes. This is followed by the rapid development of a painful red or purple rash that spreads and blisters, affecting both the skin and mucous membranes of the mouth, eyes, nose, and genitals. SJS can lead to serious complications, including dehydration, sepsis, eye damage, and acute respiratory failure, and often requires hospitalization-sometimes in an intensive care or burn unit. Without prompt treatment, SJS can be fatal.

Among high-risk drugs, NSAIDs, such as ibuprofen, have been identified as potential triggers for SJS. It occurs in approximately 1 to 6 individuals per million annually.[393]

Case Report

A 9-year-old child with no prior medical history developed SJS after taking ibuprofen suspension three times during the early course of an illness. The child initially exhibited symptoms of severe skin reactions, liver insufficiency, and an intestinal infection, as confirmed through liver biopsy and physical examination. [394]

Genetic testing revealed that the child carried the HLA-B*5801 allele, a genotype known to increase the risk of severe drug-induced skin reactions. This genetic variant is more commonly found in individuals of Asian descent compared to Caucasian or African populations.[394]

Upon diagnosis, the child was hospitalized in the intensive care unit. Management included immediate discontinuation of ibuprofen, supportive care with intravenous fluids to prevent dehydration. The child's condition gradually improved with these interventions, and full recovery was achieved without lasting effects.

After ruling out other potential causes, including viral infections and preexisting liver disease, researchers determined that the liver damage was likely induced by ibuprofen. While some studies suggest a link between drug-induced liver injury and genetic susceptibility, further research is needed to fully understand the relationship between ibuprofen, liver toxicity, and SJS, especially in children with this genotype.[394]

This case report highlights the importance of early recognition and aggressive management of SJS, as well as the potential role of genetic predisposition in drug-induced adverse reactions.

Conclusion

Ibuprofen can cause liver damage in SJS through a combination of toxic metabolic byproducts, immune-mediated mechanisms, and disruption of bile acid homeostasis. Excessive or prolonged use of ibuprofen has been linked to drug-induced liver injury (DILI) and hepatotoxicity. When SJS and DILI occur together, they exacerbate each other, leading to a more severe clinical course, higher rates of complications, and increased mortality. Early recognition, prompt withdrawal of the offending drug, and intensive supportive care are critical to improving outcomes in these patients.[395,396]

While further research is needed to fully understand ibuprofen's effects on individuals with varying health conditions, existing studies indicate that it can cause liver damage, particularly in those with preexisting conditions such as chronic liver disease or alcoholism (**Fig. 9.2**). However, the precise dosage threshold that triggers these effects remains unclear, as does its interaction with conditions like hepatitis B or Gilbert syndrome.

Fig. 9.2. Pre-existing factors that increase risk of side effects when taking ibuprofen

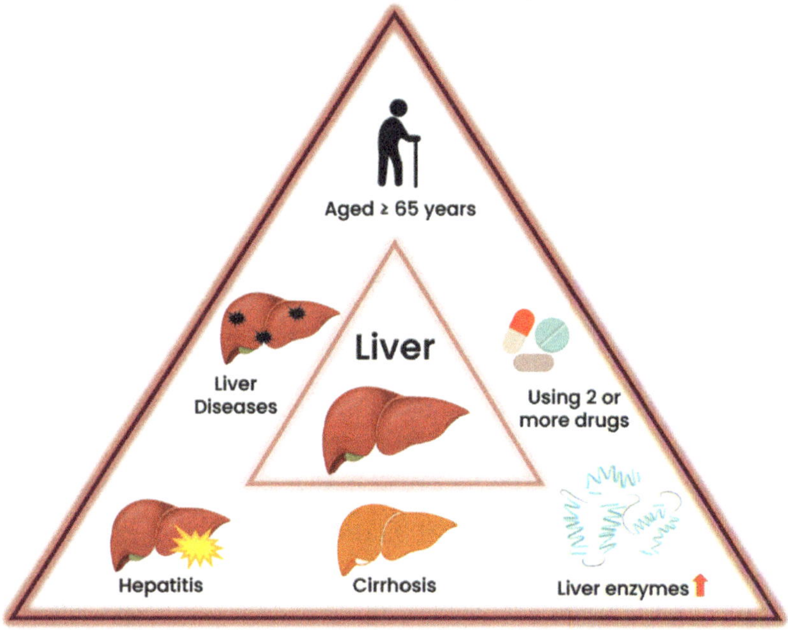

Looking Ahead

The healthcare community must continue researching these risks and raising public awareness about the safe use of ibuprofen. With better education, physicians can guide patients more effectively on its potential long-term effects, ultimately improving treatment decisions and overall health outcomes.

A deeper understanding of ibuprofen's impact is essential for ensuring its safe and effective use in medical practice, benefiting patients across diverse backgrounds and health conditions. Specifically, further research is needed to clarify the mechanisms by which ibuprofen affects liver function, including the molecular pathways involved in both acute and chronic liver injury, and to determine why these effects can vary significantly between males and females. Studies are also needed to further identify the risk factors that predispose certain individuals to ibuprofen-induced liver injury, the role of genetic and metabolic differences, and how ibuprofen interacts with other medications via liver enzyme systems such as cytochrome P450.

Key Takeaways:

- Using ibuprofen consistently increases the risk of inducing liver disease.
- Excessive ibuprofen use may cause acute liver failure.
- Drug-induced liver injury from NSAIDs is more commonly caused by diclofenac in the US and ibuprofen in Spain and India.
- Taking ibuprofen and alcohol together could negatively affect liver function.
- Chronic use of ibuprofen increases the probability of liver disease, especially for those who have a preexisting condition.

Chapter 10
When Relief Hurts: The Gastrointestinal and Renal Toll of Ibuprofen

The digestive system, also known as the gastrointestinal (GI) tract, is a complex network that includes the mouth, esophagus, stomach, small and large intestines, rectum, and anus.[397] One of the most well-documented side effects of ibuprofen and other NSAIDs is their impact on the digestive system. A quick search of the scientific literature reveals thousands of studies examining this topic, highlighting the significant concern surrounding GI complications.

Fig. 10.1. Relative risk of GI problems for different NSAIDs.[1]

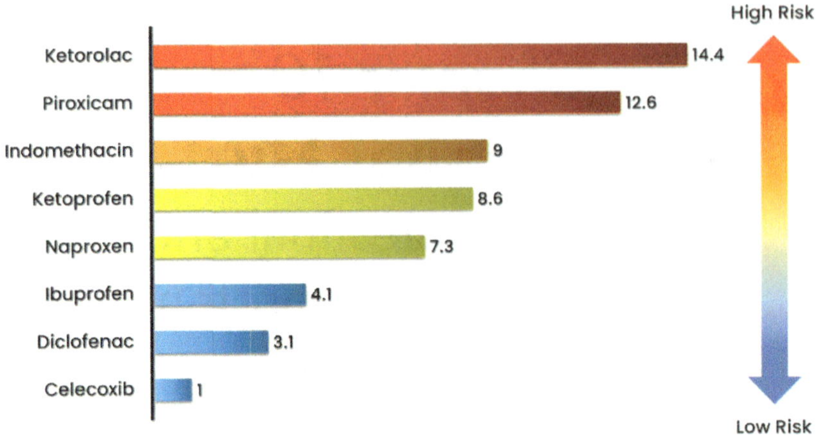

Research shows that NSAIDs, such as ibuprofen, are strongly linked to various digestive issues, including peptic ulcers in the stomach and the duodenum (the first part of the small intestine) (**Fig. 10.1**).[398,399] Even when ulcers don't develop, many people experience discomfort, such as indigestion or upper abdominal pain after taking ibuprofen. In fact, regular NSAID use can increase the risk of developing stomach or duodenal ulcers by 15-30%, as seen in endoscopic studies.[400]

Why does this happen?

Ibuprofen can irritate the stomach lining, leading to issues like bleeding, inflammation, and, in severe cases, stomach perforation. If you've ever struggled with heartburn, acid reflux, or an ulcer, you know how painful and disruptive these conditions can be.[144,398,401,402] Alarmingly, NSAID-induced damage to the intestinal lining is believed to contribute to 10-15% of iron deficiency anemia cases, often due to unnoticed small intestine bleeding.[403]

Additionally, certain individuals with preexisting conditions are more prone to developing stomach ulcers from taking ibuprofen and other NSAIDs. Those with gastritis are more likely to develop stomach ulcers from taking ibuprofen due to the weakening of the stomach lining.[404] Additionally, individuals suffering from alcoholism are also at greater risk for gastric bleeding and stomach ulcers when taking NSAIDs.[405]

The good news is that these complications are often reversible. In most cases, simply stopping NSAID use allows the body to heal on its own. Doctors may also prescribe proton pump inhibitors (PPIs), a type of medication that reduces stomach acid and helps protect the stomach lining while using NSAIDs.[406]

So, why does ibuprofen cause these issues in the first place? It all comes down to how the drug works. Ibuprofen blocks two key enzymes in the body: COX-1 and COX-2. COX-1 plays an essential role in protecting the stomach lining by producing substances like prostaglandins PGE2 and PGI2, which help maintain a strong mucosal barrier. When ibuprofen inhibits COX-1, this protective barrier weakens, making the stomach more susceptible to damage, irritation, and ulcers (**Fig. 10.2**).

COX-2, on the other hand, is mainly responsible for inflammation and pain. Since blocking COX-2 doesn't significantly affect the stomach lining, scientists have developed selective COX-2 inhibitors that relieve pain while reducing the risk of stomach irritation. However, traditional NSAIDs, like ibuprofen, block both COX-1 and COX-2, which is why they pose a higher risk of digestive issues.

Research has found that 15-30% of people who use NSAIDs regularly have ulcers, which can be seen via endoscopy.[407,408] *However, this is likely to be an underestimation, as up to 70% of NSAID users show stomach lining damage during endoscopy.*[398] *It is also important to know that when stomach lining damage occurs, such as when erosions are detected, about 90% of patients have no symptoms of heartburn or stomach discomfort.*[398]

So, why does ibuprofen cause these issues in the first place? It all comes down to how the drug works by blocking enzymes in the digestive system that interfere with its function. Ibuprofen blocks two key enzymes in the body: COX-1 and COX-2. COX-1 plays an essential role in protecting the stomach lining by producing substances like prostaglandins PGE2 and PGI2, which help maintain a strong mucosal barrier. When ibuprofen inhibits COX-1, this protective barrier weakens, making the stomach more susceptible to damage, irritation, and ulcers (**Fig. 10.2**).

COX-2, on the other hand, is mainly responsible for inflammation and pain. Since blocking COX-2 doesn't significantly affect the stomach lining, scientists have developed selective COX-2 inhibitors that relieve pain while reducing the risk of stomach irritation. However, traditional NSAIDs like ibuprofen block both COX-1 and COX-2, which is why they pose a higher risk of digestive issues.

To prevent ulcers and bleeding, it's often necessary to look beyond standard ibuprofen. One option is switching to selective COX-2 inhibitors like Bextra and Celebrex, which are specifically designed to reduce pain and inflammation while minimizing stomach damage. Another alternative is natural pain-relieving supplements (see Chapter 14 for more on these).[409]

Fig. 10.2. How ibuprofen causes stomach problems

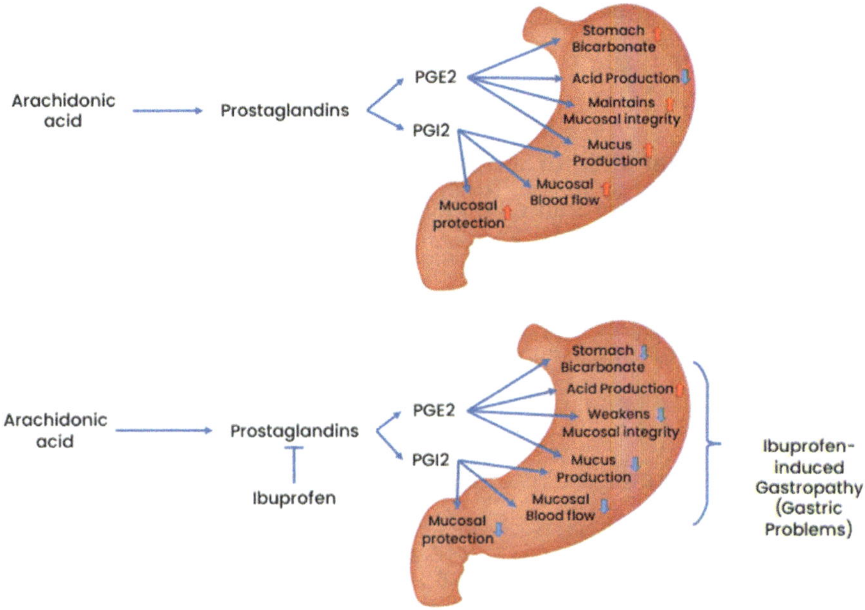

Unlike ibuprofen, which blocks both COX-1 and COX-2 enzymes, COX-2 inhibitors target only COX-2, the enzyme responsible for pain and inflammation. This selective action helps relieve discomfort while sparing COX-1, which plays a key role in protecting the stomach lining. As a result, these medications significantly lower the risk of ulcers and GI bleeding compared to traditional NSAIDs.

However, COX-2 inhibitors aren't risk-free. Research shows they may increase the likelihood of heart attacks, strokes, and kidney complications with long-term use.[410,411] Considering this, it's important to use them under a doctor's supervision to ensure the benefits outweigh the risks for your individual health needs, especially if you are at higher risk of developing severe side effects.

If you're thinking about switching to a COX-2 inhibitor or trying natural alternatives, talk to your doctor to find the safest and most effective pain-relieving option for you.

Disrupting the Gut's Natural Balance

Did you know that ibuprofen can change the balance of bacteria in your gut? This community of microorganisms, known as the gut microbiota, plays a vital role in digestion, metabolism, and immune function. However, research shows that ibuprofen can significantly reduce both the number and variety of these beneficial microbes.[412]

In addition to ibuprofen's direct harmful effect on the gut through COX-1, it can also harm the balance of bacteria in your gut. This community of microorganisms, known as the gut microbiota, plays a vital role in digestion, metabolism, and immune function. However, research shows that ibuprofen can significantly reduce both the number and variety of these beneficial microbes.

Why does this matter? A healthy gut microbiota helps break down food, produce essential nutrients, and keep the immune system in check. Different areas of the digestive tract have their own unique microbial populations. For example, the colon is home to trillions of bacteria, while the stomach, jejunum, and duodenum contain far fewer microbes due to their acidic and oxygen-rich environments.

Why does it happen?

Prostaglandins help maintain the gut mucosal barrier and regulate immune responses. The reduction in prostaglandin synthesis caused by its inhibition of COX increases gut permeability, making the intestine more susceptible to inflammation and bacterial translocation.[413] Besides this, ibuprofen and other NSAIDs can increase the production of more harmful types of bile acids. Normally, gut bacteria help process these bile acids, but when the balance of gut bacteria is disturbed (dysbiosis), this process is disrupted. As a result, the toxic effects of bile acids increase, contributing to NSAID-induced enteropathy (intestinal injury).[413] When ibuprofen disrupts this balance, it can lead to digestive issues, inflammation, and even long-term health consequences. But what exactly happens to the gut microbiota after repeated ibuprofen use? Let's explore this further.

Scientists have long suspected a link between NSAIDs like ibuprofen and gut health. In fact, research dating back to 1977 revealed a surprising discovery: rats without gut bacteria were resistant to intestinal damage caused by NSAIDs. This study by Robert and Asano suggested that the gut microbiota plays a key role in how these drugs affect the digestive system.[414]

More recent studies by Wang et al. and Rogers et al. confirmed this connection. They found that ibuprofen, celecoxib, and aspirin can shift the balance of gut bacteria, increasing certain bacterial families like *Enterobacteriaceae* and *Acidaminococcaceae* when compared to non-users.[413,415] In humans, ibuprofen use has been linked to a measurable rise in these bacteria, altering the gut microbiome's natural composition.

Changes in gut bacteria can affect how ibuprofen is processed, influencing both its effectiveness and potential side effects. For example, some gut bacteria produce enzymes like β-glucuronidase, which can increase the drug's exposure in the small intestine. This, in turn, can lead to intestinal damage (a condition called enteropathy).[416]

Understanding these gut interactions is crucial, especially for those who take ibuprofen regularly. But is there a way to protect the gut while using NSAIDs? Let's explore some potential solutions.

NSAIDs and Microscopic Colitis: A Hidden Risk?

Did you know that regular ibuprofen use may increase the risk of microscopic colitis with concomitant use of proton pump inhibitors.[417] This chronic inflammatory bowel disease (IBD) causes persistent inflammation in the colon's inner lining, leading to symptoms like chronic watery diarrhea but without bleeding. While anyone can develop microscopic colitis, it's most common in older adults and women.

Surprisingly, proton pump inhibitors (PPIs), medications commonly used to reduce stomach acid, pose an even higher risk. Studies show that people taking PPIs are over three times more likely to develop microscopic colitis than those who don't use these medications.[417,418] In addition, when used in conjunction with NSAIDs, the risk of developing microscopic colitis is greatly increased, so discuss any new medication use with your doctor.[417]

Ibuprofen increases the risk of microscopic colitis by weakening the gut's protective barrier, altering the gut microbiota, and promoting immune-mediated inflammation.[417,419] The risk is dose- and duration-dependent, and is further increased when combined with other medications affecting gut health.[417]

How Is It Diagnosed?

Since symptoms like diarrhea can be caused by many conditions, a biopsy is often required to confirm microscopic colitis. Doctors check for persistent inflammation in the lamina propria—the layer of connective tissue beneath the colon's inner lining. (See **Fig. 10.3** for a summary of ibuprofen's effects on the GI tract).

Fig. 10.3. Ibuprofen's effect on the GI Tract

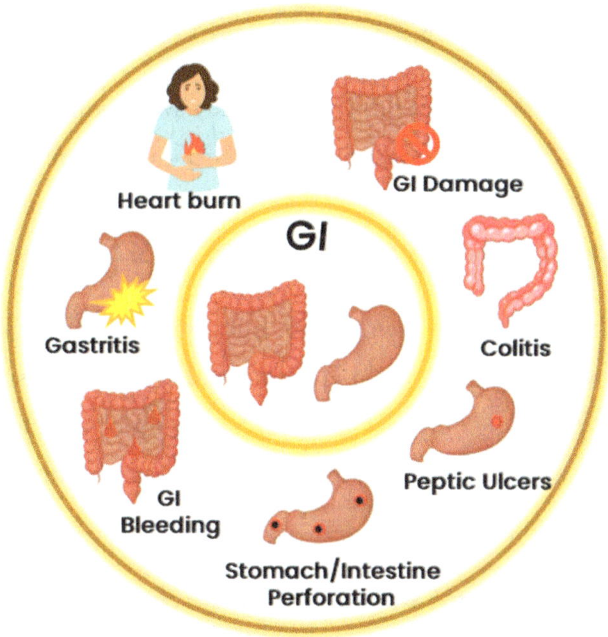

Managing and Preventing NSAID Complications

To reduce the risks associated with ibuprofen, follow these key precautions:

- Limit use to the shortest duration possible, as long-term use increases the likelihood of GI complications.

- Monitor for symptoms. If you're over 55 and experiencing frequent indigestion or stomach discomfort, it's time to check in with your doctor.

- Get regular screenings. Exams like gastroscopy and endoscopy can detect early signs of damage before serious complications arise.

By staying informed and proactive, you can make safer choices when it comes to pain management.

For younger individuals experiencing difficulty swallowing (dysphagia), or unexplained weight loss, a gastroscopy is strongly recommended. These symptoms may indicate serious conditions like esophageal or stomach cancer, so early screening is essential regardless of NSAID use.

If you don't have these symptoms but are experiencing digestive discomfort, your doctor might recommend a non-invasive test for Helicobacter pylori (*H. pylori*)—a common bacterial infection linked to ulcers. If H. pylori is present, stopping NSAID use might be advised to prevent further complications.

Protecting Your Stomach During Long-Term Ibuprofen Use

If long-term ibuprofen use is necessary, taking it alongside a proton pump inhibitor (PPI) can help protect your stomach. PPIs work by reducing stomach acid, lowering the risk of:

- Indigestion (dyspepsia)
- Ulcers
- Upper gastrointestinal bleeding
- Other stomach injuries

People with a history of ulcers, bleeding, or stomach perforations, or those taking aspirin regularly for heart health, should consult a doctor about using a PPI for added protection.

Fig. 10.4. Known GI pre-existing risk factors for ibuprofen

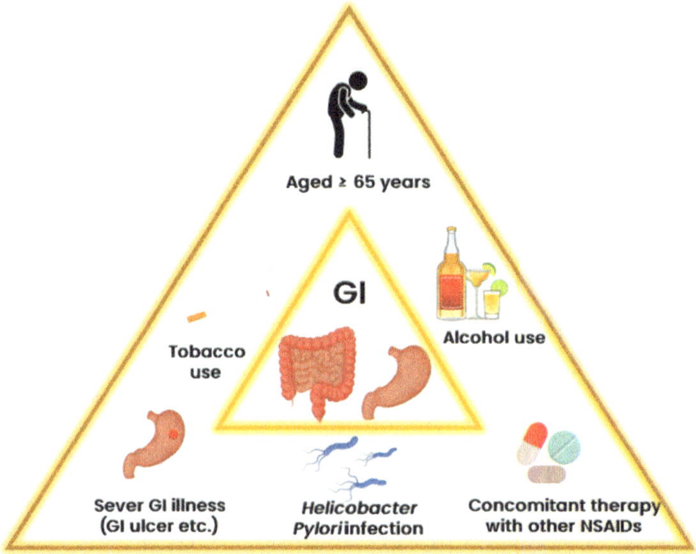

It's important to note that PPIs are not a universal solution and come with their own risks. In a study involving 1,211 patients with microscopic colitis and 6,041 controls with a mean age of 63.4 years, exposure to NSAIDs, PPIs, or selective serotonin reuptake inhibitors (SSRIs) for 4-12 months (long-term use) was found to increase the risk of microscopic colitis.[417] The use of NSAIDs and PPIs together showed the highest risk of microscopic colitis. Long-term PPI use has also been associated with an increased risk of bacterial infection and chronic kidney disease, so anyone considering taking PPIs should also consult with their doctor regarding these risks.[420]

Who Is at Higher Risk for GI Side Effects from Ibuprofen?

While ibuprofen is often considered safer than other pain relievers like diclofenac and naproxen in terms of bleeding risks, it still carries a potential for serious side effects, especially related to the GI system. Certain factors can make some people more vulnerable to these issues, such as bleeding from peptic ulcers or upper GI perforation (**Fig. 10.4**). Below are the key factors that increase the risk of GI complications when using ibuprofen:

1. **Age:** As we age, our bodies become more sensitive to medications like ibuprofen. People over 65 are particularly at risk for GI problems such as bleeding and ulcers. Younger people generally have lower risks of these issues.[421]

2. **Use of Certain Medications:** Some medications can heighten the risk of GI complications when taken alongside ibuprofen. These include corticosteroids, anticoagulants (blood thinners), selective serotonin reuptake inhibitors (SSRIs, used for depression), and antiplatelet drugs like aspirin. Long-term use of these drugs, along with ibuprofen, can significantly increase the chances of experiencing side effects.[422]

3. **Alcohol Consumption:** Drinking alcohol irritates the lining of the stomach. When combined with ibuprofen, this can raise the risk of stomach bleeding and other GI problems, even with moderate drinking.[423]

4. **Diabetes:** People with diabetes can have impaired blood flow to the stomach and intestines, which can make these areas more susceptible to injury from ibuprofen. This means that diabetics may be at higher risk for GI side effects.[398] In addition, diabetes-related

nerve and blood vessel damage, specifically diabetic neuropathy and microvascular disease, can impair healing in the GI tract, increasing the risk of ulcers.

Cardiovascular Disease and High Blood Pressure: Ibuprofen can cause the body to retain fluid, leading to swelling (edema) in the arms and legs. This fluid retention can worsen conditions like high blood pressure and heart disease, and might increase the chances of more serious complications in people already dealing with these issues.[424]

Strategies to Minimize GI Effects from Ibuprofen

If you experience moderate to severe GI symptoms, it's important to consult a doctor right away. However, if your symptoms are mild or manageable, adopting the following strategies may help reduce GI discomfort and improve overall gut health:

Adopt a Healthier Diet:

- **Cut back on carbonated and sugary beverages:** These can contribute to bloating and discomfort in the stomach.
- **Incorporate probiotics:** Foods like yogurt, kombucha, sauerkraut, and kimchi contain beneficial bacteria that support gut health and digestion by restoring the composition of gut bacteria and introducing beneficial functions to bacterial communities.[425]
- **Eat more fruits and vegetables:** These provide fiber, vitamins, and minerals that support a healthy digestive system. However, it's important to note that individuals with certain digestive issues, like IBD, may be sensitive to certain vegetables that may exacerbate inflammation.

- **Stay hydrated:** Drinking plenty of water is essential for digestive health and can help prevent dehydration, which may worsen GI symptoms. Some sources recommend drinking a full glass of water (8 oz) with each dose of an NSAID.[426]

- **Limit processed foods and junk food:** These foods often contain unhealthy fats and additives that can irritate the digestive tract.

- **Choose whole grains and nuts:** These are nutrient-rich options that provide fiber and help maintain gut health.

Other Healthy Lifestyle Changes:

- **Quit smoking:** Smoking irritates the GI tract and can exacerbate symptoms like heartburn and indigestion. When combined with ibuprofen, it can dramatically increase ulcer risk.

- **Get regular exercise:** Physical activity promotes digestion and can reduce the risk of constipation and bloating.

- **Limit red and processed meats:** These foods can be harder on the digestive system and may contribute to inflammation.

By following these dietary and lifestyle changes, you can reduce the risk of GI issues and support your overall digestive health while taking ibuprofen.

Ibuprofen and Your Kidneys: What You Need to Know

Ibuprofen, like other NSAIDs (such as naproxen and high-dose aspirin), can negatively impact kidney function when used frequently or in high doses.[427] The reason? NSAIDs interfere with prostaglandins—hormone-like compounds that help regulate:

- Salt and water balance[428]
- The release of essential kidney enzymes[428]
- Blood flow within the kidneys[428]

Since ibuprofen inhibits prostaglandin production, it can disrupt these critical processes, potentially leading to:

- Decreased kidney function
- Fluid retention and swelling
- Imbalances in urinary electrolytes

If you rely on ibuprofen for chronic pain management, it's essential to monitor kidney health and discuss alternative pain relief strategies with your doctor, especially if you have pre-existing kidney conditions or other risk factors.

Who Is at Risk?

Research suggests that young, healthy individuals have a low risk of developing kidney issues from NSAID use. However, while rare, acute kidney injury (AKI) and chronic kidney disease (CKD) can still occur, even in those without pre-existing conditions. Many studies indicate that short-term, non-prescription NSAID use does not significantly increase the risk of kidney disease in the general population. However, the risk rises with prolonged use or higher prescription-strength doses, particularly without proper medical oversight.[429]

For example, a 2019 study examined data from 764,228 U.S. Army soldiers, primarily men (85.8%), with an average age of 28.6. Researchers categorized soldiers into three groups based on their NSAID usage over the previous six months:

- No NSAID use (65.8%)[430]
- Light use (1-7 daily doses per month) – 17.9%[430]
- Frequent use (more than 7 daily doses per month) – 16.3%[430]

The study found that 2,356 soldiers developed acute kidney injury (AKI), while 1,634 were diagnosed with chronic kidney disease (CKD). Those who took more than seven doses of ibuprofen per month faced a 20% higher risk of developing AKI or CKD compared to non-NSAID users.

To put this into perspective: For every 100,000 individuals who take ibuprofen for more than seven days per month, an additional 17.6 cases of AKI and 30 cases of CKD may occur. [430] While the overall risk remains small, these findings highlight the potential dangers of prolonged NSAID use, even among otherwise healthy individuals.

While ibuprofen is generally safe for short-term use in healthy individuals, certain groups are more vulnerable to kidney-related complications (**Fig. 10.5**).

Older Adults (65+)

Adults over 65 face a significantly higher risk of kidney damage due to age-related declines in kidney function. The effects of ibuprofen can compound these changes, making them more susceptible to acute and chronic kidney injuries. One study found that ibuprofen increased the risk of acute kidney disease by 73% in the general population, but for older adults, the risk surged to 151%.[431]

Fig. 10.5. Known kidney disease pre-existing risk factors for ibuprofen

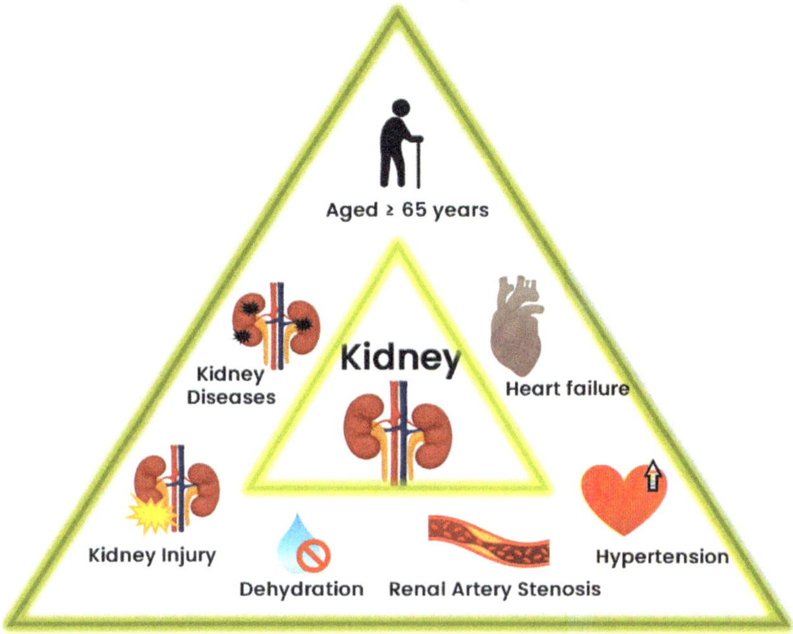

Similarly, a Taiwanese study of 31,976 individuals with hypertension revealed that NSAID use significantly increased the risk of developing chronic kidney disease, with longer durations of use correlating with even higher risks.[432]

Medication Interactions

People taking certain medications are at even higher risk when combining them with NSAIDs. Specifically, renin-angiotensin blockers (e.g., ACE inhibitors), diuretics, and NSAIDs together create a dangerous interaction that can drastically increase the likelihood of acute kidney failure. These drugs alter fluid and electrolyte regulation, amplifying ibuprofen's effects on kidney function.

One case report illustrates this risk: A 30-year-old woman was admitted to the emergency room with seizures and diagnosed with ibuprofen-induced syndrome of inappropriate diuresis, a condition that leads to dangerously low sodium levels. She had ingested 8 grams of ibuprofen (far exceeding the recommended dose) two days before her hospitalization. Although she was successfully treated with intravenous saline, she temporarily developed acute kidney injury as a result.[433]

Children

Even younger populations are not immune to these risks. A study of 50,420 children hospitalized with acute kidney injury found that 11% had used ibuprofen, and the risk of injury increased with higher doses.[434] This underscores the importance of cautious NSAID use in children, particularly at elevated doses.

Whether for older adults, those with chronic conditions, or children, understanding these risks is crucial. Those at risk should monitor kidney health and seek medical guidance before starting ibuprofen or other NSAIDs to avoid potential complications.[435]

Even younger populations are not immune to these risks. A study of 50,420 children hospitalized with acute kidney injury found that 11% had used ibuprofen, and the risk of injury increased with higher doses.[434] The median dose taken was around 12.13 mg/kg /dose, which is close to the recommended 10 mg/kg/dose. This underscores the importance of cautious NSAID use in children, particularly at elevated doses.

Whether for older adults, those with chronic conditions, or children, understanding these risks is crucial. Those at risk should monitor kidney health and seek medical guidance before starting ibuprofen or other NSAIDs to avoid potential complications.[435]

How Ibuprofen Can Harm the Kidneys

Prolonged use of NSAIDs, including ibuprofen, can impair kidney function and disrupt the body's fluid balance (**Fig 10.6**). One significant consequence is the production of concentrated urine, which increases the risk of kidney stone formation. This risk is further heightened by dehydration, a common but preventable factor.

Staying hydrated is essential for kidney health and overall well-being. Water is one of nature's simplest yet most powerful remedies. So, the next time you consider skipping a glass, remember that hydration is a simple step toward better health.

Although the precise mechanisms through which ibuprofen and other NSAIDs contribute to kidney damage remain unclear, they can be generally classified into three primary processes:

Fig. 10.6. Potential effect of ibuprofen on the kidney

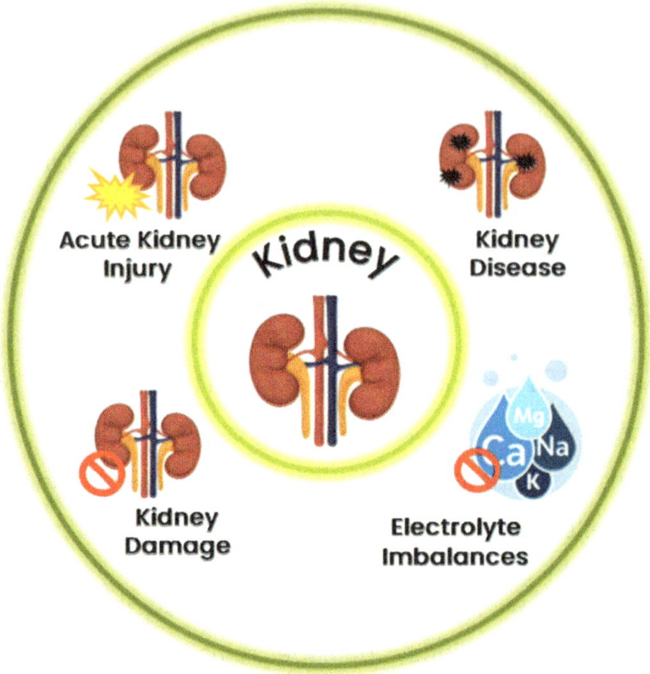

- **Direct Toxicity:** Ibuprofen can directly harm the kidneys by reducing glutathione and/or damaging proteins and lipids.

- **Immune Responses:** Ibuprofen leads to responses that cause the accumulation of immune complexes in parts of the kidney called the glomeruli, leading to kidney damage.[436]

- **Reduced Blood Flow:** Ibuprofen's inhibition of COX enzymes results in decreased glomerular filtration rate (the rate of kidney filtering blood) and reduced kidney blood flow. Chronic NSAID use can also contribute to kidney stones that reduce blood flow due to fluid imbalances, altered urine composition, and changes in calcium and oxalate levels.

The Importance of Prostaglandins

Prostaglandins, such as PGE2 and PGI2, are critical for maintaining healthy kidney function. These compounds, synthesized by the COX-1 and COX-2 enzymes, help regulate blood flow, glomerular filtration rate (GFR), and the balance of salt, water, and potassium in the body.

When ibuprofen inhibits these enzymes, it disrupts these vital processes, which can lead to complications such as acute interstitial nephritis—a form of kidney inflammation.[436] This kind of inflammation involves immune cell infiltration, which can lead to acute kidney injury and chronic kidney disease.

Interestingly, COX inhibitors have also been explored as potential treatments for nephrogenic diabetes insipidus, a condition characterized by excessive urination and thirst. NSAID inhibition of prostaglandins can enhance kidney water reabsorption in NDI patients, reducing excessive urination. In this context, these inhibitors enhance specific kidney transporters, highlighting the complex and multifaceted role of prostaglandins in renal health.[437]

Key Takeaways:

- **Short- and Long-Term Risks:** Ibuprofen can cause stomach problems like heartburn with short-term use and lead to more severe GI issues, such as ulcers, with prolonged use.
- **Protective Measures:** Proton pump inhibitors can help reduce GI damage from ibuprofen, and maintaining hydration is crucial for minimizing risks to kidney function.

- **Lifestyle Adjustments Matter:** A healthier diet, avoiding alcohol, quitting smoking, and limiting processed foods can significantly reduce ibuprofen's adverse effects on the GI tract and kidneys.

Chapter 11
Ibuprofen in Our Waters: A Silent Pollution Crisis

Commonly used drugs like ibuprofen are often praised for their ability to alleviate pain and inflammation. But have you ever considered what happens to this common medication once it leaves our bodies? Ibuprofen, together with its breakdown products, and other pharmaceuticals can make their way into our waterways, transforming them from everyday remedies into silent pollutants. This pollution can present significant risks to our aquatic ecosystems and compromise the quality of our drinking water.

To understand the full scope of this issue, let's start by testing our knowledge with a few questions about ibuprofen's role and impact on our ecosystems.

1. **Which of the following is an appropriate disposal method for ibuprofen to use at home if a take-back program is not available?**
   A) Dissolve it in hot water and pour it outside

   B) Mix it with cat litter or spent coffee grounds and seal it in a leakproof bag

   C) Crush the pills and scatter them in the garden

   D) Flush it down the toilet

2. **Which of the following is a reason ibuprofen may be detected in rivers and lakes?**
    A) Runoff from pharmaceutical manufacturing plants
    B) Residue from wastewater treatment plants that do not entirely remove ibuprofen
    C) People dumping it directly into water bodies
    D) All of the above
3. **What specific property of ibuprofen makes it difficult for common wastewater treatment plants to remove it from water sources completely?**
    A) High water solubility
    B) Low biodegradability
    C) High volatility
    D) Strong adsorption to organic particles
4. **Studies show that ibuprofen acts as an endocrine disruptor in some aquatic species. The endocrine refers to the glands and organs that create and release hormones into the blood. Which of the following describes a potential effect of ibuprofen on marine organisms?**
    A) Increased ability to reproduce
    B) Alteration of hormonal systems affecting reproduction and development
    C) Enhanced growth rates due to anti-inflammatory properties
    D) Decreased sensitivity to pollutants in water

5. **What is a potential long-term ecological risk associated with chronic exposure of aquatic ecosystems to ibuprofen residues, even at low concentrations?**
   A) Bioaccumulation leading to toxic levels in larger predators

   B) Complete degradation of ibuprofen in food chains

   C) Adaptation of aquatic species to tolerate higher pollution levels

   D) Reduced competition among species leading to increased biodiversity

Answers:

1. B) Mix it with cat litter or spent coffee and seal it in a leakproof bag. This makes the medication less appealing and reduces the risk of accidental ingestion by humans or animals.
2. D) All of the above.
3. B) Low biodegradability.
4. B) Alteration of hormonal systems affecting reproduction and development.
5. A) Bioaccumulation leading to toxic levels in larger predators.

How Ibuprofen Contaminates Our Water

Most people are unaware that the medications they take can end up in the environment, as commonly used drugs often make their way into rivers, groundwater, and wastewater treatment plants. As one of the most widely used over-the-counter and prescription medications, ibuprofen's pervasive presence has contributed to significant environmental concerns (**Fig. 11.1**).[438]

Fig. 11.1. How ibuprofen gets into the environment

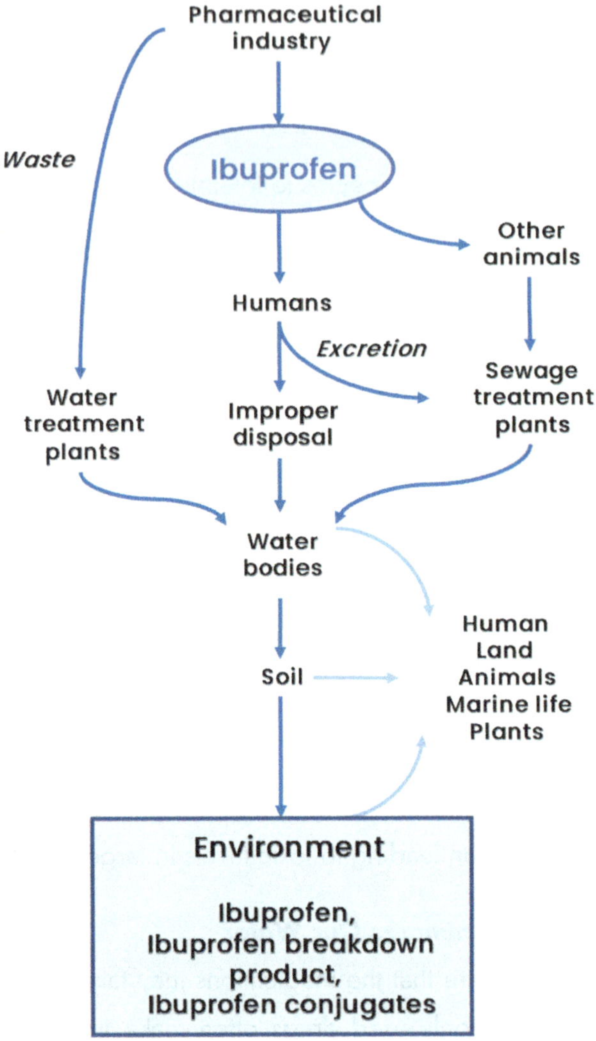

When people take ibuprofen, a portion is excreted from their bodies, entering wastewater. Additionally, improper disposal, such as flushing pills down the toilet or tossing them in the trash, contributes to contamination. Studies show that wastewater treatment plants often fail to remove pharmaceutical residues completely, allowing ibuprofen to remain detectable in treated water.[439] As a result, traces of the drug have been detected in lakes, rivers, and even groundwater and drinking water supplies. This raises serious questions about the long-term impact on both human health and the environment.[440]

How Much Ibuprofen Is in the Environment?

The presence of ibuprofen in the environment is a growing global concern. Studies have detected alarming concentrations in various regions, highlighting the widespread nature of the issue.

- In Lahore, Pakistan, wastewater from the pharmaceutical industry along Sheikhupura Road contained 1,673 µg/L of ibuprofen, with 6,046 µg/kg in solid waste and 610 µg/kg in soil samples.[441]
- In the Lake Erie basin of North Ohio, ibuprofen levels reached 2.8 µg/L.[442]
- In South China's Pearl River Delta, researchers found 1.4 µg/L of ibuprofen.[443]
- In South Africa's KwaZulu-Natal Province, river water contained up to 19.2 µg/L.[444]
- In Greece, surface water samples showed concentrations ranging from 1.0 to 67 µg/L.[445]
- Taiwan, China, reported levels between 5.0 and 280 µg/L.[445]
- Korea recorded concentrations from less than 15 to 414 µg/L.[445]

However, these numbers likely underestimate the actual amount of ibuprofen in the environment. When we take ibuprofen, our bodies break it down into other chemicals known as metabolites, which are often not measured in environmental studies.[446] These metabolites may pose an even greater risk to aquatic life than ibuprofen itself.[447]

While no universally established safe thresholds exist for ibuprofen in freshwater ecosystems, research suggests several risks at even trace concentrations (0.1 μg/L) as discussed in the next section.[448]

Why Is Ibuprofen an Environmental Concern?

The presence of ibuprofen in the environment raises serious ecological concerns, particularly due to its harmful effects on aquatic life. Even at low concentrations in rivers and lakes, ibuprofen can be toxic to marine organisms (**Fig. 11.2**). Research has shown that it can disrupt growth, reproduction, and behavior in fish, algae, and invertebrates.[449] Additionally, ibuprofen acts as an endocrine disruptor, interfering with hormone regulation in fish and amphibians, which can negatively impact their reproductive systems.[450]

Fig. 11.2. Ibuprofen's effect on marine life

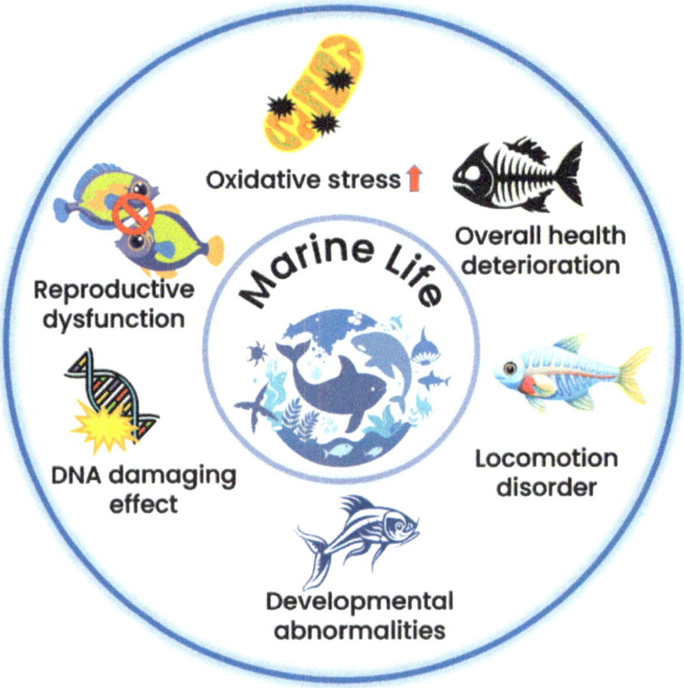

Bioaccumulation of ibuprofen in fish (0.01-15 µg/g) was as much as 3000 times what was found in the water.[451] Besides having a major negative effect on fish health, if the levels of ibuprofen in our waters increase, the bioaccumulation of ibuprofen in fish can result in therapeutic doses of ibuprofen for those who frequently eat highly contaminated fish.

Studies have also linked ibuprofen exposure to:

- Hormonal disturbances – It decreases aromatase activity (essential for sexual differentiation and brain function), reduces testosterone production, and increases 17-β estradiol levels.[452,453]
- Cellular damage – Just 0.1 µg/L of ibuprofen can decrease lysosomal membrane stability and increase oxidative stress in

aquatic organisms. At 5 μg/L, it triggers lipid peroxidation (a process that damages cell membranes), and at 10 μg/L, it causes DNA damage.[454]

- Delayed development – Exposure to 0.1 μg/L can delay fish embryo hatching, and even lower levels (1–100 ng/L) have been shown to reduce the activity of *Gammarus pulex*, a key species in freshwater ecosystems.[454,455,456,444]

Disruption of fish reproduction can alter predator-prey dynamics and undermine the stability of the entire food web within the ecosystem.

Antibiotic Resistance and Long-Term Exposure

While ibuprofen is not classified as an antibiotic, studies suggest that its presence in water can contribute to antibiotic resistance. It triggers bacterial stress responses, leading to significant shifts in bacterial diversity in aquatic environments.[457]

Although ibuprofen does not accumulate in the environment as much as pollutants like nitrates from agricultural runoff, its continuous release results in chronic exposure, disrupting entire ecosystems over time. Ibuprofen can also bioaccumulate in crops irrigated with contaminated water or grown in soils fertilized with sewage sludge, introducing them into the food chain.[458] While not well studied, consumption of contaminated fish or crops could lead to prolonged low-dose exposure, compounding risks for vulnerable populations such as those with preexisting heart, kidney, or liver problems.[458]

What Can Be Done?

To address these concerns, a combination of individual action and systemic improvements is required. Further research is needed to understand the long-term effects of ibuprofen pollution and develop strategies for reducing its environmental impact, such as more efficient and environmentally friendly degradation methods. Equally important is raising public awareness about the proper disposal of medications, to prevent unnecessary contamination.

Fig. 11.3. Ibuprofen's effect on plants

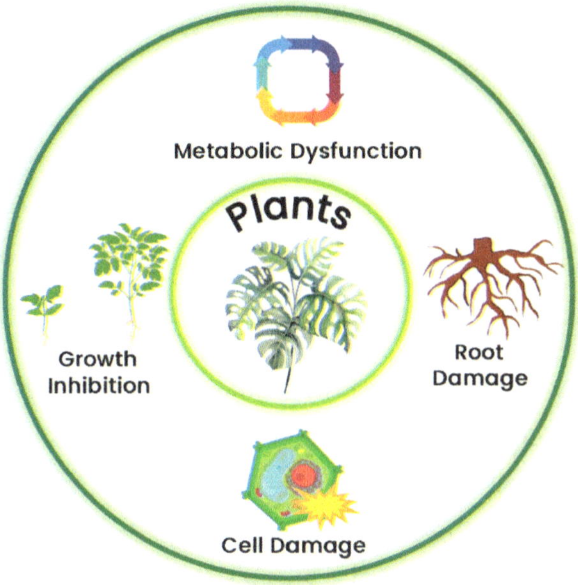

Ibuprofen and Plants

Ibuprofen doesn't just impact animals and marine life, it also affects plants (**Fig. 11.3**). Ibuprofen contamination in soil is widespread and not limited to a single type of environment.[438] When ibuprofen enters the soil, it can:

- Cause plant cell damage
- Disrupt metabolic pathways essential for plant growth
- Inhibit root development and overall plant health

These effects highlight the broader environmental consequences of pharmaceutical pollution, extending beyond aquatic ecosystems to agricultural and natural landscapes.[459,460] For humans, improper disposal increases the risk of accidental poisoning in children and pets, who may ingest discarded pills.[447] Additionally, unsecured medications can be accessed and abused, contributing to the growing problem of prescription drug misuse.

How to Properly Dispose of Ibuprofen

Unfortunately, most people dispose of unused or expired medications incorrectly, leading to environmental contamination and accidental ingestion by animals.[461-463] The safest way to dispose of ibuprofen is through drug take-back programs, which help prevent pharmaceutical waste from entering water supplies and ecosystems.[464]

The availability of drug take-back programs varies widely depending on your location. Some areas offer year-round, government-funded programs at pharmacies, hospitals, or police stations, while others rely on periodic events like the U.S. Drug Enforcement Administration's (DEA) National Prescription Drug Take-Back Day or local initiatives. In some countries, take-back programs are managed nationally, while in others, they are run by individual pharmacies or community organizations.

To find a local drug take-back site in the United States:

- Use the **FDA's Drug Disposal Locator** by searching "drug disposal near me" or "medication disposal near me" in Google Maps.[465]

- Visit the **DEA's year-round authorized collector locator** on their Diversion Control Division website or call 1-800-882-9539 for assistance.[466]
- Try the **Safe.Pharmacy Drug Disposal Locator Tool** at safe.pharmacy/drug-disposal, which lists over 10,000 permanent disposal locations nationwide.[467]

For those outside the U.S., check your local pharmacy, municipal website, or national health authority for information on available take-back programs.

What if there's no take-back site nearby?

If a drug take-back program isn't accessible, the FDA and Environmental Protection Agency (EPA) recommend checking whether your pharmacy offers mail-back envelopes for medication disposal.[468] If that's not an option, follow these steps for safe disposal at home:

1. Remove all personal information from the medication container.
2. Take the ibuprofen from its original container and put it into a disposable container with a lid (first choice) or in a sealed plastic bag (second choice). A disposable container with a tight-fitting lid is preferred over a plastic bag because it provides better protection against accidental exposure and environmental contamination.
3. Then, mix the ibuprofen with an unappealing substance like used coffee grounds, cat litter, or dirt. This lowers the threat of accidental ingestion by animals.

4. Once the ibuprofen is mixed with the unappealing substance and sealed in a leakproof container, it can be placed in the trash.[468]

Lastly, there are a few disposal practices you should always avoid:

1. **Flushing ibuprofen down the toilet:** This can lead to higher concentrations of ibuprofen in wastewater treatment plants, which often fail to fully remove pharmaceuticals, resulting in pollution of rivers, lakes, and even drinking water—harmful to aquatic life and ecosystems.

2. **Crushing ibuprofen pills before disposal:** Crushing increases the risk of accidental inhalation of the powder during disposal. Additionally, handling crushed tablets exposes the skin to the active drug, potentially causing irritation or allergic reactions.[469]

3. **Disposing of pills without a leakproof container:** Placing ibuprofen directly into a trash bag or bin can expose children and pets to the risk of accidental ingestion. Remember, ibuprofen is dangerous for pets, particularly dogs and cats, due to their increased sensitivity to its toxic effects.[470] Over time, pills in landfills that are not in leakproof containers may also leach ibuprofen into the environment. Ibuprofen in landfills can dissolve in rainwater or landfill waste, allowing active drug ingredients to seep into the soil and contaminate groundwater or nearby water sources, threatening aquatic ecosystems and drinking water.

Key Takeaways:

- The increasing presence of ibuprofen in the environment, in our water bodies and soil at levels that can harm aquatic life and disrupt ecosystems, underscores the urgent need for better wastewater treatment, public awareness, and safer disposal practices. Research into its long-term ecological impact is crucial to protecting ecosystems and reducing contamination.

- You can make a real difference: By choosing proper disposal methods, such as returning unused or expired medications to pharmacy take-back programs or following local guidelines for safe disposal, each of us plays a key role in reducing pharmaceutical waste and safeguarding our environment.

THE UNEXPECTED

Chapter 12
Ibuprofen's Secrets:
What the Label Doesn't Tell You

While researching how NSAIDs like ibuprofen impact molecular pathways, we discovered some surprising and lesser-known effects beyond their well-known role as a pain reliever.

Does the Coating on Ibuprofen Tablets Matter?

Yes! The coating on ibuprofen tablets significantly affects how the medication is absorbed, released, and tolerated by the body. Different coatings serve specific purposes, and their composition can vary by manufacturer.[471,472]

- **Sugar-Coated Tablets**: These have a sweet outer layer that improves taste and helps the tablet dissolve quickly in the stomach. While the sugar coating enhances user experience, it has minimal impact on how ibuprofen is absorbed or distributed in the body.

- **Film-Coated Tablets**: This coating protects the ibuprofen from environmental factors like light, air, and moisture, ensuring the medication remains stable. Similar to sugar-coated tablets, they dissolve easily in the stomach and provide fast relief.

- **Enteric-Coated Tablets**: These are designed to dissolve only in the more neutral environment of the small intestine, bypassing the acidic stomach. This protects the stomach lining and reduces the risk of irritation, but it also delays the onset of the drug's action. This delayed release might not be ideal if fast relief is needed.[472]

Understanding the different types of coatings can help you choose the right ibuprofen for your needs, whether you prioritize fast relief or reduced stomach irritation.

Do Additives in Ibuprofen Matter?

Yes! In addition to coatings, inactive ingredients are included in tablets to aid in manufacturing, stability, and absorption. The so-called "inactive ingredients" in ibuprofen tablets can be more important than you might think. The next time you check the label, you'll notice a list of compounds that may seem unrelated to pain relief but play crucial roles in the tablet's formulation and effectiveness nonetheless. While most additives are considered safe, some are controversial and others are restricted in certain countries.[58]

These ingredients include:

- **Colorants:** Substances like titanium dioxide and iron oxides give the tablets their characteristic appearance.

- **Binding Agents:** Microcrystalline cellulose, polyvinyl alcohol, and polyethylene glycols help hold the tablet together.

- **Lubricants:** Compounds like magnesium stearate and talc prevent the tablets from sticking to machinery during manufacturing.

- **Disintegrants:** Additives like croscarmellose sodium and cornstarch help the tablet break down efficiently in your stomach.
- **Sweeteners and Flavor Enhancers**: Some chewable ibuprofen tablets, especially those for children, include phenylalanine to improve taste.

While these ingredients are generally safe, some individuals may experience sensitivities or mild side effects. For example, polyvinyl alcohol and polyethylene glycols can cause mild GI discomfort in sensitive individuals.[473] Similarly, the sweetener phenylalanine is harmless for most people but can be dangerous for those with phenylketonuria (PKU), a rare genetic disorder affecting phenylalanine metabolism.[474] If you have allergies, sensitivities, or medical conditions, reviewing the inactive ingredients in ibuprofen is a good precaution.

Hidden Ingredients in Supplements

The FDA has repeatedly warned consumers about over-the-counter supplements marketed for pain relief that contain undisclosed ingredients.[475] This is especially concerning for those using ibuprofen or other NSAIDs, as hidden additives can increase the risk of harmful drug interactions.[476-478]

For example, Arth-Q, a supplement promoted for pain relief, was found to contain ibuprofen without proper labeling.[477] Similarly, Tepee Herbal Tea included piroxicam, another NSAID. If someone unknowingly takes these supplements alongside ibuprofen, they could face a higher risk of adverse effects such as GI damage, kidney issues, or cardiovascular problems.

Beyond NSAIDs, some supplements have been found to contain undisclosed pharmaceuticals. Products like Dream Body Extreme Gold and

Natural Max Slimming were found to contain sibutramine (a banned weight-loss drug), fluoxetine (an antidepressant), and sildenafil (the active ingredient in Viagra).[478] While these substances aren't directly related to ibuprofen, they highlight the broader issue of unlisted ingredients in supplements and the dangers of unintended drug interactions.

These hidden additives pose serious health risks and emphasize the importance of purchasing supplements from reputable brands. Always check for third-party testing and certifications to ensure the safety and transparency of the products you use. If possible, verify the safety of any supplement you use through specific resources like NSF International, USP Verified, or ConsumerLab.com.

Does It Matter When You Take Ibuprofen?

The timing of ibuprofen use might seem important, but its impact on effectiveness isn't fully understood.

One animal study using a mouse tibia (leg bone) fracture model found that ibuprofen was most effective for pain relief and healing when taken during the daytime.[479] In contrast, ibuprofen given at night appeared to impair bone healing significantly. The study used doses equivalent to 500 mg in humans every 8 hours.

Researchers suggest that this difference is linked to the body's circadian rhythm, our internal biological clock. During the day, the body is in its active phase, which may allow ibuprofen to work more effectively with natural healing processes.

What Does This Mean for Humans?

While this research is intriguing, it's important to remember that these findings are based on animal studies and specifically focus on bone healing. For most people, taking ibuprofen at night is not a concern, especially if it's needed for general pain relief. However, if you're recovering from a bone fracture, taking ibuprofen during the day may be more beneficial. This recommendation is supported by the preclinical evidence in mice discussed above showing that daytime administration aligns with circadian rhythms, enhancing anti-inflammatory effects.[479] In these studies, bone healing speed was increased 30–50% compared to nighttime use.[12]

Two human studies show no significant delay in fracture healing with ibuprofen use.[480,481] However, no human studies have looked at the effect of daytime or nighttime administration of ibuprofen. The specific benefits of daytime administration are only theorized for bone healing. For most pain relief, dosage and frequency are more important than the time of day.

Does Posture Affect Ibuprofen Absorption?

Most of us don't consider our posture when taking ibuprofen, but could it make a difference?

The most important factor is taking ibuprofen with plenty of water. Without enough liquid, the pill can get stuck at the top of the esophagus, causing irritation or a burning sensation. Once in the stomach, ibuprofen dissolves quickly, but studies suggest traces of the drug can remain in the stomach for up to seven hours.[482]

Sitting or standing upright provides a similar absorption speed as lying flat on your back.[483] If you don't usually experience stomach discomfort, waiting 30 minutes before lying flat is generally fine. However, if ibuprofen tends to upset your stomach, waiting longer before lying down may help reduce discomfort or acid reflux.

Can Different Positions Change How Fast Ibuprofen Works?

A Johns Hopkins study explored whether body position affects how quickly ibuprofen dissolves and reaches the small intestine for absorption.[483] Researchers tested four postures:

1. Leaning Right
2. Sitting or Standing Upright
3. Leaning Back
4. Leaning Left

The results? Leaning right allowed the pill to settle quickly in the lower part of the stomach, leading to faster dissolution within 10 minutes. The right-leaning position enables faster dissolution of ibuprofen, mainly due to the anatomical shape and natural asymmetry of the stomach, as well as due to gravity. The slowest position was leaning left, where it took up to 100 minutes for the pill to start breaking down.

While more studies are needed to confirm these findings in real-life scenarios, these insights suggest small adjustments in posture could optimize how quickly ibuprofen takes effect.

Now that we've explored the mechanics of ibuprofen, let's dive into some of its unexpected effects on the body.

NSAID Use and Prolonged Back Pain

A 2016 study analyzing randomized controlled trials revealed a surprising finding: NSAIDs provided little long-term benefit over a placebo in reducing lower back pain. Even more concerning, clinical studies have shown that NSAIDs come with adverse effects that may outweigh their benefits for certain types of pain.[484]

Recent research has also challenged the long-held belief that NSAIDs are the go-to solution for ongoing pain relief. In a study involving mice, scientists found that while the NSAID diclofenac initially reduced pain, it ultimately led to prolonged pain over time.[485] This suggests that NSAIDs may offer short-term relief but could contribute to chronic pain in the long run.

Human studies support this idea. A study analyzing data from 98 patients with low back pain found that frequent NSAID use was linked to an increased risk of developing chronic pain after the initial acute phase.[485] This means that for individuals relying on NSAIDs for back pain relief, regular use could unintentionally turn temporary pain into a long-term problem.

Another issue is the potential for developing a "tolerance" to NSAIDs, where the same dose becomes less effective over time. A meta-analysis of 10 trials found that NSAIDs provided only modest pain relief after one to four years of use.[486] As a result, some individuals may take higher doses, which could complicate pain management further.

Additionally, observational data suggest that long-term NSAID use is associated with worsened osteoarthritis progression in some patients.[487] While NSAIDs can provide temporary relief, these findings suggest they may not be the best choice for long-term pain management. Exploring alternative pain relief methods could be essential for those dealing with prolonged back pain. For example, combining topical NSAIDs with physiotherapy would reduce systemic exposure to the body.

Ibuprofen and Spinal Cord Injury

Early-stage animal studies suggest that ibuprofen may aid recovery after a spinal cord injury. Researchers have conducted both *in vitro* (outside a living organism) and *in vivo* (inside a living organism) experiments to determine whether ibuprofen can promote nerve growth and reduce tissue loss.[488]

One of the main obstacles to spinal cord recovery is a protein called Ras homolog family member A (RhoA), which helps organize actin filaments—structures essential for cell shape and function. Ibuprofen appears to block lysophosphatidic acid receptors, which activate RhoA, stabilize actin cytoskeletons, and block axon growth. By doing so, ibuprofen may promote nerve regeneration and improve recovery.[488,489]

Laboratory tests on chick spinal nerve cells found that ibuprofen prevented the collapse of growth cones, structures necessary for axonal growth. More growth cones mean a greater chance for neurons to regenerate. Similarly, in a study involving 48 female rats with spinal cord injuries, those treated with small doses of ibuprofen via a mini-pump showed better motor function recovery, lower RhoA activity, and higher scores on a motor behavior scale. By the end of the study, some rats could even support themselves on their hind limbs.[488]

Further experiments in mice with severe spinal injuries showed similar results.[490] Mice treated with ibuprofen regained movement in their hind ankles, and researchers observed improved fiber regeneration in serotonin-releasing neurons, an essential neurotransmitter for mood and movement.

Despite these promising findings, it remains unclear whether ibuprofen will have the same effect in humans as it did in mice. While it shows potential for aiding spinal cord recovery, comprehensive clinical data from well-designed human trials are necessary before drawing any definitive conclusions about ibuprofen's safety or effectiveness in spinal cord injury recovery.

Can Ibuprofen Cause Hair Loss?

In 1979, a physician published a letter in the *Journal of the American Medical Association (JAMA)*, suggesting a possible link between ibuprofen use and hair loss (alopecia). While this observation gained attention, it was not part of a formal, peer-reviewed study.[491]

Since then, various online sources have claimed that NSAIDs, including ibuprofen, can cause hair loss.[11] However, many of these online references lack proper citations, with only a few sites referencing the one study specifically addressing ibuprofen's role in hair loss.[491]

If ibuprofen were to contribute to hair loss, one possible explanation is its inhibition of prostaglandin synthesis. Prostaglandins like PGE2 play a crucial role in hair follicle cycling and hair growth. By interfering with this process, ibuprofen could potentially disrupt the natural hair growth cycle.[492,493]

As of now, the connection between ibuprofen and hair loss remains inconclusive. If you're concerned about hair loss while using ibuprofen, consider consulting your doctor to explore alternative medications or investigate other underlying causes.

Ibuprofen and Muscular Dystrophy

Nitric oxide is vital for enhancing circulation through the dilation (relaxation) of blood vessels. Researchers have discovered that combining NO with ibuprofen may offer therapeutic benefits for certain types of muscular dystrophy. In mouse studies, administering ibuprofen (50 mg/kg per day) alongside NO enhanced muscle regeneration, reduced necrotic damage, and alleviated muscle inflammation.[494] These findings suggest that this combination therapy could help counter some of the debilitating effects of muscular dystrophy.

NO and ibuprofen contribute to muscle regeneration through complementary mechanisms, which include NO protecting myoblasts and regenerating fibers from apoptosis, and ibuprofen's anti-inflammatory action preventing increased cytokine levels that impair NO bioavailability.[494,495] NO, as a vasodilator, enhances blood flow to damaged areas, improving oxygen and nutrient supply critical for repair, while ibuprofen reduces prostaglandin-mediated inflammation, preventing excessive immune cell infiltration that reduces regeneration.[494]

To put this into human context, due to differences in metabolism and body surface area, a 50 mg/kg dose in mice translates to approximately 4 mg/kg in humans. For a person weighing around 62 kg (136 pounds), this equates to a 250 mg dose of ibuprofen, which is a typical over-the-counter amount.[496]

However, not all muscular dystrophies may benefit from ibuprofen. Dysferlinopathy, a rare type of muscular dystrophy characterized by progressive muscle weakness and atrophy due to a deficiency in the protein dysferlin, responds differently. In mouse models of dysferlinopathy, low doses of ibuprofen (30 mg/kg per day, or approximately 2.5 mg/kg in humans) led to negative effects. These mice experienced a 40% reduction in treadmill endurance, indicating a decline in muscle function.[497]

Ibuprofen's differing effects in muscular dystrophies may be due to molecular processes that lead to the development and progression of the dystrophies. Dysferlin deficiency disrupts the repair of the muscle cell membrane (sarcolemma) and interferes with the normal trafficking of repair vesicles, compromising the cell's ability to recover from injury. In contrast, the absence of dystrophin weakens the structural stability of muscle cells, making them much more susceptible to damage during muscle contraction.

While research on ibuprofen and NO therapy for muscular dystrophy is still in its early stages, these results present an exciting opportunity for further investigation. However, clinical trials will be necessary to determine safety, effective dosing, and specific conditions where this therapy may be beneficial or potentially harmful.

Ibuprofen and Tinnitus

Tinnitus, often described as ringing, buzzing, or hissing sounds in the ears, can result from various factors, including exposure to loud noise, sinus infections, and, in some cases, the use of NSAIDs like ibuprofen.

A 2022 large-scale study explored the potential link between NSAIDs and tinnitus by tracking 69,455 women (aged 31-48) over two decades (1995-2017). By the study's end, 10,452 participants (about 15%) had developed persistent tinnitus.[498] The findings indicated that frequent use of non-aspirin NSAIDs or acetaminophen (4-5 days per week) was associated with an 8-

17% increased risk of developing tinnitus. For participants taking NSAIDs for 6-7 days each week, they had a 7-20% higher risk.

Researchers suggest that prolonged use of ibuprofen and acetaminophen may reduce blood flow to the cochlea, the inner ear structure responsible for sound processing. This reduced oxygen supply (cochlear hypoxia) could lead to cellular damage and diminished cochlear function, ultimately resulting in tinnitus.

Since it is possible that pre-existing conditions, such as age or lifestyle factors (e.g., smoking or alcohol use), could contribute to the risk, tinnitus-prone individuals should monitor ibuprofen use and explore alternative pain management options when possible.

The good news? Tinnitus caused by ibuprofen is typically reversible once the medication is discontinued or its dosage is reduced. However, the long-term effects of chronic NSAID use on the inner ear remain uncertain. Further research is needed to determine whether prolonged ibuprofen use could cause permanent hearing damage.

Pediatric Ibuprofen Hypersensitivity

Ibuprofen is a widely used NSAID for relieving pain and reducing fever in children. However, it is also the most common cause of drug hypersensitivity reactions in pediatric patients.[290,499] This means that some children experience immune system reactions after taking ibuprofen, ranging from mild skin issues to more severe symptoms.

Between January 2017 and March 2024, researchers prospectively studied 82 children with confirmed ibuprofen hypersensitivity (median age: 5.9 years) using drug provocation tests, which are the diagnostic gold standard for confirming hypersensitivity reactions. Drug provocation tests (DPTs) were positive in 22% of the 82 children. As a result of this study, they developed a risk stratification tool to help identify children at low risk of hypersensitivity. This tool may reduce unnecessary ibuprofen avoidance in cases where it is still safe to use.

Identified Risk Factors

Angioedema (2 points): Most common symptom (60% of cases in related studies).[500]

Anaphylaxis history (1 point): Linked to severe reactions during DPTs.

Age ≥10 years (1 point): Older children had higher reaction risks.

Risk Stratification:

- Low-risk (score <3): 94.7% negative predictive value (NPV), with only a 3.5% anaphylaxis rate during drug provocation tests.
- High-risk (score 3–4): 11.4x higher reaction risk vs. low-risk, 36% anaphylaxis rate during drug provocation tests.

Some of the common symptoms of ibuprofen hypersensitivity include:

- **Urticaria (Hives):** Raised, red, and itchy welts on the skin.[499]
- **Angioedema:** Swelling, particularly around sensitive areas like the face, lips, or eyes.[499]
- **Respiratory Symptoms:** While less common, hypersensitivity can aggravate breathing issues, including nasal congestion, wheezing, or shortness of breath in children with asthma or respiratory conditions (known as NSAID-exacerbated respiratory disease).[499]

Reactions to ibuprofen can occur within minutes of taking the medication or may take several hours to develop. This makes it essential for parents to stay alert after administering ibuprofen, especially if their child has a history of allergies or sensitivities to other medications.

If hypersensitivity is suspected, a pediatrician may recommend allergy testing to confirm the diagnosis and identify safe treatment options. While ibuprofen hypersensitivity is relatively rare, understanding the risks and recognizing symptoms can help ensure a child's safety.

While most children tolerate ibuprofen well, rare but serious allergic reactions can occur. Parents should watch for signs such as difficulty breathing, swelling of the face or throat, hives, or severe rash. If any of these symptoms develop, seek immediate medical attention.

Fig. 12.1. Effect of ibuprofen on male and female fertility

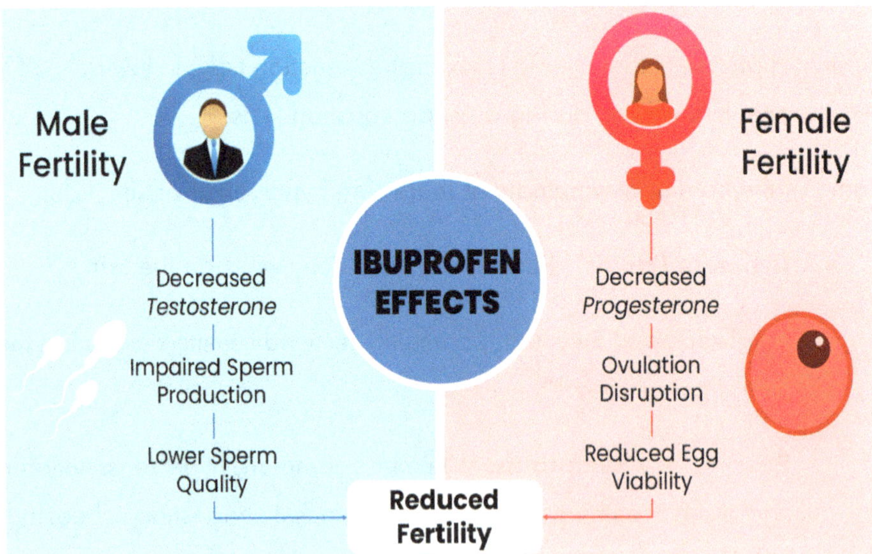

Ibuprofen and Female Reproductive Health

i. Impact on Fertility

Research suggests that ibuprofen and other NSAIDs can negatively affect female fertility by disrupting ovulation and altering hormone levels essential for conception (**Fig. 12.1**).

A 2015 study examined 39 women who took diclofenac, naproxen, or a selective COX-2 inhibitor (etoricoxib) daily for 10 days at recommended doses. The results showed a dramatic decline in ovulation across all groups, with the most significant reduction observed in the diclofenac group, where only 6% of women ovulated.[106] Additionally, all treatment groups exhibited a significant drop in prostaglandin and progesterone levels compared to the control group.

Prostaglandins play a key role in triggering ovulation, and their inhibition by NSAIDs can delay or even prevent it. Similarly, progesterone, a hormone crucial for preparing the body for pregnancy, was found to be significantly reduced, further impairing fertility.

Beyond ovulation, ibuprofen may also impact ovarian health. A 2018 study exposed human fetal ovaries to low doses of ibuprofen for 2, 4, or 7 days. This exposure led to reduced ovarian cell numbers, decreased cell proliferation, increased apoptosis (cell death), and a decline in germ cells. These findings suggest potential disruptions in ovarian development, though it's important to note that the study was conducted in a lab environment, which may not fully reflect effects in the human body.[105]

Current evidence suggests that ibuprofen and other NSAIDs not only reduce ovulation rates but may also affect egg viability and hormone levels critical for conception. [5,501] While more *in vivo* studies are needed, these findings highlight the need for caution when using ibuprofen while trying to conceive.

ii. Ibuprofen Use During Pregnancy

Pregnancy is a critical period, and ibuprofen use can pose risks to both the mother and developing baby. Research provides insights into the potential dangers, particularly in the later stages of pregnancy.

A large-scale study involving 90,417 pregnant women from the Norwegian Mother and Child Cohort Study found that 5.9% of participants reported using ibuprofen during pregnancy.[502] The study revealed that ibuprofen use in the third trimester was associated with an increased risk of structural heart defects in newborns. Additionally, use during the second and third trimesters was linked to a higher likelihood of asthma development in children by 18 months of age.

Further supporting these findings, a longitudinal study of 1,490 mother-infant pairs found an association between ibuprofen use during pregnancy and persistent wheezing and asthma in early childhood, though this effect did not persist into mid-childhood (ages 7–10).[503]

A separate large-scale study analyzing 185,617 mother-child pairs from the Danish and Norwegian Mother and Child Cohort Studies investigated a potential link between ibuprofen use during pregnancy and cerebral palsy. While 4% of mothers use ibuprofen, the study found no significant association between prenatal ibuprofen exposure and cerebral palsy after adjusting for confounders.[504] This absence of a significant link is noteworthy as it suggests that, within the studied population, ibuprofen use during pregnancy does not appear to increase the risk of cerebral palsy. However, the study relied on maternal recall, which could introduce bias, and most participants came from higher socioeconomic backgrounds, potentially limiting the generalizability of the findings.

Other Potential Risks of Ibuprofen Use During Pregnancy

Other potential risks of ibuprofen use during pregnancy include neurodevelopmental effects. For example, a study of 1,225 mother-child pairs found that prenatal and early postnatal exposure to ibuprofen was associated with diminished executive function and behavioral issues in children.[505] However, it is important to note that such studies often rely on maternal recall and may be affected by socioeconomic factors, which can limit the generalizability and accuracy of the findings. The observational design and potential for confounding variables mean that these results should be interpreted with caution, and more robust research is needed to confirm any causal relationship.

Additionally, though rare, neonatal kidney failure has been reported following as little as two days of in-utero ibuprofen exposure, with 35 cases and 8 deaths linked to COX inhibitors and related complications.[506] Most cases occur after 20 weeks of gestation, when the fetus becomes more reliant on its own kidneys to produce amniotic fluid. Notably, in 11 cases, amniotic fluid levels returned to normal after discontinuing NSAIDs, indicating the condition can be reversible if detected early.

Due to these risks, the FDA has issued a warning against the use of NSAIDs, including ibuprofen, after 20 weeks of pregnancy. Potential complications include reduced amniotic fluid levels, which can lead to kidney problems in the fetus, and, after 30 weeks, risks of heart-related defects.[506] While ibuprofen is generally considered safe in early pregnancy, its use in later stages requires caution. If ibuprofen is deemed necessary in late pregnancy, healthcare providers may recommend monitoring amniotic fluid levels via ultrasound if treatment extends beyond 48 hours.

iii. Ibuprofen and Miscarriage Risk

Beyond concerns about ibuprofen use during pregnancy, research suggests that NSAIDs like ibuprofen may also increase the risk of early miscarriage.

A prospective study of 1,097 pregnant women found that NSAID use around the time of conception was associated with an 89% higher risk of miscarriage, even after controlling for factors such as smoking, age, multivitamin use, caffeine consumption, and previous miscarriage history.[507]

Notably, the risk appeared to be influenced by body mass index (BMI). Women with a BMI of 25 or lower who used ibuprofen were more than three times as likely to experience a miscarriage compared to women of similar BMI who did not use NSAIDs. In contrast, overweight women were less likely to experience early miscarriage under similar conditions. Inhibition of COX enzymes results in decreased PGE2 levels, which facilitates embryo adhesion by increasing uterine vascular permeability and stromal decidualization.[508] Researchers hypothesized that higher prostaglandin levels in individuals with obesity might help counteract the harmful effects of NSAIDs on pregnancy.[507]

Additionally, a dose-dependent relationship was observed: higher NSAID doses (measured per kilogram of body weight) were linked to greater miscarriage risk. Since NSAIDs inhibit prostaglandin production, which plays a key role in pregnancy maintenance, underweight individuals may be particularly vulnerable to these effects.

While further research is needed to fully understand the underlying mechanisms, current evidence suggests that avoiding ibuprofen and other NSAIDs during conception and early pregnancy may help reduce the risk of miscarriage.

Ibuprofen and Neurodevelopmental Outcomes in Children

Prenatal exposure to ibuprofen and its potential long-term neurodevelopmental effects remains a topic of ongoing research, but the *Project Viva* cohort study (involving 1225 mother-child pairs) found that prenatal ibuprofen use (≥10 times) was associated with a significant increase in parent-rated poorer executive function and behavior by age 8.[505] Infant exposure (≥6 doses in the first year) correlated with similar deficits. A different study involving 6,876 pregnant women with prenatal exposure to NSAIDs found that these parents reported their children had more attention problems at younger ages, such as age 3.; however, teachers reported that these children showed no significant difference from those not exposed to NSAIDs prenatally.[509] These results suggest potential reporting bias by parents.

Ibuprofen and Male Reproductive Health

i) Fertility

Emerging research suggests that ibuprofen and other NSAIDs may negatively impact male reproductive health. A 2018 clinical trial involving 31 young men (ages 18-35) examined the effects of ibuprofen use at a dosage of 600 mg twice daily for six weeks.[510] The study found that ibuprofen use led to "compensated hypogonadism," a hormonal imbalance typically seen in older men and linked to reproductive disorders, including reduced sex drive, erectile dysfunction, and infertility. Compensated hypogonadism is characterized by normal testosterone levels but elevated luteinizing hormone, due to the testes starting to work less efficiently.

The researchers discovered that ibuprofen altered levels of testosterone and luteinizing hormone, both of which are crucial for sexual development and testicular function. Additionally, experiments on adult human testis tissues exposed to ibuprofen showed a suppression of testosterone production, suggesting that ibuprofen may interfere with the pituitary gland and other essential reproductive processes.[510]

Animal studies further support these findings. A meta-analysis of studies on adult male mice and *in vitro* sperm treatments revealed consistent declines in sperm motility, viability, count, and DNA integrity after ibuprofen exposure.[511] These effects were observed both after prolonged treatment (approximately 35 days) and within minutes in laboratory settings. Researchers propose that ibuprofen's and other NSAIDs' impact on male fertility may be due to:

- Disruption of testosterone and prostaglandin synthesis
- Inhibition of nitric oxide production, which is essential for healthy sperm motility

Although further research is needed, the current evidence highlights potential reproductive risks associated with ibuprofen use. Men trying to conceive may want to limit their ibuprofen intake and consult a healthcare professional for alternative pain management options.

ii) Erectile Dysfunction

Erectile dysfunction (ED) is a common condition, with over 330 million men worldwide expected to experience it by 2025.[512] Could ibuprofen, a widely used over-the-counter pain reliever, be contributing to this rising concern? Some studies suggest that regular ibuprofen use may increase the risk of developing ED.[513]

While the exact mechanisms are still being explored, several possible explanations have been proposed:

- Decreased blood delivery to the penis, which is essential for both starting and upholding an erection.
- Interference with prostaglandins, molecules essential for erectile function.
- Impact on nitric oxide levels, a key compound that relaxes blood vessels and facilitates erections.
- Ibuprofen may be interacting with other medications or pre-existing health conditions, as NSAID users often have underlying inflammatory conditions (arthritis) that independently impair vascular health.

To understand the importance of nitric oxide, consider how medications like Viagra work: they increase nitric oxide, which helps improve blood flow and sustain erections. Interestingly, ibuprofen appears to have a complex relationship with nitric oxide. In some cases, it reduces nitric oxide levels, particularly by inhibiting an enzyme called inducible nitric oxide synthase.[514] A reduction in nitric oxide might impair blood vessel dilation, leading to difficulty in achieving or maintaining an erection. A study on 12 individuals taking 2400 mg of ibuprofen showed decreased nitric oxide levels compared to a placebo group.[180]

Several large-scale studies have examined the link between NSAIDs and erectile dysfunction:

- A study of Finnish men (ages 50-70) found that those who regularly used ibuprofen had a 160% higher risk of developing ED compared to non-users.[513]

- A 2017 study of 4,726 men from the Prostate Cancer Prevention Trial linked non-aspirin NSAID use to an increased risk of mild to moderate ED. The authors speculated that the connection might stem from underlying conditions (such as arthritis or atherosclerosis) rather than NSAID use alone. However, they also noted that aspirin use was linked to more severe ED.[515]

In a notable case from Saudi Arabia, a 26-year-old man experienced a temporary increase in libido and improved erectile function after taking a single 600 mg dose of ibuprofen following dental surgery.[516] This dosage aligns with common short-term prescription use (typically 400-800 mg per dose), though it exceeds standard over-the-counter recommendations of 200-400 mg every 4-6 hours (max 1,200 mg/day). His improved erectile function occurred again after taking a second dose the following day. While intriguing, this isolated case does not suggest that ibuprofen can be used as an ED treatment, and its effects on erectile function remain complex and inconsistent.

Takeaways:

- Regular or long-term ibuprofen use (6 or more weeks) at high doses (1,200 mg/day or more) may contribute to ED by disrupting blood flow, prostaglandin production, and nitric oxide levels.

- Short-term use (<10 days) at OTC doses shows minimal ED risk in most populations. However, more research is needed to clarify its effects, as the risk is likely to vary between individuals.
- Men experiencing ED who regularly take ibuprofen should consult a healthcare provider before making any changes to their medication regimen.

While ibuprofen remains a commonly used pain reliever, these findings suggest caution in long-term or frequent use, particularly for men concerned about fertility and sexual health.

Does Ibuprofen Affect Sleep Patterns?

Sleep is regulated by complex processes, including the role of prostaglandins like prostaglandin D2 (see Chapter 3), which promotes sleep. Since ibuprofen inhibits COX enzymes, reducing prostaglandin production, it may impact normal sleep patterns. However, conflicting findings exist across studies, with some reporting insomnia and others noting improved sleep quality.

A 1994 study examined this connection by analyzing sleep in 37 young adults (average age 20) over two nights in a sleep lab. Participants who took ibuprofen or aspirin experienced reduced sleep efficiency, more frequent awakenings, and delayed onset of deep sleep compared to those given a placebo. They also spent more time awake during the night. In contrast, acetaminophen had no significant effect on sleep. The study used a total daily dose of 400 mg of ibuprofen or 650 mg of aspirin/acetaminophen, administered at 11 p.m., 8:15 a.m., and again at 11 p.m. before sleep monitoring.[517]

However, a 2006 study with 30 participants (average age 28.6) found no significant sleep disturbances with ibuprofen use. Participants took 400 mg doses at 3 p.m., 7 p.m., and 11 p.m. (totaling 1200 mg daily), resulting in only a 1.2% change in sleep efficiency and a mean increase of 3 minutes in wake time, neither reaching statistical significance ($p > 0.05$). Unlike the previous study, researchers allowed participants to acclimate to the sleep environment before measuring baseline sleep patterns. This improved study design found no notable changes in sleep quality, though two participants reported mild side effects.[518]

One possible explanation for these differing results is that ibuprofen may influence both prostaglandin D2 (which promotes sleep) and prostaglandin E2 (which is linked to wakefulness), potentially balancing out any sleep disruptions.[519] For those concerned about sleep disturbances, it's important to use ibuprofen responsibly and consult a healthcare provider for guidance.

For individuals seeking alternatives, non-pharmacological approaches such as practicing good sleep hygiene, cognitive behavioral therapy for insomnia, and relaxation techniques may be helpful. Other over-the-counter pain relievers, such as acetaminophen, generally have less impact on sleep architecture and may be considered as alternatives-though these too should be used under medical supervision. Always discuss any ongoing sleep or pain concerns with a healthcare professional to determine the safest and most effective treatment plan for your individual needs.

Is Ibuprofen Use Linked to Depression?

While ibuprofen and other NSAIDs are generally considered neutral or even beneficial for brain health (see Chapter 5), concerns have been raised about their effects on individuals with mental health conditions. A 1996 report documented four psychiatric outpatients (one with schizophrenia and three with affective disorders) who developed moderate to severe depression after beginning NSAID treatment for pain, with one case of paranoia. The NSAIDs involved included ibuprofen, naproxen, and diclofenac.[520] The symptoms diminished upon discontinuation and reappeared with rechallenge, suggesting a pharmacological mechanism rather than due to random occurrence. These results imply a possible link between NSAIDs and mood changes. Affective disorders, such as bipolar disorder and depression, affect emotional regulation, making these findings particularly noteworthy. A possible mechanism is that inhibition of COX enzymes by ibuprofen decreases PGE2 levels, which may disrupt dopamine transmission in limbic regions.[521]

However, this study had significant limitations, including a very small sample size and potential confounding factors such as concurrent medications. The study also lacked control for illness duration, treatment adherence, or comorbid medical conditions. Since then, no large-scale studies have further explored the relationship between NSAID use and mental health disorders, leaving this topic largely understudied. Further research with larger, more rigorous studies and updated diagnostic criteria could help clarify whether NSAIDs have an impact on mental health in vulnerable populations.[520]

The Complex Patterns of NSAID Use and Misuse

I) Unfilled Prescriptions

A recent study in Finland (2020-2022) revealed that 13.3% of prescriptions remained unfilled two years after being written. Among the most commonly unfilled medications were paracetamol, ibuprofen, and salbutamol.[522] This finding raises critical questions: Are physicians overprescribing medications like ibuprofen, or are patients neglecting necessary treatments? For individuals who genuinely need these medications but fail to take them, the issue highlights a significant communication gap between healthcare providers and patients.

II) The Dark Side of Misuse

The misuse of ibuprofen has severe consequences, particularly among young people. Data indicate that ibuprofen was the third most common drug linked to mortality in patients aged 10-24 following hospital discharge for a non-lethal, intentional overdose.[523] This statistic underscores the urgent need for greater awareness about the potential dangers of over-the-counter medications like ibuprofen. Although widely perceived as safe, improper use can have life-threatening repercussions.

III) NSAIDs in Sports: Common but Controversial

NSAID use is widespread in both recreational and professional sports, often occurring without medical supervision.[524] These medications were among the most frequently dispensed at major athletic events, including the Olympic and Paralympic Games, where acetaminophen and NSAIDs led medication usage at the Winter 2018 and Summer 2020 Games.[525,526] Similarly, FIFA's monitoring of international soccer players found that over half used NSAIDs, with up to one-third taking them routinely before every match, regardless of participation.[527]

In the United States, NSAID usage among athletes is similarly high. Studies reveal that 30% of NFL players use NSAIDs daily, a practice associated with increased systolic blood pressure and body weight. Disturbingly, many athletes begin habitual NSAID use in high school, long before their bodies are fully developed.[528]

Much like the general population, many athletes remain unaware of the potential risks of NSAIDs. Surveys indicate that many users never read the warning labels on ibuprofen bottles. Among runners, this trend persists. A UK survey of 806 runners (average age 48.4 years) found that 87.8% were frequent NSAID users, with ibuprofen being the most common. Alarmingly, 23.5% of these runners reported taking ibuprofen for eight or more days in the month preceding the survey. About one-third experienced adverse reactions, predominantly GI issues.[96,529]

Despite their widespread use, many athletes express a desire for better education about the benefits and risks of NSAIDs.[530] This pattern reflects systemic issues in sports medicine and adolescent health literacy, rather than individual recklessness or clinical mismanagement. Both athletes and the general public should be aware that while NSAIDs can provide short-term pain relief, long-term use carries significant risks that may outweigh the benefits, particularly when used without medical supervision.[71] This underscores the urgent need for improved awareness, regulation, and oversight. Ensuring proper prescription practices and raising awareness about potential side effects are essential steps toward promoting safer NSAID use and protecting public health.

Key Takeaways:

- While NSAIDs are widely used, there are still gaps in knowledge regarding their long-term health impact.

- Research suggests ibuprofen may negatively affect both male and female fertility, making it a potential concern for individuals trying to conceive.

- Ibuprofen should be avoided in late-stage pregnancy unless medically supervised, as it poses risks such as reduced amniotic fluid and fetal heart complications.
- If you experience unexpected side effects after taking ibuprofen or other NSAIDs, report them to the FDA's MedWatch program. Your report can help identify potential issues with specific medication batches and contribute to public safety.

Chapter 13
Drugs That Don't Play Nice with Ibuprofen

In 2021, around 65% of Americans over the age of 18 consumed prescription drugs, with the average increasing with age.[531] Furthermore, the percentage of Americans consuming multiple prescription drugs concurrently also rises with age, with more than 76% of those aged 60+ using two or more prescription drugs at once and more than 37% using five or more. Given that ibuprofen is one of the most commonly bought over-the-counter medications, many people unknowingly consume it alongside other medications, unaware of the potential risks.[532] In some cases, the interaction between ibuprofen and other drugs can result in harmful side effects. This section reviews some of the most concerning drug interactions with ibuprofen.

Serious Adverse Effects

Several well-known drugs have been clinically shown to cause significant harmful side effects when used with ibuprofen, including aspirin, lithium, naproxen, and warfarin. A summary of many of the known ibuprofen-drug interactions is provided in **Table 13.1**.

Fig. 13.1. Commonly used compounds that interact with ibuprofen

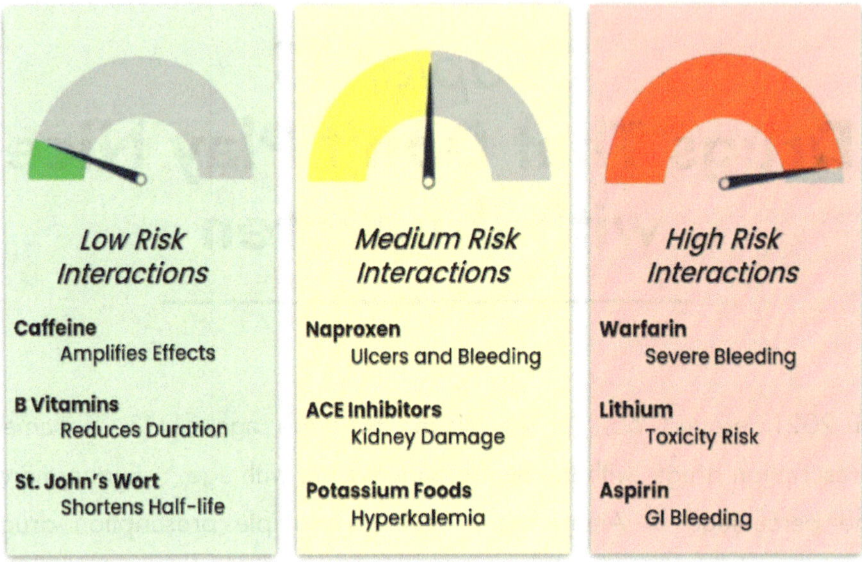

When Pain Relief Meets Mood Stabilizers: Ibuprofen and Lithium at Odds

Lithium is a metal that is typically consumed through food or medications. Lithium has been found to be associated with mood stabilization and is often used to treat mental illnesses, including mania, bipolar disorder, and major depressive disorder.[533] Although the prescription of lithium drugs has declined over the past few decades, it is still used due to more than 60 years of evidence supporting its effectiveness in managing symptoms. and preventing relapse in various psychiatric conditions, such as bipolar disorder.[534] However, regular monitoring of lithium levels is essential for individuals on lithium therapy, especially if they are prescribed or use ibuprofen.

Ibuprofen can significantly increase blood levels of lithium in patients, leading to secondary effects, such as nausea, diarrhea, and ataxia (the loss of muscle control).[535] Furthermore, ibuprofen has been shown to reduce the kidneys' ability to filter out lithium, thereby contributing to elevated blood lithium levels.[536] If left untreated and unmonitored, elevated levels of blood lithium can lead to lithium intoxication, which can sometimes be fatal, and may even require hospitalization.[537] Lithium intoxication can lead to serotonin syndrome (a condition in which there is too much serotonin being produced in your brain), brain damage, coma, and in some cases, even death.[538]

Warfarin's Frenemy: The Ibuprofen Factor

NSAIDs, like ibuprofen, can increase the risk of bleeding when taken with oral anticoagulants (blood thinners), including warfarin, by decreasing the levels of a substance in the blood called prothrombin.[539] Prothrombin plays a critical role in blood clotting, helping to prevent excessive bleeding following an injury. The interaction between warfarin and ibuprofen can cause hemorrhagic peptic ulcer disease and result in fatalities. Some other effects include GI irritation and inhibition of platelet adhesion, which stops clot formation.[539] Additionally, various NSAIDs have also been shown to change the movement of warfarin in the body and other anticoagulants, resulting in increased prothrombin time (blood takes longer to clot).

Note that warfarin is a derivative of coumarin, which is found in high concentrations in cinnamon. An observational study on a population of coumarin consumers, which took place over one year, found that there is a risk of bleeding complications associated with the use of NSAIDs.[540] Coumarin derivatives are also found in many common foods and other substances, including Tonka beans, fennel, green tea, carrots, and licorice root, among others.[541] Despite this, no studies have directly examined interactions within these foods, so the effects of taking ibuprofen alongside them remain unclear.

Hence, our current scientific understanding is inconclusive, and more research is needed to fully understand the potential risks associated with these combinations.

Ibuprofen and Aspirin: Friends or Foes?

Studies have shown that the effectiveness of taking aspirin to prevent heart attacks or strokes can be reduced with frequent or regular use of ibuprofen.[542] Aspirin is a common drug often used to treat pain and inflammation. In addition, it is prescribed to heart failure patients due to its heart-protective qualities. Studies show that regular or frequent use of ibuprofen can reduce the protective qualities of aspirin against heart attacks or strokes.[542] This interaction is particularly significant for individuals taking low-dose aspirin to prevent cardiovascular events.

While aspirin and ibuprofen both inhibit the COX-1 enzyme, they do so in different ways. Aspirin binds COX-1 irreversibly (providing long-lasting antiplatelet effects), while ibuprofen's inhibition is reversible and short-lived.[543] When taken together, ibuprofen can block aspirin's access to COX-1, reducing aspirin's effectiveness in preventing blood clots and heart attacks.

Combining aspirin with ibuprofen can also increase the risk of developing ulcers, bleeding, and perforation in the GI tract.[544] A study was conducted on seven rheumatoid arthritis patients who were given both ibuprofen and aspirin. The results showed an average of 56% reduced ibuprofen levels in these patients without a change in the excretion rate. It was also found that there was no change in the rate at which ibuprofen was broken down inside the body.[545] This suggests that ibuprofen, when taken with aspirin, was binding to something, such as proteins, instead of being broken down or excreted at a faster rate. To prevent this from happening, ibuprofen should not be taken with aspirin.

Ibuprofen and Naproxen: A Risky NSAID Affair

Combining naproxen, another NSAID, with ibuprofen is not recommended because they work in similar ways and have overlapping side effects. Using these NSAIDs together can increase the risk of side effects in the GI tract, such as inflammation, bleeding, ulceration, and perforation of the esophagus, stomach, or intestines.[546] Gastrointestinal perforation is a serious adverse effect characterized by the formation of holes in the stomach or intestine and can be fatal.

Ibuprofen and Antihypertensive Drugs (Blood Pressure Medications)

Ibuprofen can reduce the effectiveness of several types of blood pressure medications, including ACE inhibitors, angiotensin receptor blockers, beta-blockers, diuretics, and alpha-blockers.[364] Ibuprofen's effect is due to its inhibition of prostaglandin synthesis, which reduces renal blood flow and counteracts the blood pressure-lowering effect of these medications. Prolonged use of ibuprofen with antihypertensives can lead to elevated blood pressure and, in some cases, an increased risk of heart attack, stroke, or kidney damage, especially when combined with diuretics and renin-angiotensin system inhibitors.[547]

Table 13.1. Summary of other ibuprofen-drug interactions[548]

Effect of combined use with Ibuprofen	Drugs
It may increase the risk or severity of bleeding.	Abciximab, Anagrelide, Apixaban, Betrixaban, Cangrelor, Caplacizumab, Cilostazol, Clopidogrel, Defibrotide, Dipyridamole, Epoprostenol, Eptifibatide, Icosapent ethyl, Lexapro, Omacetaxine mepesuccinate, Pentoxifylline, Prasugrel, Sertraline, Sulfinpyrazone, Ticagrelor, Ticlopidine, Tirofiban, Triflusal, Treprostinil, Vorapaxar, Zidovudine
It may reduce the therapeutic efficacy (the ability of the drug to perform its intended function) of the drug.	Ambrisentan, Aprocitentan, Bendroflumethiazide, Benzthiazide, Bepridil, Bethanidine, Bimatoprost, Bosentan, Bretylium, Bumetanide, Chlorothiazide, Chlorthalidone, Clonidine, Cryptenamine, Cyclopenthiazide, Cyclothiazide, Dasiglucagon, Debrisoquine, Deserpidine, Diazoxide, Dihydralazine, Dinoprost, Doxazosin, Etacrynic acid, Fenoldopam, Furosemide, Guanabenz, Guanadrel, Guanethidine, Guanfacine, Guanoxan, Hydroflumethiazide, Indapamide, Indoramin, Lacidipine, Latanoprost, Latanoprostene bunod, Lercanidipine, Levamlodipine, Lofexidine, Macimorelin, Macitentan, Manidipine, Mecamylamine, Methyldopa, Metyrosine, Mifamurtide, Minoxidil, Moxonidine, Muzolimine, Nimodipine, Nisoldipine, Nitrendipine, Nitroprusside, Nitroglycerin, Nicorandil, Pentolinium, Phenoxybenzamine, Phentolamine, Piretanide, Prazosin, Quinethazone, Reserpine, Riociguat, Selexipag, Sitaxentan, Trimethaphan, Trichlormethiazide, Travoprost, Torasemide, Tolazoline, Unoprostone

The risk of severity of gastrointestinal bleeding may be increased.	Amitriptyline, Amitriptylinoxide, Amoxapine, Apixaban, Butriptyline, Citalopram, Clodronic acid, Clomipramine, Deferasirox, Deflazacort, Desipramine, Desvenlafaxine, Dibenzepin, Dosulepin, Doxepin, Duloxetine, Escitalopram, Etidronic acid, Fluoxetine, Fluvoxamine, Ibandronate, Imipramine, Methylprednisolone, Milnacipran, Nortriptyline, Pamidronic acid, Paroxetine, Pargyline, Prednisone, Prednisone acetate, Prednisolone, Prednisolone acetate, Prednisolone phosphate, Protriptyline, Risedronic acid, Sibutramine, Trazodone, Tiludronic acid, Trimipramine, Zoledronic acid, Zimelidine
The risk or severity of gastrointestinal irritation may be increased.	Beclomethasone dipropionate, Betamethasone, Betamethasone phosphate, Budesonide, Ciclesonide, Clobetasol propionate, Corticotropin, Corticotropin zinc hydroxide, Cortisone acetate, Desoximetasone, Dexamethasone, Dexamethasone acetate, Difluocortolone, Ethanol, Fludrocortisone, Flumethasone, Flunisolide, Fluocinolone acetonide, Fluocinonide, Fluocortolone, Fluorometholone, Fluprednisolone, Fluticasone, Fluticasone furoate, Fluticasone propionate, Hydrocortisone, Hydrocortisone acetate, Hydrocortisone butyrate, Hydrocortisone cypionate, Hydrocortisone succinate, Methylprednisolone aceponate, Methylprednisolone hemisuccinate, Meprednisone, Mometasone furoate, Tixocortol, Triamcinolone, Trilostane, Vamorolone
The risk or severity of peptic ulcer (sores in the stomach or small	Deferasirox

intestine) may be increased.	
It may increase the risk of severity of angioedema (swelling of deep layers of the skin and/or mucous membranes).	Alogliptin, Alteplase, Anistreplase, Icatibant, Pregabalin, Reteplase, Sacubitril, Sirolimus, Streptokinase, Temsirolimus, Urokinase, Vildagliptin
Ibuprofen metabolism may be increased (i.e., ibuprofen is removed more quickly from the body).	Abatacept, Adalimumab, Alogliptin, Anakinra, Apremilast, Asciminib, Avatrombopag, Bimekizumab, Carbamazepine, Canakinumab, Certolizumab pegol, Desogestrel, Emapalumab, Ergotamine, Etanercept, Ethinylestradiol, Golimumab, Ifosfamide, Ivosidenib, Lamotrigine, Metreleptin, Mitapivat, Mitotane, Nirogacestat, Peginterferon alfa-2b, Pentobarbital, Phenobarbital, Primidone, Rifabutin, Rifampin, Rifapentine, Rilonacept, Secobarbital, Secukinumab, Siltuximab, St. John's Wort, Tecovirimat, Vildagliptin
Ibuprofen metabolism may be decreased (i.e., ibuprofen remains longer in the body).	Abatacept, Abiraterone, Abrocitinib, Acetyl sulfisoxazole, Acyclovir, Adenine, Agomelatine, Almotriptan, Alosetron, Amiodarone, Amodiaquine, Amprenavir, Apomorphine, Aprepitant, Armodafinil, Atazanavir, Avapritinib, Azelastine, Adagrasib, Berotralstat, Bexarotene, Bezafibrate, Boceprevir, Bortezomib, Buprenorphine, Cabozantinib, Cannabidiol, Ceritinib, Cerivastatin, Chenodeoxycholic acid, Ciprofloxacin, Cisapride, Clarithromycin, Clevidipine, Clozapine, Conivaptan, Curcumin, Cyclizine, Cyclophosphamide, Dacomitinib, Danazol, Dapsone, Darunavir, Dasabuvir, Delavirdine, Diacerein, Dicoumarol, Diethylstilbestrol, Diltiazem, Diosmin, Doconexent,

	Donepezil, Dronedarone, Efavirenz, Eltrombopag, Elvitegravir, Encorafenib, Epinephrine, Etravirine, Favipiravir, Felbamate, Felodipine, Fenofibrate, Flecainide, Floxuridine, Fluconazole, Flunitrazepam, Fluvastatin, Fosnetupitant, Fostamatinib, Fusidic acid, Gemfibrozil, Ginkgo biloba, Glecaprevir, Indinavir, Isavuconazole, Isavuconazonium, Isoniazid, Isradipine, Itraconazole, Ketoconazole, Lansoprazole, Leflunomide, Letermovir, Levoketoconazole, Levothyroxine, Linagliptin, Lonafarnib, Loperamide, Lopinavir, Medroxyprogesterone acetate, Methimazole, Methylene blue, Metronidazole, Mephenytoin, Miconazole, Midostaurin, Modafinil, Montelukast, Morphine, Mycophenolate mofetil, Nabilone, Nefazodone, Nelfinavir, Netupitant, Nevirapine, Nicardipine, Norgestimate, Noscapine, Nilotinib, Nilutamide, Nilvadipine, Olanzapine, Ombitasvir, Ondansetron, Oritavancin, Oxandrolone, Oxybutynin, Paramethadione, Paritaprevir, Peginterferon alfa-2b, Phenobarbital, Pirfenidone, Pirtobrutinib, Piperaquine, Pioglitazone, Pibrentasvir, Pyrimethamine, Posaconazole, Propofol, Promethazine, Progesterone, Primaquine, Pralsetinib, Quizartinib, Quinidine, Regorafenib, Repaglinide, Repotrectinib, Resmetirom, Rilpivirine, Ribociclib, Rosiglitazone, Rucaparib, Rupatadine, Salmeterol, Saquinavir, Secobarbital, Secukinumab, Siltuximab, Simvastatin, Simeprevir, Sildenafil, Sulfadiazine, Sulfapyridine, Sulfamethazole, Sulfamethizole, Sulfaphenazole, Sulfisoxazole, Tamoxifen, Terbinafine, Teriflunomide, Tazarotene, Tenecteplase, Teniposide, Telaprevir, Telithromycin, Tepotinib, Theophylline, Thalidomide, Troleandomycin, Trimethadione,

	Trimethoprim, Triclabendazole, Tranylcypromine, Tocilizumab, Tipranavir, Urokinase, Venlafaxine, Venetoclax, Vemurafenib, Verapamil, Viloxazine, Vildagliptin, Zafirlukast, Zileuton, Zolpidem, Ziprasidone
Drug metabolism may be decreased.	Acenocoumarol, Amlodipine, Anastrozole, Artemether, Asunaprevir, Atovaquone, Atorvastatin, Benzyl alcohol, Brigatinib, Cabazitaxel, Daprodustat, Domperidone, Elagolix, Enasidenib, Erdafitinib, Erlotinib, Estradiol acetate, Estradiol benzoate, Estradiol cypionate, Estradiol dienanthate, Estradiol valerate, Estrone sulfate, Eszopiclone, Etrasimod, Finerenone, Fluindione, Fluorouracil, Fosphenytoin, Fruquintinib, Glasdegib, Halofantrine, Hydroxychloroquine, Idarubicin, Iptacopan, Istradefylline, Ketamine, Lacosamide, Lapatinib, Lynestrenol, Mestranol, Niclosamide, Olodaterol, Ospemifene, Ozanimod, Paclitaxel, Pazopanib, Proguanil, Roxadustat, Selumetinib, Testosterone cypionate, Testosterone enanthate, Thiamylal, Trabectedin, Tucatinib, Vardenafil, Velpatasvir, Vemurafenib, Voxilaprevir, Voxelotor, Vortioxetine, Ximelagatran, Zopiclone
This may result in a decreased excretion rate of the drug (resulting in higher concentrations of the drug in the blood and therefore a greater chance of experiencing side effects).	Abacavir, Acamprosate, Aclidinium, Acrivastine, Albutrepenonacog alfa, Aldesleukin, Allopurinol, Almasilate, Alprazolam, Alprostadil, Amantadine, Aminohippuric acid, Amoxicillin, Amikacin, Ampicillin, Amrinone, Ancestim, Antihemophilic factor (recombinant) PEGylated, Antithrombin III human, Arsenic trioxide, Auranofin, Aurothioglucose, Avanafil, Avibactam, Azacitidine, Azathioprine, Azelaic acid, Aztreonam, Baclofen, Benserazide, Benzatropine, Benznidazole,

	Benzylpenicillin, Bepotastine, Bicisate, Bismuth subgallate, Bisoxatin, Bleomycin, Brivaracetam, Bromazepam, Bupropion, Butabarbital, Capreomycin, Carbidopa, Carmustine, Cefaclor, Cefazolin, Cefdinir, Cefotiam, Ceftibuten, Ceftizoxime, Ceftolozane, Cephalexin, Cevimeline, Chloral hydrate, Chlorzoxazone, Cholic Acid, Choline C 11, Choline salicylate, Chromic chloride, Chromic nitrate, Chromium, Chromium gluconate, Chromium nicotinate, Chromous sulfate, Cimetidine, Cisplatin, Clobazam, Clofarabine, Clonazepam, Clorazepic acid, Clove oil, Colchicine, Colistin, Conjugated estrogens, Corifollitropin alfa, Dabigatran etexilate, Dacarbazine, Dalfampridine, Daptomycin, Deferiprone, Deutetrabenazine, Dexpanthenol, Dexrazoxane, Dextran, Diatrizoate, Diazepam, Dichlorobenzyl alcohol, Dicyclomine, Didanosine, Dienogest, Dimercaprol, Dimethyl sulfoxide, Dinoprostone, Disopyramide, Doripenem, Doxacurium, Doxycycline, Dyphylline, Edoxaban, Edrophonium, Eluxadoline, Ertapenem, Estazolam, Estradiol, Ethambutol, Etonogestrel, Eucalyptus oil, Ezogabine, Fenofibric acid, Fesoterodine, Fexofenadine, Flavoxate, Florbetaben F-18, Florbetapir F-18, Flucytosine, Fludeoxyglucose (18F), Flumazenil, Fluorescein, Flurazepam, Flutamide, Folic acid, Fomepizole, Fondaparinux, Formestane, Fosfomycin, Gabapentin enacarbil, Gadobenic acid, Gadodiamide, Gadofosveset trisodium, Gadopentetic acid, Gadoteric acid, Gadoteridol, Ganciclovir, Gemcitabine, Gentamicin, Gimeracil, Glycerol phenylbutyrate, Golodirsen, Goserelin, Hydromorphone, Hydrochlorothiazide, Hydroxocobalamin, Hydroxyethyl Starch, Ibutilide, Idarucizumab,

	Idebenone, Indigotindisulfonic acid, Inosine pranobex, Inositol, Iobenguane sulfate I-123, Iodixanol, Ioflupane I-123, Iopromide, Iothalamic acid, Ioversol, Ioxilan, Ipecac, Ipilimumab, Isosorbide mononitrate, Isosulfan blue, Isotretinoin, Ixazomib, Kanamycin, Ketazolam, Lamivudine, Ledipasvir, Lenalidomide, Lesinurad, Leucovorin, Leuprolide, Levobupivacaine, Levocarnitine, Levomilnacipran, Liothyronine, Lithium carbonate, Lithium citrate, Lithium hydroxide, Lixisenatide, Lorazepam, Lorcaserin, Lorpiprazole, Lubiprostone, Magnesium carbonate, Magnesium chloride, Magnesium hydroxide, Magnesium trisilicate, Mangafodipir, Maprotiline, Megestrol acetate, Memantine, Meperidine, Mepivacaine, Mercaptopurine, Meropenem, Methylnaltrexone, Methyltestosterone, Metyrapone, Midazolam, Migalastat, Milrinone, Mycophenolic acid, N-acetyltyrosine, Naldemedine, Nalmefene, Naloxone, Nateglinide, Nedaplatin, Nedocromil, Netilmicin, Nitric Oxide, Octinoxate, Opium, Oseltamivir, Oxacillin, Oxybenzone, Oxyquinoline, Oxytetracycline, Oxazepam, Palonosetron, Pantoprazole, Patent Blue, Pegaptanib, Peginesatide, Pemetrexed, Pentaerythritol tetranitrate, Pentastarch, Pentetic acid, Pentostatin, Permethrin, Pholcodine, Phosphoric acid, Phylloquinone, Picosulfuric acid, Piperacillin, Piracetam, Plazomicin, Plerixafor, Polythiazide, Pomalidomide, Pralatrexate, Pravastatin, Pralidoxime, Pramipexole, Procainamide, Procaine benzylpenicillin, Propantheline, Prucalopride, Pyrantel, Pyrazinamide, Pyrazinamide, Ramelteon, Ranitidine, Ranolazine, Relebactam, Resorcinol, Ribavirin, Ribostamycin, Rivaroxaban, Roflumilast, Ropivacaine, Rosuvastatin, Ruxolitinib, Salmon

	calcitonin, Saxagliptin, Seladelpar, Selenious acid, Selenium, Sevelamer, Sitagliptin, Sodium acetate, Sodium fluoride, Sodium sulfate, Sofosbuvir, Sorbitol, Stavudine, Streptomycin, Strontium chloride, Succinic acid, Sucralfate, Sulbactam, Synthetic Conjugated Estrogens, A, Synthetic Conjugated Estrogens, B, Tamsulosin, Tasimelteon, Taurocholic acid, Tazobactam, Technetium Tc-99m exametazime, Technetium Tc-99m mebrofenin, Technetium Tc-99m oxidronate, Technetium Tc-99m pyrophosphate, Teduglutide, Telavancin, Temazepam, Temozolomide, Tenofovir alafenamide, Testolactone, Testosterone, Tetracycline, Tetradecyl hydrogen sulfate (ester), Thiabendazole, Thiethylperazine, Tinidazole, Tiopronin, Tiotropium, Tobramycin, Tocopherol, Tolcapone, Tolterodine, Topiramate, Topotecan, Tositumomab, Tramadol, Trametinib, Triazolam, Triethylenetetramine, Trifluridine, Trimetrexate, Tropisetron, Vaborbactam, Vadadustat, Valaciclovir, Valbenazine, Valganciclovir, Vancomycin, Varenicline, Warfarin, Zalcitabine, Zaleplon, Zanamivir
The excretion rate of ibuprofen may be increased, resulting in lower serum levels.	Acetazolamide, Bromotheophylline, Diclofenamide, Isosorbide, Meticrane, Methazolamide, Satralizumab
The excretion rate of ibuprofen may be decreased, resulting in higher serum levels.	Metaxalone, Metformin, Methadone, Methoxsalen, Probenecid
Serum concentration of the drug may increase (the concentration of the	Ampicillin, Amrinone, Ancestim, Antihemophilic factor (recombinant) PEGylated, Antithrombin III human, Arsenic trioxide, Baclofen, Baricitinib,

drug in the blood increases).	Benserazide, Benzatropine, Benznidazole, Bepotastine, Bicisate, Bismuth subgallate, Bisoxatin, Bleomycin, Brivaracetam, Bromazepam, Bupropion, Butabarbital, Capreomycin, Carbidopa, Carmustine, Ceftolozane, Cevimeline, Chloral hydrate, Chlorzoxazone, Choline C 11, Choline salicylate, Chromic chloride, Chromic nitrate, Chromium, Chromium gluconate, Chromium nicotinate, Chromous sulfate, Cisplatin, Clobazam, Clonazepam, Clorazepic acid, Clove oil, Colchicine, Colistin, Corifollitropin alfa, Dabigatran etexilate, Dacarbazine, Dalfampridine, Daptomycin, Deferiprone, Deutetrabenazine, Dexpanthenol, Dexrazoxane, Dextran, Diatrizoate, Diazepam, Dichlorobenzyl alcohol, Dicyclomine, Didanosine, Dienogest, Digoxin, Dimercaprol, Dimethyl sulfoxide, Disopyramide, Doxacurium, Doxycycline, Dyphylline, Edoxaban, Edrophonium, Ertapenem, Estazolam, Ethambutol, Etonogestrel, Eucalyptus oil, Ezogabine, Fenofibric acid, Fesoterodine, Flavoxate, Florbetaben F-18, Florbetapir F-18, Flucytosine, Fludeoxyglucose (18F), Flumazenil, Flurazepam, Flutamide, Folic acid, Fomepizole, Fondaparinux, Formestane, Fosfomycin, Gabapentin enacarbil, Gadobenic acid, Gadodiamide, Gadofosveset trisodium, Gadopentetic acid, Gadoteric acid, Gadoteridol, Ganciclovir, Gemcitabine, Gentamicin, Gimeracil, Glycerol phenylbutyrate, Golodirsen, Goserelin, Haloperidol, Hydromorphone, Hydroxocobalamin, Hydroxyethyl Starch, Ibutilide, Idarucizumab, Idebenone, Indigotindisulfonic acid, Inosine pranobex, Inositol, Iobenguane sulfate I-123, Iodixanol, Ioflupane I-123, Iopromide, Iothalamic

	acid, Ioversol, Ioxilan, Ipecac, Ipilimumab, Isosorbide mononitrate, Isosulfan blue, Isotretinoin, Ixazomib, Kanamycin, Ketazolam, Lamivudine, Ledipasvir, Lenalidomide, Lesinurad, Leuprolide, Levobupivacaine, Levomilnacipran, Liothyronine, Lithium carbonate, Lithium citrate, Lithium hydroxide, Lixisenatide, Lorazepam, Lorcaserin, Lorpiprazole, Lubiprostone, Magnesium carbonate, Magnesium chloride, Magnesium hydroxide, Magnesium trisilicate, Mangafodipir, Maprotiline, Megestrol acetate, Memantine, Meperidine, Mepivacaine, Meropenem, Methylnaltrexone, Phenytoin, Vadadustat
Serum concentration of the drug may decrease (the concentration of the drug in the blood decreases).	Imatinib
Serum concentration of ibuprofen may increase (the concentration of ibuprofen in the blood increases).	Abametapir, Capecitabine, Epcoritamab, Erythromycin, Fedratinib, Glofitamab, Ivacaftor, Linzagolix, Methotrexate, Mifepristone, Ritlecitinib, Ritonavir, Selpercatinib, Voriconazole
Serum concentration of ibuprofen may decrease (the concentration of ibuprofen in the blood decreases).	Alpelisib, Apalutamide, Cenobamate, Dabrafenib, Enzalutamide, Isosorbide, Lumacaftor, Mavacamten, Omaveloxolone, Sotorasib, Telotristat ethyl
It may increase the risk of severity of renal failure (when your kidneys are unable to	Aliskiren, Amiloride, Azilsartan medoxomil, Benazepril, Candesartan cilexetil, Canrenoic acid, Captopril, Cilazapril, Cyclosporine, Enalapril, Enalaprilat, Eplerenone, Eprosartan, Fosinopril,

properly filter waste from your blood and produce urine).	Irbesartan, Lisinopril, Losartan, Moexipril, Olmesartan, Perindopril, Quinapril, Ramipril, Rescinnamine, Sodium phosphate monobasic, Spirapril, Tacrolimus, Telmisartan, Trandolapril, Triamterene, Valsartan, Zofenopril
It may increase the risk or severity of adverse effects.	Aceclofenac, Acemetacin, Alclofenac, Alendronic acid, Antipyrine, Antrafenine, Azficel-T, Balsalazide, Bendazac, Benorilate, Benoxaprofen, Benzydamine, Betulinic Acid, Bromfenac, Bufexamac, Bumadizone, Carprofen, Celecoxib, Choline magnesium trisalicylate, Dexibuprofen, Dexketoprofen, Diclofenac, Diflunisal, Etodolac, Etoricoxib, Fenbufen, Fenoprofen, Floctafenine, Flurbiprofen, Glycol salicylate, Icosapent, Indomethacin, Isoxicam, Ketoprofen, Ketorolac, Lornoxicam, Loxoprofen, Lumiracoxib, Meclofenamic acid, Mefenamic acid, Meloxicam, Menthyl salicylate, Nabumetone, Naproxen, Nepafenac, Nimesulide, Oxaprozin, Oxyphenbutazone, Parecoxib, Phenylbutazone, Piroxicam, Pitolisant, Polymyxin B, Rofecoxib, Salicylamide, Salicylic acid, Salsalate, Sparsentan, Sulfasalazine, Sulindac, Suprofen, Tenoxicam, Tiaprofenic acid, Tolfenamic acid, Tolmetin, Trolamine salicylate, Valdecoxib
The risk of the severity of hypertension may be increased.	Albuterol, Alfentanil, Aliskire, Amiloride, Aminophenazone, Amphetamine, Arbutamine, Arformoterol, Aripiprazole, Aripiprazole lauroxil, Asenapine, Atomoxetine, Atropine, Benazepril, Benzphetamine, Brexpiprazole, Bromocriptine, Buspirone, Cabergoline, Candesartan cilexetil, Canrenoic acid, Captopril, Cariprazine, Chlorpromazine, Cilazapril, Clenbuterol, Cyclosporine, DL-Methylephedrine, Desflurane, Desmopressin, Dexmedetomidine,

	Dexmethylphenidate, Dextroamphetamine, Diethylpropion, Dihydroergocornine, Dihydroergocristine, Dihydroergotamine, Dobutamine, Dopamine, Dopexamine, Doxapram, Droperidol, Droxidopa, Dutasteride, Eletriptan, Enalapril, Enalaprilat, Ephedrine, Eplerenone, Eprosartan, Ergoloid mesylate, Ergometrine, Esketamine, Etafedrine, Etilefrine, Etomidate, Fenoterol, Fentanyl, Finasteride, Flibanserin, Flupentixol, Formoterol, Fosinopril, Halothane, Iloperidone, Indacaterol, Iofetamine I-123, Irbesartan, Isocarboxazid, Isoetharine, Isoflurane, Isometheptene, Isoprenaline, Isoxsuprine, Levonordefrin, Levosalbutamol, Linezolid, Lisdexamfetamine, Lisinopril, Lisuride, Losartan, Lurasidone, Mephentermine, Metamfetamine, Metaraminol, Metergoline, Methotrimeprazine, Methoxamine, Methoxyflurane, Methoxyphenamine, Methylergometrine, Methylphenidate, Methysergide, Mianserin, Midodrine, Minaprine, Mirabegron, Mirtazapine, Moclobemide, Moexipril, Moxisylyte, Naphazoline, Naratriptan, Naxitamab, Nialamide, Nicergoline, Nitrous oxide, Norepinephrine, Nylidrin, Olmesartan, Orciprenaline, Oxymetazoline, Paliperidone, Pergolide, Periciazine, Perindopril, Phendimetrazine, Phenelzine, Phenmetrazine, Phentermine, Pirbuterol, Pizotifen, Propiomazine, Propiverine, Quetiapine, Quinapril, Quinupramine, Racepinephrine, Ramipril, Rasagiline, Remifentanil, Rescinnamine, Risperidone, Ritodrine, Rizatriptan, Safinamide, Sevoflurane, Siponimod, Solifenacin, Spirapril, Sufentanil, Sumatriptan, Tadalafil, Tafluprost, Telmisartan, Terazosin, Terbutaline, Tetryzoline, Thioridazine, Trandolapril, Triamterene, Trichloroethylene, Trifluoperazine, Valsartan,

	Vilanterol, Vilazodone, Xamoterol, Yohimbine, Zofenopril, Zolmitriptan, Zuclopenthixol
The risk or severity of nephrotoxicity (kidney damage due to toxins, chemicals, medications, etc.) may be increased.	Adefovir dipivoxil, Amphotericin B, Bacitracin, Carboplatin, Cefadroxil, Cefalotin, Cefamandole, Cefapirin, Cefditoren, Cefepime, Cefmenoxime, Cefmetazole, Cefonicid, Cefoperazone, Ceforanide, Cefotaxime, Cefotetan, Cefoxitin, Cefpiramide, Cefpirome, Cefpodoxime, Cefprozil, Cefradine, Ceftaroline fosami, Ceftazidime, Ceftobiprole, Ceftriaxone, Cefuroxime, Cephaloglycin, Cidofovir, Colistimethate, Dihydrostreptomycin, Foscarnet, Framycetin, Frovatriptan, Givosiran, Inotersen, Latamoxef, Loracarbef, Mannitol, Mesalazine, Metamizole, Nalidixic acid, Neomycin, Olsalazine, Oxaliplatin, Paromomycin, Pentamidine, Phenazopyridine, Solriamfetol, Tenofovir disoproxil
A decrease in antihypertensive activities could occur.	Acebutolol, Atenolol, Betaxolol, Bisoprolol, Carvedilol, Celiprolol, Esmolol, Hydralazine, Labetalol, Landiolol, Levobetaxolol, Metoprolol, Nadolol, Nebivolol, Oxprenolol, Penbutolol, Pindolol, Practolol, Propafenone, Propranolol, Sotalol, Timolol
It may decrease the antiplatelet activities of the drug (reduces the ability of the drug to prevent blood clots from forming).	Acetylsalicylic acid (Aspirin)
It may decrease protein binding of the drug.	Acetohexamide, Chlorpropamide, Gliclazide, Glimepiride, Glipizide, Gliquidone, Glyburide, Tolbutamide, Valproic acid

The risk or severity of hyperkalemia (when there is too much potassium in the blood) increases when ibuprofen is combined with the drug.	Amiloride, Ammonium chloride, Ardeparin, Bemiparin, Benazepril, Canagliflozin, Candesartan cilexetil, Canrenoic acid, Captopril, Certoparin, Cilazapril, Cinnarizine, Cyclandelate, Dalteparin, Danaparoid, Dantrolene, Dipotassium phosphate, Drospirenone, Enalapril, Enalaprilat, Enoxaparin, Eplerenone, Eprosartan, Estetrol, Ethosuximide, Fish oil, Flunarizine, Fluspirilene, Fosinopril, Heparin, Irbesartan, Levomenthol, Lidoflazine, Lisinopril, Losartan, Magnesium sulfate, Mannitol busulfan, Methsuximide, Moexipril, Monopotassium phosphate, Nadroparin, Nifedipine, Nitrofurantoin, Olmesartan, Parnaparin, Perhexiline, Perindopril, Pinaverium, Potassium, Potassium Iodide, Potassium acetate, Potassium alum, Potassium bicarbonate, Potassium carbonate, Potassium cation, Potassium chloride, Potassium citrate, Potassium gluconate, Potassium guaiacolsulfonate, Potassium hydroxide, Potassium lactate, Potassium nitrate, Potassium perchlorate, Potassium sulfate, Prenylamine, Quinapril, Ramipril, Rescinnamine, Reviparin, Spirapril, Spironolactone, Succinylcholine, Sulodexide, Telmisartan, Tinzaparin, Tolvaptan, Trandolapril, Triamterene, Trimebutine, Valsartan, Valsartan, Zofenopril, Zofenopril, Zonisamide, Zonisamide
Ibuprofen may increase the neuroexcitatory (increasing stimulation and excitation of the neurons) activities of the drug.	Cinoxacin, Delafloxacin, Enoxacin, Gatifloxacin, Gemifloxacin, Grepafloxacin, Levofloxacin, Lomefloxacin, Moxifloxacin, Norfloxacin, Ofloxacin, Pefloxacin, Rosoxacin, Sparfloxacin, Trovafloxacin, Trovafloxacin

The risk or severity of elevated intracranial pressure may be increased when ibuprofen is combined with the drug.	Tretinoin
It can cause a decrease in the absorption of ibuprofen.	Cholestyramine, Colesevelam, Colestipol
The risk or severity of hyponatremia (when sodium level is low in the blood) may be increased.	Desmopressin
The risk or severity of water intoxication (when there is too much water in the body, leading to decreased sodium levels and swelling of the cells) may be increased.	Desmopressin

Ibuprofen and Drug Interactions

While the ibuprofen-drug interactions table (**Table 13.1**) is comprehensive, it does not include every possible interaction. Factors such as whether a medicine is taken with or without food or alongside alcohol can influence its effects. To ensure safety, always read the manufacturer's package information and consult a healthcare professional (doctor or pharmacist) before adding a new drug to your routine.

Ibuprofen's Interactions with Food

Since many medications are derived from natural compounds, food can sometimes influence their effects. According to the National Health Service (NHS), ibuprofen should be taken with a meal or snack.[549]

Taking ibuprofen with food helps protect the stomach lining and reduces the risk of GI side effects, such as bleeding. However, food can also delay ibuprofen absorption. Despite the NHS stating there are no known food interactions, some research suggests otherwise.[550]

Foods That May Interact with Ibuprofen

One potential concern is potassium-rich foods, including chicken, dairy, salmon, tuna, spinach, avocado, sweet potatoes, and broccoli. Potassium is also used as a sodium replacement in some salt alternatives for individuals with hypertension.[548] Taking ibuprofen alongside high-potassium foods or supplements may increase potassium levels in the blood, potentially leading to hyperkalemia, a condition that can cause kidney damage, muscle paralysis, or even cardiac arrest.[551]

Ibuprofen influences potassium regulation through three key mechanisms: reduced potassium excretion by the kidneys, suppressed aldosterone (a hormone that promotes potassium excretion), and reduced kidney blood flow that decreases the kidneys' ability to filter and excrete potassium.[427,552]

Interestingly, one study found that ibuprofen absorption increases when taken with Coca-Cola, likely due to caffeine, which has a similar effect.[553] This suggests that consuming ibuprofen with Coca-Cola or other caffeinated beverages might enhance its absorption, potentially requiring a lower dosage.[554] Supporting evidence suggests that a combination of 400 mg of ibuprofen and 100 mg of caffeine significantly increased ibuprofen's peak plasma concentration by 13%.[555]

Ibuprofen and Alcohol

Ibuprofen also interacts with ethanol (alcohol). Alcohol consumption is already linked to liver damage, and taking ibuprofen alongside alcohol can amplify this effect. Both substances are processed by the liver, and when used together, they can cause more harm than either one alone.[392] This is because both ibuprofen and alcohol increase oxidative stress in liver cells, making it harder for the liver to repair itself and clear toxins. It is best to avoid alcohol while using ibuprofen, especially for individuals who drink regularly or have liver concerns.[392]

Ibuprofen and Vitamins

Certain vitamins may also interact with ibuprofen. Studies suggest that NSAIDs, when taken with B vitamins, may have a reduced duration of action, shortening their effectiveness by up to 50%.[551]

Ibuprofen and Herbal Supplements

Herbal medicines often go unreported in medical consultations and are less regulated by the FDA. While research on ibuprofen's interaction with herbal supplements is limited, some herbs may amplify its effects.[556,557,558]

- **St. John's Wort**: Reduces the time S-ibuprofen (the more active form) stays in the body.[559]

- **Ginkgo biloba**: One report links Ginkgo and ibuprofen to a fatal brain hemorrhage that resulted in a coma, suggesting a possible increased bleeding risk.[558] A review suggests that Ginkgo is used by more than 2% of the adult population and found that six reports found that patients with bleeding including intracranial bleeding who stopped using Ginkgo had no reoccurring bleeding.[560]

Since NSAIDs already reduce prostaglandin production, which plays a role in blood clotting, combining ibuprofen with herbs that have antiplatelet activity can further increase the risk of excessive bleeding. These include:

Ginkgo, garlic, ginger, bilberry, feverfew, turmeric, meadowsweet, willow, and ginseng. Additionally, herbs containing coumarin, a natural anticoagulant, may also interact with ibuprofen. Some examples include: Motherwort, chamomile, horse chestnut, red clover, and fenugreek.

Although these herbs are suspected of interacting with ibuprofen, clinical evidence remains limited. Users should also be aware that "natural" does not mean "safe"—some herbal supplements can cause adverse effects and may be contaminated or mislabeled, as they are not individually monitored by the FDA.[561] It is important to consult a doctor or pharmacist before using herbal supplements with medications like ibuprofen to avoid harmful herb-drug interactions and side effects.

Managing Ibuprofen Interactions

When ibuprofen interacts with a concurrently used medication, careful attention to dosing schedules is essential. Drug interactions depend on factors like half-life (the time it takes for half the drug to leave the body) and absorption rates. While some interactions can be minimized by taking medications 2-6 hours apart, others, such as those involving drugs with long half-lives, may require 24 hours or more to avoid harmful effects.[562,563]

Caution: Taking ibuprofen with blood thinners increases bleeding risk. If both must be used, there is no safe timing interval to fully prevent interaction; close monitoring is required, and bleeding time should be checked a few days after starting ibuprofen. Discontinue ibuprofen if bleeding time is prolonged.[539] Similarly, the interaction between ibuprofen and blood pressure medications typically develops after more than five days of concurrent use, so simply spacing doses apart does not prevent the reduction in the effectiveness of the blood pressure medications.[364]

For safe medication use, consult your healthcare provider. They can recommend alternative treatments or advise on proper timing based on the latest clinical research.

Key takeaways:

- Ibuprofen interacts with many drugs. Check any new medication you are taking against the database of known interactions between ibuprofen and other medicines.[564]
- Interactions between ibuprofen and other drugs could lead to unexpected side effects and, in rare occurrences, can be fatal.

Most important takeaway

- Verify drug interactions and connect with your medical provider before consuming ibuprofen with any other drug.

MOVING FORWARD

Chapter 14
Beyond Pills:
Strategies to Reduce Painkillers

Extensive research has explored ways to reduce or prevent the risk of chronic diseases, and the findings point to three key lifestyle factors: exercise, diet, and stress management. Studies show that poor habits in these areas can increase the risk of painful conditions, such as chronic back pain, fibromyalgia, rheumatoid arthritis, cardiovascular disease, and type 2 diabetes. Even osteoarthritis, a degenerative joint disease, has been linked to inadequate exercise and poor nutrition. However, the good news is that adopting healthy habits can not only prevent these conditions but also help manage pain if they develop.[565,566]

Irrespective of your age, if you're not currently experiencing significant pain, now is the perfect time to take preventative steps to protect your long-term health. If you already experience daily pain, making therapeutic lifestyle changes can help reduce your discomfort. The best part? Many preventative and therapeutic measures are the same, meaning it's never too early or too late to start making a difference in your health.

Lifestyle Changes and Ibuprofen Use

Lifestyle changes, such as adopting a healthy diet and engaging in regular exercise, can significantly reduce the need for painkillers like ibuprofen in managing chronic pain. It does this by empowering individuals to manage pain more effectively and safely. Regular physical activity not only improves joint flexibility and mobility but also stimulates the production of endorphins (your body's pain-relieving chemicals). Endorphins act similarly to opioids by binding to pain receptors in the brain, reducing the perception of pain and often leading to less need for pharmaceutical painkillers.[567]

Fig. 14.1. Three powerful ways to reduce pain and improve quality of life

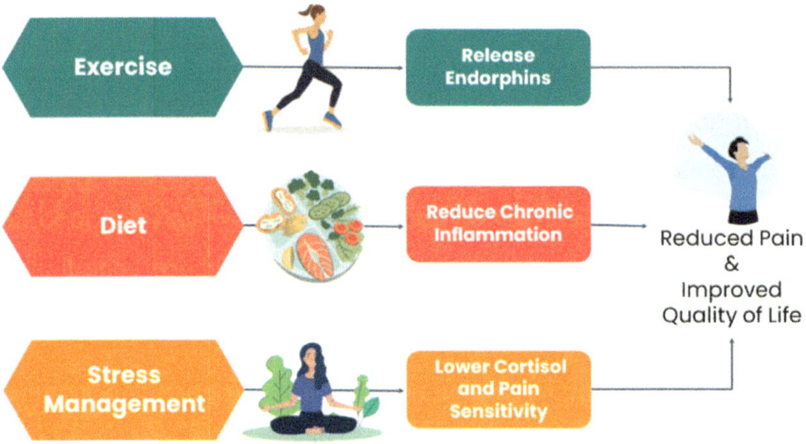

Just moving more has its benefits. Movement increases blood flow, delivers nutrients to joint tissues, and promotes the circulation of synovial fluid in joints, which lubricates joints and reduces stiffness. Improved joint function and reduced inflammation mean less pain and, consequently, less need for medications like ibuprofen.

An anti-inflammatory diet can lower systemic inflammation, a key driver of chronic pain. Reducing inflammatory foods (like processed foods and sugars) helps soothe pain and can decrease reliance on anti-inflammatory drugs.[568]

Three Key Steps to Prevent or Manage Chronic Pain (Fig. 14.1):

1. Move Your Body More: The Power of Regular Physical Activity

The evidence is clear: regular physical activity, including aerobic exercise, strength training, yoga, and Pilates, can significantly reduce chronic pain.[569-571] But why is exercise so powerful in preventing and managing chronic diseases?

Exercise addresses the root causes of chronic conditions, such as inflammation, metabolic dysfunction, and stress, while also enhancing the body's natural repair mechanisms.[572] This makes physical activity one of the most effective and accessible lifestyle interventions available.

Exercise as a Natural Pain Reliever

Beyond disease prevention, exercise has a direct impact on pain relief. When we move, our bodies produce endorphins, natural painkillers that also act as mood boosters.[573] This release of endorphins contributes to the well-known "runner's high" and helps alleviate pain naturally.

Additionally, physical activity improves joint flexibility, posture, and muscle strength, reducing the likelihood of injuries and pain.[574-577] While exercise alone is unlikely to fully resolve chronic pain, it has many benefits independent of other methods. For optimal pain reduction, a holistic approach is the most effective way to manage pain—one that combines lifestyle changes, exercise, proper medication, and often physical therapy.

The Indirect Benefits of Exercise for Pain Reduction

Exercise also improves factors that aren't always directly linked to pain relief, including:

i. **Better Sleep –** A 2023 meta-analysis found that regular, moderate-intensity exercise improves sleep quality, sleep duration, and sleep onset time. [578] However, engaging in high-intensity workouts close to bedtime can disrupt sleep. Since sleep plays a crucial role in pain perception, inflammation control, and healing, poor sleep can contribute to chronic pain conditions, including joint pain.

ii. **Reduced Stress & Better Mental Health –** Exercise helps regulate stress hormones, reducing anxiety and depression, which are often linked to chronic pain.[579]

iii. **Improved Circulation & Strengthened Joints –** Increased blood flow nourishes tissues, reduces stiffness, and enhances recovery, helping prevent pain before it starts.

A 2024 meta-analysis reinforced this connection, showing that sleep disturbances are strongly linked to persistent musculoskeletal pain.[580] By improving sleep and reducing stress, exercise provides both immediate and long-term pain relief.

Examples of Moderate Physical Activity

Always check with your healthcare provider before starting any new exercise routine. If you are suffering from limited mobility, a physical therapist can design a safe, personalized exercise program to strengthen muscles around the joints, improve flexibility, and reduce pain. In general, individuals with joint pain may benefit from low-impact exercises like swimming, cycling, and walking, which are gentle on the joints. Resistance exercises (using bands or light weights) and balance activities (like tai chi or yoga) help strengthen bones and muscles, improve stability, and reduce fall risk. Braces or supports may help after fractures or during recovery, but prolonged use can weaken muscles, so follow your doctor's guidance on when to start strengthening exercises.

Moderate physical activity is any movement that raises your heart rate while still allowing you to carry on a conversation. Here are some excellent options:

I. **Brisk Walking –** If you're new to exercise, walking is one of the best ways to start moving. Begin at 2 mph and gradually increase to 3.5–4 mph. Aim for 30 minutes, 5 times per week or 1 hour, 3 times per week. Be sure to wear proper footwear and comfortable clothing.

II. **Gardening & Yard Work –** Activities like raking leaves, mowing the lawn, or pulling weeds provide a great workout while keeping your outdoor space tidy.

III. **Dancing –** Whether you're dancing socially or for fun at home, it's a fantastic way to stay active while enjoying yourself.

IV. **Swimming –** Just 10 minutes or more of swimming offers a full-body workout that strengthens muscles and improves cardiovascular health.

V. **Cycling –** Riding a bike at 5–8 mph on level ground or slight hills is a great way to incorporate movement into your routine.

VI. Other moderate activities include tennis, hiking, and even household chores like mopping and scrubbing floors.

Don't Forget Muscle-Strengthening Activities!

In addition to aerobic exercise, adults should engage in muscle-strengthening activities at least twice per week.[581] Strength training is crucial for maintaining muscle mass, joint stability, and bone health.

A meta-analysis of 44 clinical trials found that therapeutic exercise reduced knee pain in people with osteoarthritis and improved their quality of life with benefits lasting up to 6 months after stopping exercise.[582]

Examples of Muscle-Strengthening Activities

Bodyweight exercises – Push-ups, planks, squats, lunges

Yoga & Pilates – Builds strength, flexibility, and balance

Daily activities – Carrying groceries, climbing stairs, shoveling

Sports & Martial Arts – Karate, kickboxing, gymnastics, rock climbing

Weight training – Lifting free weights (dumbbells, barbells)

How to Know If You're Exercising at Moderate Intensity

A simple test:

You should be able to talk but not sing while doing moderate activity.

It is important to listen to your body and avoid pushing yourself too hard, especially if you are new to exercise or already experiencing pain.

World Health Organization (WHO) Recommendations

Children & Adolescents (Ages 5–17)

- At least 60 minutes of moderate to vigorous-intensity physical activity daily.[583]

- More than 60 minutes per day provides additional health benefits.[583]

Adults (Ages 18 and Older)

- At least 150 minutes of moderate-intensity exercise per week **OR** 75 minutes of vigorous-intensity exercise per week. [581,583]
- For greater health benefits, aim for 300 minutes (5 hours) per week.

Physical activity is widely recognized as an effective strategy for managing chronic pain and reducing inflammation. Exercise helps balance pro-inflammatory and anti-inflammatory cytokines, normalize neuroinflammation by downregulating pro-inflammatory mediators in the central nervous system and upregulating factors that counteract inflammation and pain sensitization.[584,585]

2. Eat for Less Pain: The Power of a Healthy Diet

What you eat plays a crucial role in managing pain—a diet rich in anti-inflammatory foods such as omega-3 fatty acids (found in fish, flaxseeds, and walnuts), fruits, vegetables, and whole grains can help combat chronic inflammation, a key contributor to pain conditions like arthritis and muscle pain. Maintaining a healthy weight also reduces stress on joints, particularly weight-bearing ones, which can help ease discomfort.

Scientific research supports the benefits of an anti-inflammatory diet. In a study involving 100 patients with Relapsing-Remitting Multiple Sclerosis (MS), those who followed an anti-inflammatory diet for 12 weeks reported improved fatigue levels and overall quality of life.[586] Another well-established anti-inflammatory eating pattern is the Mediterranean diet, which has been found to reduce pain, stiffness, and markers of cartilage damage.[587] Beyond its anti-inflammatory effects, the Mediterranean diet also promotes gut health, which is increasingly recognized as a critical factor in overall well-being.[588]

If transitioning to a full Mediterranean-style diet feels overwhelming, start small. Gradually incorporating more anti-inflammatory foods into your meals can still offer significant benefits. Other diets, including plant-based, vegetarian, and anti-inflammatory diets can have similar benefits to the Mediterranean diet in reducing inflammation and supporting overall health.[589-591]

Five Anti-Inflammatory Foods That Are Easy to Find

i. Olive Oil (Extra Virgin)

A staple of the Mediterranean diet, olive oil contains oleocanthal, a compound with strong anti-inflammatory properties.[592] A long-term study tracking 92,383 adults over 28 years found that consuming just 7 grams (about half a tablespoon) of olive oil daily reduced the risk of dementia-related mortality by 28% regardless of the rest of the diet.[593] Additionally, olive oil has been linked to potential anti-cancer benefits.[594]

ii. Ginger

Ginger is well-known for its anti-inflammatory, antioxidant, and immune-boosting effects.[595] Studies show that ginger supplementation can help reduce pain and improve quality of life, especially for individuals with chronic conditions.[596] Beyond pain relief, ginger also supports gut health and has been shown in animal studies to reduce amyloid plaque buildup in the brain, which is associated with neurodegenerative diseases like Alzheimer's.[597]

iii. Green Tea

Green tea contains epigallocatechin-3-gallate (EGCG), a powerful antioxidant with anti-inflammatory properties.[598] In a 2018 study on knee osteoarthritis patients, those who took green tea extract (alongside a standard pain medication) experienced significant pain reduction and improved physical function within just four weeks.[599] This suggests that green tea may enhance conventional pain management approaches.

iv. Curcumin (Found in Turmeric)

Curcumin, the active compound in turmeric, has been extensively studied for its pain-relieving properties.[600] A meta-analysis of 12 studies on curcumin's effects on knee osteoarthritis found that patients taking around 1,000 mg per day for 4 to 16 weeks experienced significant improvements in pain and joint function.[596] While it may not have dramatically altered overall quality of life in all cases, its impact on reducing discomfort was clear.[596]

vi. *Boswellia Serrata* (Indian Frankincense)

Boswellia serrata, though less commonly known, is widely available in capsule, tablet, and powder form at health food stores and online. A review of nine studies found that Boswellia was effective in managing symptoms of knee osteoarthritis, making it a promising natural alternative for joint pain relief.[601]

For all of these compounds, it is important to note that not everyone experiences the same level of benefit, so results are not guaranteed for everyone, and it may be most beneficial as part of a broader pain management plan. Few, if any, compounds have no side effects, but these compounds are all generally well tolerated when used at recommended amounts, with mild and infrequent side effects.

1. Chronic Stress is Your Enemy: Managing Stress with Mindfulness

Chronic stress negatively affects both the body and mind, leading to issues such as anxiety, sleep disturbances, cardiovascular problems, digestive issues, muscle tension, skin conditions, reproductive complications, and chronic diseases like type 2 diabetes. [602,603] Studies even suggest that stress can heighten pain perception. For example, individuals with fibromyalgia report increased pain levels during periods of heightened stress.[604] A 2021 commentary titled "Stress Kills" underscores just how dangerous prolonged stress can be.[605]

Some stress is preventable

While stress is sometimes unavoidable, we can manage it effectively. Research shows that mindfulness meditation helps reduce stress-related pain, including tension headaches and migraines. A 2018 review analyzing previous studies on mindfulness and headaches found that mindfulness meditation significantly decreased pain intensity. [606] An eight-week mindfulness program, in particular, demonstrated a strong positive impact on headache and migraine pain.

A 2021 meta-analysis of 16 studies involving 1,058 patients found that mindfulness-based stress reduction (MBSR) and cognitive behavioral therapy (CBT) both improved pain levels and overall quality of life.[607] In this study, participants with chronic low back pain affecting at least 12% of adults experienced reduced pain after practicing mindfulness techniques.[607]

Why does this work?

Stress triggers the body's "fight-or-flight" response, activating the sympathetic nervous system and releasing cortisol and adrenaline.[608] These hormones increase muscle tension and pain sensitivity, preparing the body to react to threats.[609,610] Mindfulness, on the other hand, engages the parasympathetic nervous system, which promotes relaxation by lowering heart rate, blood pressure, and stress levels. Additionally, mindfulness helps regulate pain by altering brain activity in pain-processing centers and reducing inflammation.[611,612]

However, it's important to note that the effectiveness of mindfulness for pain relief varies from person to person and may depend on the specific pain condition. For example, studies show mindfulness-based interventions are particularly helpful for conditions like fibromyalgia and chronic low back pain, but results can be more modest for other types of pain.[613-615]

As individuals respond differently to mindfulness techniques, it's useful to try different mindfulness practices or combine them with other therapies to determine what works best for you.[616]

Practical Mindfulness Exercises:

Body Scan: Lie down comfortably, close your eyes, and slowly focus your attention on each part of your body from head to toe, noticing sensations without judgment.[617]

Breath Awareness: Sit quietly and focus on your breathing, gently bringing your attention back whenever your mind wanders.

Mindful Movement: Practices like mindful walking or gentle yoga can also help manage pain.

If mindfulness meditation isn't for you, deep breathing exercises offer another effective way to manage stress. Controlled breathing activates the parasympathetic nervous system, encouraging relaxation. In one study, participants who practiced diaphragmatic breathing for eight weeks (20 sessions of 15-minute deep breathing exercises) reported lower stress levels and improved focus compared to those who did not participate. [618]

By incorporating mindfulness meditation or deep breathing exercises into daily life, you can reduce the emotional and physical toll of stress, ultimately improving overall well-being and minimizing chronic pain.[619]

Key Takeaways:

- Many chronic diseases can be prevented or delayed with proactive lifestyle choices. Prioritizing physical activity, a balanced diet, and stress management can reduce dependence on painkillers and enhance overall well-being.
- If you experience chronic pain, making adjustments to your diet, exercise routine, and stress management strategies can help you manage symptoms more effectively.

Chapter 15
Exploring Natural Alternatives to Ibuprofen

While ibuprofen and similar drugs are widely used for pain relief, their potential side effects—especially with moderate to long-term use—highlight the need for safer alternatives. Many natural products are marketed for pain relief, but clinical evidence supporting their effectiveness remains limited. However, some natural remedies have shown promising results in reducing pain and inflammation.

The Best Alternatives for Pain and Inflammation Relief

1) Tart Cherries

Prunus cerasus, commonly known as tart cherries, has gained recognition as a natural remedy for inflammation, a key factor in many chronic diseases. Their effectiveness stems from their high concentration of anthocyanins, powerful antioxidants that combat oxidative stress, a major driver of inflammation.[620] These compounds directly influence key inflammatory pathways, including COX-1 and COX-2, which are commonly targeted by pain-relief medications.

How Tart Cherries Help Athletes

Research highlights tart cherries' ability to reduce exercise-induced inflammation. In a 2022 study, 54 runners were divided into two groups, with one consuming 355 milliliters of tart cherry juice twice daily for a week before running 16 miles, while the other received a placebo.[621] After the run, pain levels were assessed using a Visual Analog Scale. The tart cherry group reported three times less pain than the placebo group simply by drinking tart cherry juice!

Tart Cherries and Muscle Recovery

Beyond pain relief, tart cherries also aid in muscle recovery. A 2006 study on college athletes found that those who drank tart cherry juice before performing eccentric elbow flexion contractions lost only 12% of their baseline muscle strength, compared to a 30% loss in the placebo group.[620] Remarkably, after four days, the tart cherry group even experienced a slight increase in muscle strength. This suggests tart cherries can accelerate post-workout recovery.

Stress and Inflammation Reduction

Another benefit of tart cherries beyond reducing pain is inflammation reduction. In a 2021 study, men who took tart cherry extract for seven days exhibited significantly lower biomarkers of skeletal and cardiac oxidative stress after intense training, such as heavy squats.[622] Adding tart cherries to your routine may provide extra support for recovery and overall well-being.

However, tart cherries aren't just for athletes. A 2019 study on older adults (ages 65-80) found that drinking tart cherry juice for 12 weeks improved DNA repair activity and reduced inflammation markers.[623] This suggests tart cherries may help combat age-related inflammation.

Tart Cherries and Arthritis

Tart cherries may also benefit individuals with arthritis. A study by Martin and Coles examined serum uric acid levels, a key indicator of inflammatory arthritis in 26 overweight and obese adults. After consuming tart cherry juice for four weeks, participants experienced a 19.2% reduction in uric acid levels and a 19.4% decrease in overall inflammation.[624]

A Simple Step for Better Health

Tart cherries provide a multifaceted approach to pain relief, muscle recovery, and inflammation reduction. Incorporating them into your diet, whether through juice or supplements, can be a simple yet effective way to enhance overall health and well-being. In fact, several members of the Gomes Lab use tart cherry juice or pills as part of their wellness routine.

Unfortunately, peer-reviewed articles exploring the side effects of supplements are limited, and we currently have to rely on reputable websites such as WebMD, which suggests that tart cherry may cause diarrhea in some people.[625]

2) Sweet Cherries

Sweet cherries (*Prunus avium L.*) are more than just a delicious treat; they are potent natural anti-inflammatory agents. Packed with anthocyanins and phenolic compounds, these fruits combat inflammation and oxidative stress while directly influencing key inflammatory pathways.

Tart and sweet cherries, while similar in appearance, differ in taste, nutrient composition, and potential health benefits. Like tart cherries, sweet cherries also contain anthocyanins and phenolic compounds, but in slightly lower concentrations. However, sweet cherries tend to be richer in natural sugars, making them a more palatable option for regular snacking. Those looking to manage inflammation, aid post-exercise recovery, or support sleep may benefit more from tart cherries, while individuals seeking a nutritious, antioxidant-rich fruit to enjoy may prefer sweet cherries.

Sweet Cherries and Inflammation

A study by the University of California, Davis, explored the anti-inflammatory effects of sweet cherries. Eighteen participants (2 men and 16 women) consumed 45 sweet cherries daily for 28 days. Blood tests before and after the study revealed a 21% to 25% reduction in key inflammatory markers.[626] This significant decrease suggests that sweet cherries may provide natural relief from inflammation.

Another study directly compared sweet cherries' anti-inflammatory properties to ibuprofen. Researchers isolated anthocyanins from sweet cherries and tested their effect on COX-1 and COX-2 pathways. At a concentration of 125 μg/ml, sweet cherry anthocyanins inhibited COX-1 by 45% and COX-2 by 47%, showing anti-inflammatory effects comparable to ibuprofen and naproxen at 10 μM concentrations.[627] This suggests that sweet cherries may offer natural pain relief similar to NSAIDs, without their potential side effects.

While sweet cherries have demonstrated promising anti-inflammatory properties in preliminary studies, the extent of their effectiveness is not yet fully understood. More comprehensive studies are needed to determine the specific contexts in which sweet cherries may be beneficial and to what degree they can be considered a reliable treatment option.

Sweet Cherries and Gout Relief

Sweet cherries don't just reduce general inflammation; they may also help with gout, a painful condition caused by uric acid buildup. A 2012 study by Zhang et al. examined 633 individuals diagnosed with gout. The results were remarkable:

- Eating cherries for just two days was linked to a 35% lower risk of gout attacks compared to no cherry intake.
- When cherry intake was combined with allopurinol (a common gout medication), the risk of gout attacks dropped by 75%.[628]

A 2019 review by Collins et al. reinforced these findings, highlighting that cherries contain anti-inflammatory compounds that target gout-related pathways, including IL-6 and TNF-α, while also inhibiting COX-1 and COX-2 enzymes. This suggests that regular cherry consumption may reduce both the severity and frequency of gout attacks.

A Natural and Delicious Pain Relief Option

The research is clear: sweet cherries offer a natural, tasty, and effective way to reduce inflammation.[629] Whether you're dealing with exercise-related soreness, chronic inflammation, or gout, incorporating sweet cherries into your diet may provide meaningful relief all without the risks of traditional painkillers.

3) Berries: Nature's Anti-Inflammatory Superfoods

Berries are a staple in many cultures worldwide, enjoyed for their delicious taste and vibrant colors. But beyond their flavor, research shows that berries possess powerful anti-inflammatory properties, comparable to those of NSAIDs like ibuprofen. Rich in polyphenols, particularly anthocyanins, these compounds combat inflammation, reduce oxidative stress, and may even alleviate symptoms of inflammation-related illnesses.

While many berries offer these benefits, some of the most well-researched include acai berries, bilberries, blueberries, and chokeberries.

Acai Berries

Acai berries (*Euterpe oleracea*) are widely known for their deep purple color and exceptional antioxidant content. Studies show that they inhibit NF-κB signaling, reducing pro-inflammatory cytokines.[630] In 2018, researchers investigated whether acai berries could reduce inflammation in people with metabolic syndrome, a condition linked to increased risks of diabetes, heart disease, and stroke.

Study Design: 37 participants were divided into two groups, one consuming a daily acai pulp beverage (162.5g) and the other consuming a placebo for 12 weeks.

Findings: While glucose and lipid metabolism markers remained unchanged, two key inflammatory markers (IFN-γ and 8-isoprostane) were significantly reduced by 76.2% and 31.2%, respectively.[631]

Takeaway: Acai berries may be a promising natural aid for reducing inflammation in metabolic syndrome.

Bilberries

Bilberries, close relatives of blueberries, are packed with anthocyanins and have shown remarkable anti-inflammatory properties.

A study found that bilberry consumption lowered levels of IL-6, C-reactive protein, and IL-12, three key inflammation markers.[632] These results suggest that bilberries may help manage metabolic syndrome and related inflammatory conditions.

Takeaway: Regular bilberry intake may support heart health, immune function, and overall inflammation control.

Blueberries

Blueberries, like acai and bilberries, are renowned for their antioxidant and anti-inflammatory properties, particularly in exercise recovery.

Study Design: Researchers tested the effect of blueberry consumption on oxidative stress and inflammation after a 2.5-hour run.[633] Participants consumed 10.5 kg of frozen blueberries over six weeks, including 375 g before the run, while a control group maintained a normal diet.

Findings:

- Oxidative stress increased by 129% in the control group but only 55% in the blueberry group.[633]
- Antioxidant levels were significantly higher in the blueberry group.[633]
- Anti-inflammatory cytokines increased, enhancing post-exercise recovery.[633]

Takeaways: Blueberries may support athletic recovery by reducing oxidative stress and boosting antioxidant levels, particularly after intense exercise. While these findings are promising, it's important to note that individual results may vary, and more research is needed to determine whether blueberries consistently enhance performance across broader populations.

Chokeberries

Chokeberries (*Aronia melanocarpa*) are an antioxidant powerhouse, with research confirming their inflammation-fighting abilities.

A systematic review analyzed nearly 2,000 studies, focusing on 18 clinical trials that examined chokeberries' impact on human health.[634] Participants consuming chokeberry juice, extract, or powder for 4 to 13 weeks showed:

- Reduced inflammation markers (C-reactive protein and TNF-α).[634]
- Enhanced antioxidant enzyme activity, including superoxide dismutase and catalase, which protect cells from damage.[634]

Takeaway: Chokeberries are a potent natural anti-inflammatory, offering protection at the cellular level.

The Power of Berries for Everyday Health

From acai to chokeberries, these fruits are natural inflammation fighters that support heart health, immune function, and recovery. Whether you blend them into smoothies, add them to oatmeal, or eat them fresh, incorporating berries into your diet can be a delicious step toward better health.

However, while berries have shown promising anti-inflammatory effects in various studies, it's important to recognize that their benefits may not be universal. Individual responses can vary based on factors such as existing health conditions, the amount consumed, and overall diet and lifestyle. Additionally, much of the current research is based on specific dosages or controlled conditions that may not reflect everyday consumption. As such, while berries can be a valuable part of an anti-inflammatory diet, their effects may differ from person to person.

3) Turmeric

Turmeric, a spice derived from the root of *Curcuma longa*, has been used for centuries in traditional Asian medicine for its potent anti-inflammatory properties. Modern research confirms these benefits, attributing them primarily to curcumin, the bright yellow pigment in turmeric. Studies suggest curcumin may help manage conditions such as arthritis, asthma, and even digestive and oral health concerns.

Curcumin and Crohn's Disease

A 2012 study examined whether curcumin supplements could improve symptoms in patients with Crohn's Disease.[635] Five participants received 360 mg of curcumin three times daily for one month, followed by 360 mg four times daily for two additional months. By the end of the study, participants showed an average 55-point reduction in the Crohn's Disease Activity Index and decreased levels of inflammatory markers in their blood. Those who combined curcumin with their existing treatment also reported better symptom management and greater overall satisfaction. While these initial findings are promising, the very small sample size limits the ability to draw broad conclusions. Additionally, curcumin may cause GI discomfort in some individuals and can interact with medications like blood thinners, so patients should consult a healthcare provider before using it as a supplement.[636]

Turmeric and Gingivitis

Turmeric may also play a role in oral health. A 2012 study compared turmeric mouthwash to chlorhexidine (CHX) mouthwash in 60 participants with plaque-induced chronic gingivitis. Researchers evaluated plaque and gingival inflammation over three weeks.[637]

At the end of the study, both groups showed significant improvements in oral health, suggesting turmeric mouthwash could be a natural alternative to conventional antiseptic rinses like chlorhexidine for managing gingivitis and reducing oral inflammation.[637]

Curcumin and Post-Exercise Muscle Recovery

Beyond its anti-inflammatory properties, curcumin may aid in muscle recovery after intense exercise. A 2022 study assessed its effects on adolescent athletes by measuring factors like muscle soreness, fatigue, inflammatory markers, and body composition over 12 weeks.[638]

Results showed that athletes taking curcumin experienced significantly less muscle soreness and fatigue. They also exhibited lower oxidative stress markers (*8-hydroxy-2-deoxyguanosine*) and improvements in basal metabolic rate and fat-free mass.[638] These findings suggest that long-term curcumin supplementation could enhance post-exercise recovery and overall performance in athletes.

4) Boswellia

Boswellia serrata, commonly known as Indian Frankincense, is an herb native to India, Northern Africa, and the Middle East. It has been a staple in Ayurveda, a centuries-old Indian medicinal system, traditionally used to treat arthritis, fevers, sores, asthma, hemorrhoids, and dysentery.[639] While research on its full range of benefits is still developing, modern studies support its anti-inflammatory, pain-relieving, and anti-arthritic properties. It is known to inhibit NF-κB, a key regulator of inflammation, and decrease the levels of inflammatory protein molecules that are involved in tissue damage and pain.[639,640]

Boswellia and Osteoarthritis

A 2020 meta-analysis examined data from seven studies to assess the effects of *Boswellia serrata* and its active compound, Boswellic acid, on osteoarthritis.[641] Three of these studies specifically evaluated the impact of Boswellia extracts (*5-Loxin* and *Aflaxin*) in doses ranging from 100 mg to 250 mg over 4 to 12 weeks. Researchers measured pain, stiffness, and mobility using visual analog scores and the Western Ontario and McMaster Universities Osteoarthritis Index (WOMAC).

Results showed that Boswellia significantly improved pain relief, reduced stiffness, and enhanced joint function compared to control groups. While these findings highlight the potential of Boswellia as a natural aid for osteoarthritis, larger clinical trials are needed to confirm its long-term effectiveness due to limitations in sample sizes and study methods.

4) Sesame Oil

Sesame oil is widely used in cooking and seasoning, but its benefits extend far beyond the kitchen. Rich in sesamin, a bioactive compound with anti-inflammatory and pain-relieving properties, sesame oil has shown promise in supporting joint health and injury recovery.[642] While much of the research has been conducted on animals, recent clinical trials suggest similar advantages for humans.

Sesamin and Rheumatoid Arthritis

A 2019 randomized, triple-blind, placebo-controlled clinical trial investigated the effects of sesamin on rheumatoid arthritis. The study included 44 patients, randomly assigned to either an intervention group receiving 200 mg of sesamin daily or a placebo group for six weeks. Researchers measured inflammatory biomarkers such as high-sensitivity C-reactive protein (hs-CRP), TNF-α, and COX-2.[643]

The results showed a significant decrease In hs-CRP, TNF-α, and COX-2 levels in the sesamin group compared to the placebo group. Participants also reported fewer tender joints and reduced overall pain severity.[643] While these findings suggest that sesamin may help alleviate rheumatoid arthritis symptoms by reducing inflammation, the relatively small sample size and short study duration limit the strength and generalizability of the conclusions. Larger and longer-term clinical trials are needed to confirm these effects and assess the long-term safety and efficacy of sesamin supplementation.

Sesame Oil and Trauma Injuries

A 2020 study explored the effects of sesame oil on traumatic injuries. Ninety patients with upper and lower body injuries received either a topical application of sesame oil or cooking oil (as a placebo).[644] After gentle massages with the oil three times daily for two days, those treated with sesame oil experienced a significant reduction in pain, sensitivity, and discomfort compared to the placebo group.

These findings suggest that both sesamin supplements and sesame oil may serve as natural remedies for reducing pain and inflammation in conditions like arthritis and trauma-related injuries.

6) Seaweed and Red Algae

Unless you're a sushi lover or a supplement enthusiast, you may not be familiar with red algae. However, this marine-based ingredient is emerging as a powerhouse of health benefits. One key compound derived from red algae, Aquamin, is gaining attention for its potential to relieve pain, reduce inflammation, and enhance bone strength. Aquamin is a rich source of calcium, magnesium, and 72 other trace minerals, making it a unique nutrient-dense supplement. It strengthens bones by supplying key minerals and helps reduce the activity of molecules (like cytokines and NF-κB) that cause inflammation in the body. It also helps keep the gut lining healthy, which can lower overall inflammation.[389,645]

Aquamin and Osteoarthritis Relief

A 2008 study explored Aquamin's effects on knee osteoarthritis in 70 participants aged 25 to 75. Participants were divided into four groups: Aquamin, glucosamine sulfate (a widely used osteoarthritis supplement), a combination of both, and a placebo. Over 12 weeks, participants consumed three capsules three times daily, with progress measured using the Western Ontario and McMaster Universities Osteoarthritis Index (WOMAC) and six-minute walking distance tests.[646]

Results showed that the Aquamin group experienced greater improvements in pain and stiffness scores compared to the glucosamine group, with pain scores decreasing by 17.5 points versus 12.6 points, and stiffness scores dropping by 20.6 points, while the glucosamine group saw no significant change in stiffness.[646] Participants in the Aquamin group also increased their six-minute walking distance by 101 feet, compared to 56 feet in the glucosamine group. While these results are promising, larger, well-powered studies are needed to confirm whether Aquamin offers clinically meaningful advantages over established treatments. Additionally, the study did not discuss whether participants experienced withdrawal effects from reducing NSAID use, which may be an important consideration in future research.

Aquamin's Potential to Reduce NSAID Use

A 2009 follow-up study examined whether Aquamin could reduce reliance on NSAIDs.[647] The study followed 22 osteoarthritis patients who took either Aquamin or a placebo for 12 weeks. Participants in the Aquamin group reduced their NSAID intake by 50%, while still experiencing improved mobility and pain relief. This suggests that Aquamin could help osteoarthritis patients cut back on NSAID use, thereby reducing potential side effects associated with these medications.[647]

Aquamin and Inflammation Control

Research indicates that Aquamin helps reduce inflammation at the cellular level.[389] A study by O'Gorman et al. found that Aquamin inhibits Nuclear Factor Kappa B (NF-kB), a key regulator of immune response and inflammation. NF-kB controls the expression of numerous pro-inflammatory genes, including COX-2. By suppressing NF-kB activation, Aquamin may effectively reduce inflammation and related symptoms.[389]

Alternatives for Migraine Relief

Chronic inflammation is increasingly recognized as a possible contributor to various health issues, including neurological conditions like migraines.[648] Migraines affect approximately 12% of the population and can involve intense headaches, nausea, and sensitivity to light and sound [649] While there is substantial research on pharmaceutical treatments, some individuals continue to explore natural alternatives, often to reduce the side effects of current medications. In fact, migraines have been associated with a significant economic burden, with some estimates placing U.S. healthcare and productivity losses around $11 billion annually.[650] Emerging studies suggest that certain natural compounds may offer complementary support for migraine management.

Lavender Oil and Migraines

A 2012 placebo-controlled clinical trial investigated lavender essential oil as a potential migraine treatment.[651] Participants inhaled lavender oil for

15 minutes during migraine episodes, while a control group inhaled liquid paraffin. 71% of those in the lavender group reported pain relief, compared to 47% in the placebo group. These findings suggest that lavender oil may serve as a safe and effective option for managing acute migraine attacks.[651]

Basil Leaf and Migraines

Basil leaf extract (*Ocimum basilicum*) has also shown anti-migraine properties. Researchers attribute its effects to compounds such as linalool and cineole, which may have analgesic and anti-inflammatory benefits.[652] In one study, 144 migraine patients were divided into four groups: a placebo group and three treatment groups receiving 2%, 4%, or 6% basil oil, applied every eight hours for three months. All participants also took 325 mg of acetaminophen every 12 hours.[653]

Results indicated that higher doses of basil oil significantly reduced migraine frequency and severity over 12 weeks, with the 6% concentration showing the greatest improvement.[653] This suggests basil oil may be an effective natural remedy for migraine sufferers.

Ginger for Migraine Relief

Ginger is another promising alternative for migraine relief, as it targets the COX pathway similarly to NSAIDs. A 2014 double-blind study compared 250 mg of ginger rhizome to 50 mg of sumatriptan, a common migraine medication.[654] Sumatriptan users and ginger users reported similar significant pain relief within two hours, indicating comparable effectiveness.[654]

A 2019 study further examined ginger's impact on severe migraines.[655] Sixty emergency room patients were split into two groups: one received a combination of 400 mg of ginger and 100 mg of ketoprofen (an NSAID), while the other received ketoprofen alone. The ginger group reported lower pain scores over two hours, suggesting that ginger may enhance pain relief and shorten recovery time compared to NSAIDs alone.[655]

Combining Natural Alternatives for Enhanced Relief

As awareness of natural health remedies continues to grow, many people are exploring the benefits of combining different natural alternatives for greater therapeutic effects. Individual compounds like curcumin (from turmeric), boswellic acid (from Boswellia), and minerals from red algae have shown promise in managing inflammation and relieving pain. Each of these natural remedies works through distinct pathways in the body, contributing to overall pain and inflammation reduction.

Recent research suggests that combining these natural compounds can create an "additive effect," where their interaction enhances each ingredient's benefits.[390] Below, we explore studies examining how combinations of curcumin, Boswellia, red algae, and sesame oil may help manage pain more effectively, offering a natural and sustainable alternative for pain relief.

Turmeric, Boswellia, and Red Algae for Osteoarthritis

A 2021 observational, longitudinal study investigated the impact of a blend of Boswellia, turmeric, and red algae extract on knee osteoarthritis pain. The study involved 118 participants (69.5% female, average age 62.9) who took 1-4 capsules daily, each containing:

- 75 mg *Boswellia serrata*
- 175 mg turmeric (*Curcuma longa*)
- 150 mg red algae (*Porphyra umbilicalis*) extract

After 90 days, results showed a 30% reduction in visual analog pain scores, alongside a 24.1% decrease in pain intensity.[390] These findings suggest that this natural combination significantly can improve pain management while reducing reliance on conventional pain medications.

Boswellia, Turmeric, and Sesame Oil for Pain Relief

Another study examined the effectiveness of a blend of turmeric, Boswellia, and sesame oil in relieving musculoskeletal pain compared to acetaminophen. Conducted by Rudrappa et al., the study involved 88 individuals with acute musculoskeletal pain, who were assigned either the herbal blend (1,000 mg/day) or acetaminophen (1,000 mg/day) for seven days. Pain levels were assessed at 6 hours, 3 days, and 7 days using standardized pain scales.[656]

Results showed that the herbal blend provided pain relief comparable to acetaminophen. However, it was 8.57 times more effective at reducing the emotional distress associated with pain, highlighting its potential to alleviate both physical and emotional aspects of discomfort.[656]

Natural Alternatives for Reducing Fever

Many people turn to ibuprofen or acetaminophen to lower a fever, which is one of the body's natural defense mechanisms against infections and inflammation. Historically, natural remedies have been used to ease fever symptoms, though research on their effectiveness compared to NSAIDs is not scientifically convincing.

Cooling blankets and cold drinks may help reduce fever and enhance the effects of natural products. However, current data on their effectiveness is inconsistent, and results can vary.[657]

Evidence-Based Recommendations

Natural products offer a promising approach for managing mild to moderate pain, such as osteoarthritis, migraines, or inflammatory conditions. For more severe pain, they may help reduce the reliance on over-the-counter or prescription pain medications. Still, it's imperative to get advice from a healthcare provider before starting to use natural supplements as part of your routine. Avoid mixing natural products with prescription drugs, and refrain from taking them within two hours of other medications.

While natural remedies and physical cooling techniques may not completely replace fever-reducing medications, they can offer additional relief and potentially help lower the need for high-dose NSAIDs. While natural supplements can offer many benefits, everyone needs to be mindful that they may also have potential side effects.

Key Takeaways:

- Compounds like tart and sweet cherries, curcumin, and Boswellia have been shown to relieve pain, reduce inflammation, and support joint health, making them valuable options alongside traditional pain medications.
- Using a combination of natural products, such as curcumin with Boswellia or adding red algae extracts, can amplify pain-relieving and anti-inflammatory effects, especially for conditions like osteoarthritis.
- For migraines, natural options like lavender oil, basil oil, and ginger offer some relief, often with fewer side effects.

- While natural remedies are beneficial, it's essential to consult a healthcare provider before adding them to your regimen, especially if you're taking other medications, to ensure safe and effective use.

Chapter 16
The Future of Ibuprofen:
New Frontiers in Pain Relief

With a global market value of $1.43 billion in 2023 and a steady annual growth rate, ibuprofen has become a household name, sold under hundreds of brand labels.[658] One key reason for its widespread use is that doctors often prefer prescribing ibuprofen over aspirin or indomethacin due to its lower risk of stomach-related side effects. But are there safer and more effective ways to use ibuprofen?

Advances in Ibuprofen Research

Although ibuprofen is widely used and effective, current formulations have drawbacks. Poor water solubility limits how well the drug is absorbed, which can reduce pain relief and increase side effects like stomach irritation. Topical forms don't always work well because ibuprofen doesn't easily pass through the skin, and creating easy-to-take products is challenging due to issues like taste and tablet quality.

Recent research on ibuprofen has focused on improving its synthesis, production, and delivery methods. Pharmaceutical companies are also exploring innovative ways to enhance its effectiveness, including combining it with other compounds for faster and more targeted pain relief. Key advancements include:

1. Combination Formulations: Enhancing Targeted Pain Relief

Targeted Synergy. Opioid Pairings: Fixed-dose combinations with codeine (e.g., 400 mg ibuprofen + 25.6 mg codeine) show more significant pain relief compared to monotherapy, improving acute post-surgical pain management.[659]

Deep eutectic solvents (DESs): A 2025 study explored ibuprofen-based therapeutic DESs (THEDESs) to enhance the solubility of poorly soluble drugs, specifically combining ibuprofen with abiraterone acetate (a treatment for prostate cancer).[660] The simultaneous oral delivery of the two compounds may reduce the number of pills needed as well as increase the bioavailability of medicines for cancer patients.

Novel Delivery Systems

Ionic Liquid Carriers: Transdermal patches using choline-geranic acid solvents improve skin permeability by 2 to over 15 times, depending on the compound, enabling effective delivery for muscle sprains.[661,662]

Topical-Nasal Dual Delivery: Several recent studies show the development of nasal delivery formulations for ibuprofen.[663,664] A 2019 study used a thermosensitive chitosan-based nasal gel to get ibuprofen rapidly across human nasal epithelial cells.[663]

Biodegradable Microneedles: Dissolvable arrays of needles bypass first-pass metabolism, achieving 75% bioavailability in the skin of preclinical models.[665]

2. Mechanism of Action: Cellular Insights Driving Safer Therapies

ROS-Mediated Toxicity: Mitochondrial Dysfunction: Ibuprofen inhibits complex I/III in the electron transport chain, increasing superoxide production in cardiomyocytes.[348,666]

DNA Damage: Chronic use of ibuprofen correlates with higher 8-Hydroxy-2′-deoxyguanosine (8-OHdG) urinary markers, indicating oxidative nucleic acid breakdown.[667] 8-OHdG is a modified nucleoside that forms when ROS oxidize guanine bases in DNA.

Scientists, including our research team, continue to study how ibuprofen works at a cellular level. A deeper understanding of its mechanisms may lead to more precise treatments and a better grasp of potential side effects. For example, in 2015, we proposed that many NSAID-related side effects stem from reactive oxygen species (ROS) damaging proteins, DNA, and lipids inside cells.[336] Supporting this idea, our studies found that vitamin C, when taken alongside NSAIDs, reduces NSAID-induced cardiac cell death. Interestingly, vitamin C itself appears to have mild pain-relieving properties, suggesting that combining it with ibuprofen could enhance pain relief.[338] Another research group found that cotreatment with vitamin C (200–500 mg/kg) reduced ibuprofen-induced liver damage by lowering oxidative stress markers.[668] Pilot clinical trials show famotidine with ibuprofen decreases GI ulcer incidence.[669] Part of famotidine's beneficial effects may be due to its anti-oxidant properties.[670]

3. Personalized Medicine: Genetic Tailoring of Therapy

Pharmacogenomic Determinants

Advances in genetic research and pharmacogenomics are shedding light on how individual genetic factors influence responses to ibuprofen.[671] This research could lead to more personalized treatments, optimizing dosage and minimizing side effects based on a patient's genetic profile.[672] **Table 16.1** shows the effect of gene variants on ibuprofen clearance in the body. Although routine pharmacogenetic screening for CYP2C9 and CYP2C8 variants before ibuprofen therapy is not currently recommended, it may be widely practiced in the future.[673] This is especially important as 82.6% of poor ibuprofen metabolizers still self-administer standard doses despite the genetic risk.[674]

Table 16.1. Effect of CYP gene variants on ibuprofen clearance

Gene	**Variant**	**Metabolic Impact**	**Clinical Recommendation**
CYP2C9	*2/*3 alleles	70% slower clearance	50% dose reduction
CYP2C8	*3/*4 alleles	89% lower enzyme activity	Avoid >1200 mg/day
ABCB1	3435C>T	2.1X higher intestinal absorption	Monitor for renal toxicity

Future Directions

- **AI-Driven Formulations**: Machine learning models predicting optimal drug combinations based on pain etiology (neuropathic vs. inflammatory).
- **Cellular Repair Focus**: Mitochondria-targeted antioxidants (e.g., MitoQ) in clinical trials for NSAID toxicity prevention.
- **Point-of-Care Genotyping**: CRISPR-based lateral flow assays enabling CYP status determination.

Advancements in Ibuprofen Synthesis and Manufacturing

i) Classical Synthesis

The original ibuprofen synthesis, developed by Boots Pure Drug Company in 1961, involved a six-step process using toxic aluminum chloride.[675] In 1992, Hoechst Company improved this method by replacing aluminum chloride with recyclable hydrogen fluoride and simplifying synthesis through a carbon monoxide insertion technique.

ii) Continuous Flow Synthesis

Recent advancements in ibuprofen manufacturing have focused on continuous-flow synthesis, which enhances efficiency and sustainability. Notable innovations include:

- Using trifluoromethanesulfonic acid as a catalyst instead of aluminum chloride.[676]
- Direct alkylation of the benzylic anion via a 'superbase'-mediated deprotonation, which is cost-effective due to reusable mixed bases and readily available starting materials.[676] However, further refinements are needed to manage its strong basicity (ability to act as a base) for large-scale production.

Other novel synthesis approaches include:

- Iron- and titanium-catalyzed hydrocarboxylation
- Electrochemical carboxylation of quaternary ammonium bromide with CO_2
- Photochemical carboxylation of alkyl benzene using visible light and catalysts

- Regioselective carboxylation via nickel- or iridium-based catalyst systems
- Allylic oxidation, aromatic coupling, alkyne-cyanation, and asymmetric hydroaminocarbonylation

These ongoing advancements aim to make ibuprofen production faster, more cost-efficient, and environmentally sustainable.

Sustainability in Ibuprofen Synthesis

Ibuprofen production is becoming more eco-friendly. Traditional energy-intensive methods are being replaced with more sustainable alternatives, such as using solar reflectors repurposed from satellite dishes as a heat source for synthesis.[677] This shift highlights the industry's commitment to reducing energy consumption and adopting greener production processes.

BASF'S Bishop, Texas location uses four steps instead of the usual six or seven steps. Their award-winning system uses a completely closed system requiring very little human intervention that achieves **99% atom efficiency** and recycles 99.9% of anhydrous hydrogen fluoride solvent.[678] Just last year, a study coming out of Max Planck Institute found that using liquid-assisted drum milling improved the overall yield of ibuprofen produced (99% yield) after just 90 minutes of milling. This technique also eliminated solvents and cut energy use by 50%.[679]

Novel Drug Delivery Systems and Formulations

To enhance ibuprofen's therapeutic effectiveness, reduce side effects, and improve patient compliance, researchers have developed various innovative drug delivery systems (**Fig. 16.1**). These advancements aim to optimize how ibuprofen is absorbed and utilized in the body. Some of the key approaches include:

- **Liposomes:** Liposomal formulation of ibuprofen enhances bioavailability and provides sustained release, while protecting the drug from degradation.[680]
- **Microspheres:** Microspheres of ibuprofen provide extended drug release while reducing the dosing frequency, enabling a controlled release through oral administration.[680]
- **Nanoparticles:** Ibuprofen nanoparticles, lipid-based or polymeric nanoparticles enhance drug stability, solubility, and sustained release.[680,681]
- **Hydrogels:** Ibuprofen hydrogels are used on top of the skin while facilitating localized drug delivery, improving penetration, minimizing systemic side effects, and prolonging contact time.[680]
- **Transdermal patches:** Ibuprofen patches are medical patches that are still being investigated.[682,683] These provide convenient administration and bypass the GI tract, minimizing GI complications. Patches can also allow controlled release through the skin. However, skin permeability, application site, and environmental conditions (such as higher temperatures) can affect absorption rates. Some reports also suggest that they may cause skin sensitivity and the amount of drug that could be administered by patches is limited and may not be adequate amounts for patients with severe pain.

- **Solid lipid nanoparticles:** Solid-lipid nanoparticles are widely used as a chemotherapeutic agent to deliver drugs to the central nervous system.[684] Ibuprofen-loaded solid-lipid nanoparticles have improved drug stability and drug bioavailability. The controlled release of solid-lipid nanoparticles allows targeted drug delivery with various administration routes.

- **Cyclodextrin complexes:** These complexes have enhanced solubility, stability, and improved drug bioavailability.[685]

Potential Areas of Ibuprofen Research and Future Directions

The field of ibuprofen research is advancing rapidly, with scientists exploring new ways to improve its effectiveness, safety, and accessibility. Innovative studies are paving the way for breakthroughs that could enhance how ibuprofen is used in medical treatments. Below are some key areas of research that hold promise for the future of ibuprofen therapy:

- Enhanced Drug Delivery Systems: There's a growing need to explore alternative formulations like nanoparticles, liposomes, or hydrogels to improve drug stability, bioavailability, and targeted delivery.

- Mechanisms of Action: Investigating additional molecular pathways or targets contributing to ibuprofen's therapeutic effects, beyond COX enzyme inhibition.

- Long-Term Effects and Safety: Further characterization of ibuprofen's long-term effects, identification of risk factors, and development of strategies to minimize potential risks.

- Combination Therapies: Exploring synergistic effects of combining ibuprofen with other drugs or medicines to enhance pain relief and reduce ibuprofen dosage.
- Personalized Medicine: Investigating genetic variations and biomarkers to predict individual response to ibuprofen and optimize dosing for customized treatment.[673,674]
- Pediatric and Geriatric Populations: Specific research on ibuprofen's optimal dosages, safety, and age-related differences in drug metabolism and how it affects pediatric and geriatric patients.

These suggested future studies and the development of new formulations and delivery systems will take time. Before new ibuprofen formulations or delivery systems can be made available to the public, they must first undergo interaction analysis and toxicological studies initially in animals, followed by human trials (**Fig. 16.2**).

Fig. 16.2. Typical process for new formulations of ibuprofen to be made available to the public

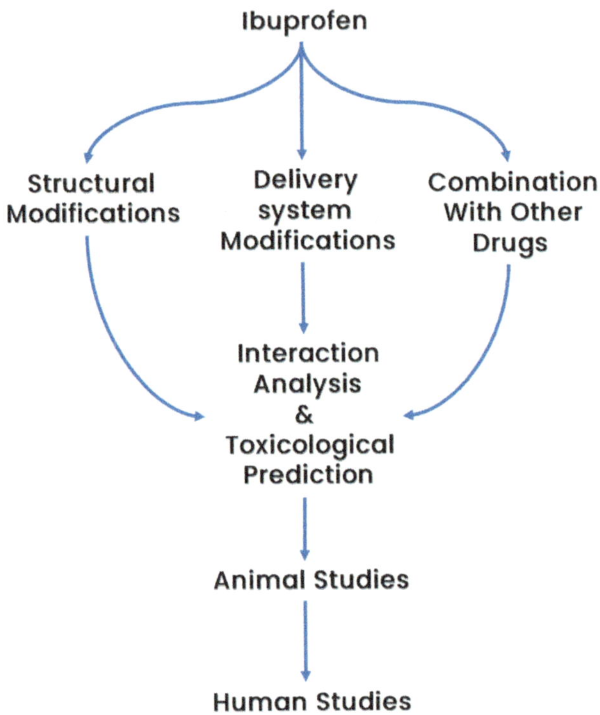

Ibuprofen Accessibility and Affordability

Ibuprofen is widely available as a relatively inexpensive OTC medication, making it a more affordable option compared to many prescription drugs. While prices vary by pharmacy, the availability of generic versions helps keep costs low, ensuring it remains an accessible and cost-effective choice for managing pain and inflammation.

However, despite its relative affordability, access to ibuprofen remains a challenge for some individuals. In many of the world's poorest and most vulnerable regions, access to essential medicines has not significantly improved since 2000, except in cases such as HIV/AIDS treatments.[686] The fragmented supply chains in vulnerable regions leave many rural areas underserved, with smaller clinics often lacking ibuprofen stocks.

On a positive note, the global ibuprofen market is projected to grow substantially, potentially leading to lower prices and wider availability in the future.[687] Some suggestions to lower ibuprofen prices are to utilize AI-driven inventory systems to optimize distribution and reduce waste, to waive import taxes on essential medicines, as proposed by WHO, and to offer tax breaks to encourage domestic ibuprofen manufacturing.

Ethical Considerations for Ibuprofen

As a widely used pain reliever, ibuprofen raises ethical considerations regarding patient safety, environmental impact, and responsible healthcare practices. Key ethical concerns include:

- **Benefits and Risks:** While recommending ibuprofen, healthcare professionals should consider individual healthcare needs, including ibuprofen's potential benefits and risks.
- **Conflicts:** Researchers should disclose any disputes to maintain transparency in prescribing practices and ibuprofen-related research.
- **Equitable Access:** More efforts are needed to confirm equitable accessibility to the drug irrespective of financial or socioeconomic factors. High out-of-pocket costs and regulatory barriers can restrict access to ibuprofen, particularly in low-income regions.
- **Responsible Use:** Long-term ibuprofen users should use the drug responsibly, considering recommended dosages accordingly and

seeking professional guidance. In some countries, a large proportion of ibuprofen is purchased without medical supervision, raising concerns about misuse, adverse effects, and lack of informed consent, especially in children.

- **Ethical drug studies:** Ethical issues arise in pediatric drug studies and use, including ensuring informed consent, balancing risks and benefits, and protecting vulnerable populations from harm or exploitation.[285,688]

- **Undertreatment and Overtreatment:** There is an ethical obligation to provide adequate pain relief, but also to avoid unnecessary or inappropriate use. Barriers such as lack of education, regulatory restrictions, and fear of side effects can lead to both undertreatment and overuse, each with ethical implications for patient well-being and justice in healthcare.[688,689]

- **Responsible Marketing:** Pharmaceutical companies have an ethical obligation to market ibuprofen responsibly, avoiding misleading claims about its effectiveness or safety. This includes clear labeling and advertising that does not downplay potential risks, especially for long-term use.[690]

- **Adverse Effects Reporting:** In case of adverse events, prompt reporting of adverse incidents is crucial for safety and ongoing assessment.

- **Voluntary Recalls when Needed:** When manufacturers produce batches that are contaminated or contain incorrect amounts of ibuprofen, it should be reported immediately, and the product recalled.[691]

- **Risks and Harms:** Responsible use and consultation with healthcare professionals is essential to reduce potential risk factors.[692]

- **Public Health Strategy**: National health agencies and healthcare providers, including pharmacists, must work together to promote campaigns that inform the public about the risks of long-term and inappropriate ibuprofen use while highlighting safe dosing practices. If requested, they should be knowledgeable and guide the public on the best alternatives.

Key Takeaway:

- While emerging trends in ibuprofen focus on novel drug delivery systems and personalized medicine to enhance effectiveness and reduce side effects, ethical responsibility remains crucial for healthcare professionals and pharmaceutical companies to ensure safer usage practices and address the specific needs of vulnerable populations.

Chapter 17 **Closing the Book:** What We've Learned

Throughout this book, we have explored the many facets of ibuprofen: its benefits, risks, and lesser-known effects that often go unnoticed. Our goal has been to provide clarity on its proper use and potential misuse, empowering readers to make informed decisions about their health.

Looking ahead, we hope the concerns and insights shared here will inspire greater awareness among manufacturers, medical professionals, and everyday users. As pain management continues to evolve, understanding the impact of commonly used medications like ibuprofen remains essential.

To wrap up, we leave you with four key takeaways—essential lessons to help you use ibuprofen safely and responsibly.

I. Awareness of Side Effects

Ibuprofen is widely regarded as safe when used as directed. However, growing research highlights potential risks associated with long-term or excessive use. As discussed in this book, ibuprofen has been linked to gastrointestinal issues, an increased risk of cardiovascular events, and potential liver and kidney damage. While severe adverse reactions are rare, they can still occur even at recommended doses.

The impact of NSAIDs, including ibuprofen, on public health is significant. NSAIDs account for approximately 30% of hospital admissions related to adverse drug reactions, primarily due to serious complications such as gastrointestinal bleeding, heart attacks, strokes, and kidney damage.[10,127] Given the millions of NSAID prescriptions issued daily, this is a concerning statistic. In fact, studies suggest that around 6% of patients prescribed NSAIDs return to their doctor within two months due to suspected adverse reactions. This could mean that over one million Americans experience NSAID-related side effects each year.[10]

Even at over-the-counter doses, ibuprofen can cause many minor side effects. For instance, if you've ever taken ibuprofen and had an episode of diarrhea, you might have attributed it to something you ate or drank. However, more than 3 in every 100 ibuprofen users report experiencing diarrhea, making it an often overlooked side effect. To further put this in context, nausea—which is a commonly occurring side effect of ibuprofen use—occurs in 3-9% of people taking ibuprofen. A list of some of ibuprofen's common and rare side effects can be found in **Fig. 17.1**.

Understanding these risks is essential for making informed decisions about ibuprofen use.

II. Awareness of Drugs Ibuprofen Interacts With

Ibuprofen interacts with more than 400 medications, including over 90 classified as major interactions that can pose serious health risks. These interactions may increase the likelihood of side effects, reduce the effectiveness of certain drugs, or even lead to dangerous complications.

Fig. 17.1. Relative occurrence of different side effects of ibuprofen

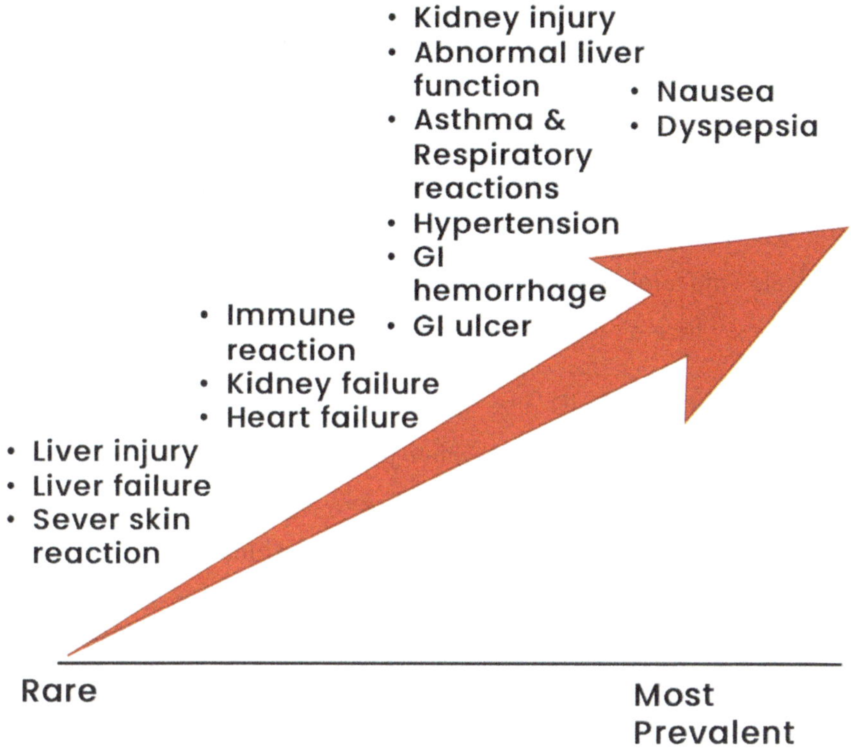

While not all interactions are fully understood, it's crucial for users to be aware of potential risks. If you regularly take ibuprofen alongside other medications or supplements, consulting a healthcare professional is always the safest approach. This ensures that you're not unknowingly putting your health at risk, and it can provide an overview of low-, moderate-, and high-risk interactions between ibuprofen and various compounds, emphasizing the importance of making informed choices when using this common pain reliever. For example, warfarin, apixaban, rivaroxaban (Xarelto), and other blood thinners can lead to severe bleeding in the brain when taken with ibuprofen. Common selective serotonin reuptake inhibitors like fluoxetine

(Prozac), sertraline, and citalopram can also increase the risk of bleeding when taken with ibuprofen.

III. Awareness of Pre-Existing Conditions That Affect Ibuprofen Use

Certain health conditions can make ibuprofen use riskier. Among young asthmatic children, the use of ibuprofen was associated with a 3.28-fold higher risk of asthma exacerbation than acetaminophen.[693] Additionally, individuals with high blood pressure, heart disease, or gastrointestinal disorders may face an increased risk of complications.

Studies show that NSAID use more than doubles the likelihood of developing acute kidney injury within just 30 days.[694] For perspective, hypertension is a major risk factor for kidney disease, with about 1 in 5 adults with high blood pressure having chronic kidney disease.[695] Since kidney function naturally declines with age, older adults are especially vulnerable to the harmful effects of ibuprofen and other NSAIDs.

Understanding how age and pre-existing conditions influence the body's response to ibuprofen can help reduce preventable health risks. Research suggests that around 10% of hospital admissions among older adults each year are due to preventable adverse drug reactions.[10] By staying informed and consulting a healthcare provider when necessary, individuals can make safer choices when using ibuprofen.

IV. We Still Don't Know A Lot About Ibuprofen

Fig. 17.2. Signaling pathways known to be affected by ibuprofen

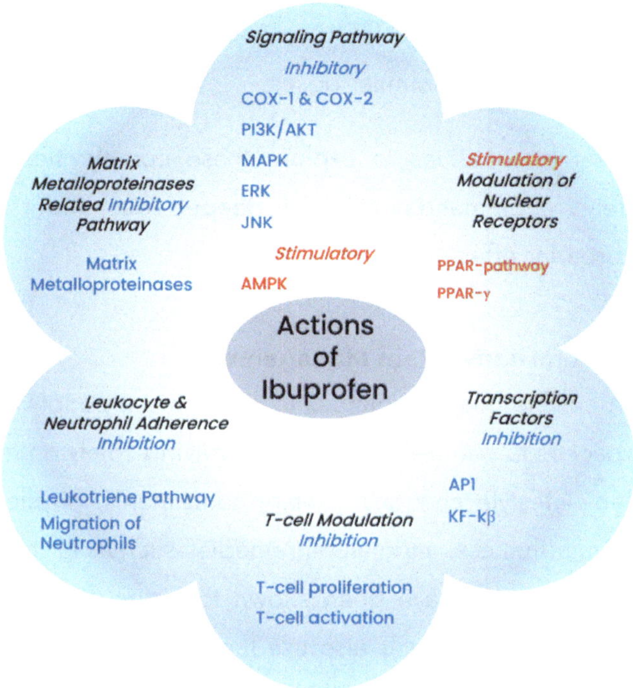

The effects of ibuprofen discussed in this book are just part of the story. Research suggests that ibuprofen influences many biological pathways (**Fig. 17.2**), but the full clinical impact of these changes remains unclear. Additionally, the way individuals respond to ibuprofen varies widely, and the reasons behind this variability are not yet well understood.

A 2022 study found that some NSAIDs, including ibuprofen and indomethacin, activate nuclear factor erythroid 2-related factor 2 (NRF2), while others do not. NRF2 is a protein that plays a key role in triggering anti-inflammatory processes in the body, which may explain why long-term NSAID use for osteoarthritis of the knee can sometimes worsen inflammation and cartilage quality.[696] NRF2 might unexpectedly worsen osteoarthritis by preventing cell death of damaged cells and disrupting cell repair mechanisms in advanced disease. These findings help clarify why different NSAIDs have varying effects on conditions like heart disease and cancer, even when taken in similar doses.

Ongoing research continues to explore these complexities, aiming to improve safety recommendations and deepen our understanding of ibuprofen's broader effects.

V. Exploring Alternative Pain Management

As interest in holistic health continues to grow, more people are seeking natural approaches to pain relief rather than relying solely on medications like ibuprofen. Lifestyle changes, dietary adjustments, physical therapy, acupuncture, mindfulness, and natural remedies such as turmeric, ginger, and omega-3 fatty acids have been shown to reduce inflammation and alleviate pain. Some individuals also use these natural options alongside ibuprofen to minimize their overall dosage and lower the risk of side effects.

In 2025, the FDA approved a new class of non-opioid analgesics, including Journavx (suzetrigine), for treating moderate to severe acute pain in adults.[697] Journavx works by disrupting a pain-signaling pathway that uses sodium channels to send pain signals from the body to the brain. The approval of new non-opioid pain relievers reflects the growing awareness of NSAID-related side effects and the need for safer alternatives. However, Journavx is only available by prescription and will only be used in certain populations that don't tolerate NSAIDs or opioids. As such, NSAIDs will remain widely used for pain relief for the foreseeable future.

Raising awareness about these natural alternatives (such as turmeric and omega-3s) and pharmaceutical advancements (such as Journavx) can have a meaningful impact on public health. By educating individuals about a wider range of pain management strategies, we can empower them to make informed choices and adopt a more balanced approach to their well-being while reducing dependence on traditional pain relievers.

The Final Message

Ibuprofen is an affordable and widely used medication that has transformed pain management for millions worldwide. However, its story serves as a powerful reminder of the delicate balance between benefit and risk, and the responsibility that comes with every prescription, every dose, and every decision to use it.

One of the most effective ways to reduce the risks associated with ibuprofen and other NSAIDs is to minimize their use in older adults whenever possible and opt for safer alternatives. Equally important is raising awareness. Educating high school students, parents, and patients can significantly reduce the risks of ibuprofen misuse. Many people remain unaware of how serious these risks can be, and also that these risks can be reduced. For example:

- GI bleeding is far more likely to be fatal in NSAID users, with a mortality rate of more than two times higher than those not taking these medications.[698] However, patients at risk for GI bleeding can significantly lower this risk by taking ibuprofen with a proton pump inhibitor such as omeprazole.[10]
- Most NSAIDs double the risk of hospitalization for heart failure. For high-dose ibuprofen, this corresponds to an additional 7–9

non-fatal and two fatal cardiovascular events for every 1,000 patients annually.[137]

How many of your friends and family know these facts? Sharing this knowledge could help prevent serious health complications and encourage safer use of ibuprofen.

As research continues to uncover the complexities of this widely used drug, we must strive for a future where scientific advancements not only deepen our understanding but also empower us to make informed choices. The story of ibuprofen is far from over, and ongoing studies will refine how we use it more effectively and safely.

Let this book serve as a reminder that even the most common medications come with profound responsibility. It is our responsibility to approach the use of these interventions with both care and caution, ensuring that the promise of relief does not come at an unintended cost. We should all advocate for healthcare policies that prioritize patient safety over profit margins and insist on comprehensive pain management approaches that extend beyond medication alone. Actively share these insights with your community, friends, and family, so that by spreading awareness, we can collectively make informed decisions.

"Ibuprofen holds the power to heal, but like a double-edged sword, its true strength lies in the wisdom of its use—misguided hands can turn a great therapy into a silent adversary."

Appendix

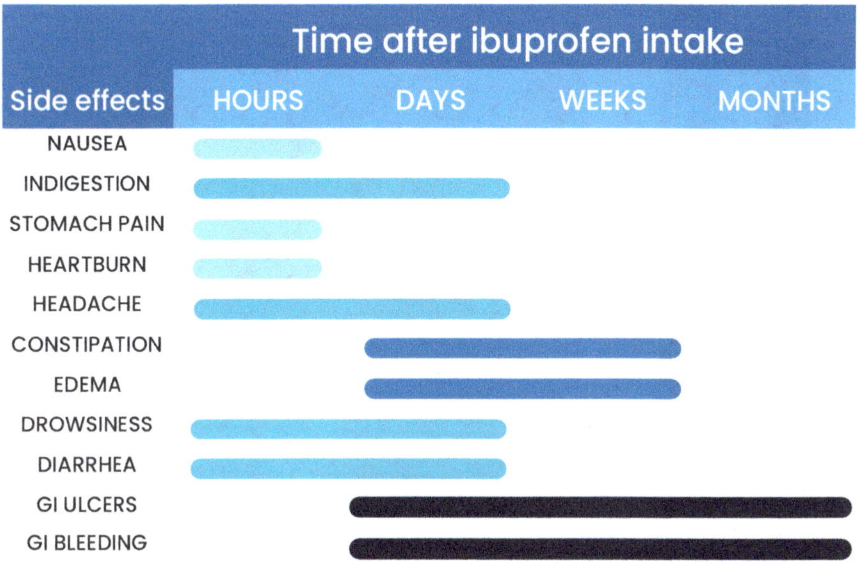

Ibuprofen Dosing information *for Adults*

For adults, the dose is not corresponded with weight nor age but whether the consumption of the drug is under a professional supervision or not.

Content	Dose	Frequency	Condition	Daily Limit
200 mg	1~2 tablets	Every 4~6 hrs.	Over The Counter	< 6 tablets/24 hrs.
200 mg	2~4 tablets	Every 6~8 hrs.	w/ Prescription	< 12 tablets/24 hrs.
400 mg	1 tablet	Every 4~6 hrs.	Over The Counter	< 3 tablets/24 hrs.
400 mg	1~2 tablet	Every 6~8 hrs.	w/ Prescription	< 6 tablets/24 hrs.

Poison Control Number in USA: 1-800-222-1222

For adults -- When should I take:

	Acetaminophen	Ibuprofen	Naproxen	Aspirin
Tension headache	✓✓	✓✓✓	✓	✓✓
Migraine	✓✓	✓✓✓	✓	✓✓
Menstrual cramps	✓	✓✓✓	✓✓✓	✓✓
Pain relief	✓✓	✓✓✓	✓✓✓	✓✓
Fever	✓✓✓	✓✓✓	✓✓	✓✓✓
Inflammation		✓✓✓	✓✓✓	✓
Sinusitis	✓✓	✓✓✓	✓✓✓	✓
Arthritis	✓	✓✓✓	✓✓✓	✓✓
Tendinitis	✓	✓✓✓	✓✓✓	✓✓
Sore muscles	✓	✓✓✓	✓✓✓	✓✓
Cardiovascular prevention				✓✓

Important Numbers

If you suspect an overdose, don't hesitate—call 911 in the U.S. Act fast and get emergency assistance immediately. Calling a helpline might use up valuable time.

If you are not seriously ill and need to contact Poison Control, call 1-800-222-1222 in the U.S. or contact local emergency services. For severe cases, seek immediate care at the nearest emergency room.

Important numbers in other countries:

India	Emergency	112
	Poison Control	(+91) 982-404-7400
China	Emergency	120
	Poison Control	(+86) 010-6609-8114
Indonesia	Emergency	112
	Poison Control	(+62) 813-1082-6879
England	Emergency	999
	Poison Control	(+44) 844-892-0111
Mexico	Emergency	911
	Poison Control	(+52) 229-932-9753

Reporting Adverse Drug Events

The FDA has implemented a website called SmartHub that allows anyone to report a product problem, including adverse drug reactions.
https://www.safetyreporting.hhs.gov/smarthub#/

If you have difficulty using the site, call *1-(888)-463-6332* or email *SRPSupport@fda.hhs.gov.*

Helpline

Substance Abuse and Mental Health Services Administration (SAMHSA)
Helpline: 1-800-662-4357.

This free helpline that can help provide advice for treatment for substance issues and mental health concerns is available 24 hours a day.

References

1 Lanas, A. *et al.* Risk of upper gastrointestinal ulcer bleeding associated with selective cyclo-oxygenase-2 inhibitors, traditional non-aspirin non-steroidal anti-inflammatory drugs, aspirin and combinations. *Gut* **55**, 1731-1738 (2006).

2 Elflein, J. *Likelihood of developing lung and bronchus cancer U.S. 2017-2019, by age and gender*, (2024). https://www.statista.com/statistics/1286377/lung-and-bronchus-cancer-probability-of-delevoping-us-age-gender/

3 *Ibuprofen: Drug Usage Statistics, United States, 2013 - 2022. ClinCalc.com*, https://clincalc.com/DrugStats/Drugs/Ibuprofen

4 Sachdeva, S. Early Treatment of Patent Ductus Arteriosus with Ibuprofen: Pediatric Cardiologist's Viewpoint. *Indian Pediatr* **61**, 573-574 (2024).

5 He, C. *et al.* Enhanced longevity by ibuprofen, conserved in multiple species, occurs in yeast through inhibition of tryptophan import. *PLoS Genet* **10**, e1004860 (2014).

6 Anderson, P. *Topical Gel Promising in Migraine*, (2015). https://www.medscape.com/viewarticle/843685

7 Bowen, B., Yuan, Y., James, C., Rashid, F. & Hunt, R. H. Time course and pattern of blood loss with ibuprofen treatment in healthy subjects. *Clin Gastroenterol Hepatol* **3**, 1075-1082 (2005).

8 Kowalski, M. L. *et al.* Classification and practical approach to the diagnosis and management of hypersensitivity to nonsteroidal anti-inflammatory drugs. *Allergy* **68**, 1219-1232 (2013).

9 Lin, B. M. *et al.* Duration of Analgesic Use and Risk of Hearing Loss in Women. *Am J Epidemiol* **185**, 40-47 (2017).

10 Davis, A. & Robson, J. The dangers of NSAIDs: look both ways. *Br J Gen Pract* **66**, 172-173 (2016).

11 *Ibuprofen Side Effects. Drugs.com*, https://www.drugs.com/sfx/ibuprofen-side-effects.html

12 Al Farii, H., Farahdel, L., Frazer, A., Salimi, A. & Bernstein, M. The effect of NSAIDs on postfracture bone healing: a meta-analysis of randomized controlled trials. *OTA Int* **4**, e092 (2021).

13 Derry, S., Wiffen, P. & Moore, A. Topical Nonsteroidal Anti-inflammatory Drugs for Acute Musculoskeletal Pain. *JAMA* **315**, 813-814 (2016).

14 *Drug Interaction Report: IBU + turmeric*, https://www.drugs.com/interactions-check.php?drug_list=1310-779,2682-0

15 *Drug Interaction Report: IBU + Ginkgo Biloba*, https://www.drugs.com/interactions-check.php?drug_list=1174-10621,1310-779

16 *Drug Interaction Report: IBU + Fish Oil*, https://www.drugs.com/interactions-check.php?drug_list=1749-3873,1310-779

17 *Drug Interaction Report: IBU + Dicumarol*, https://www.drugs.com/interactions-check.php?drug_list=874-0,1310-779

18 *Drug Interaction Report: IBU + Regorafenib*, https://www.drugs.com/interactions-check.php?drug_list=1310-779,3420-0

19 *Drug Interaction Report: IBU + Tinzaparin*, https://www.drugs.com/interactions-check.php?drug_list=1310-779,2199-0

20 Duff, W. R. *et al.* Effects of low-dose ibuprofen supplementation and resistance training on bone and muscle in postmenopausal women: A randomized controlled trial. *Bone Rep* **5**, 96-103 (2016).

21 Zheng, Z. *et al.* Potential Adverse Effect of Nonsteroidal Anti-Inflammatory Drugs (NSAIDs) on Bisphosphonate Efficacy: An Exploratory Post Hoc Analysis From a Randomized Controlled Trial of Clodronate. *J Bone Miner Res* **37**, 1117-1124 (2022).

22 van Staa, T. P., Leufkens, H. G. & Cooper, C. Use of nonsteroidal anti-inflammatory drugs and risk of fractures. *Bone* **27**, 563-568 (2000).

23 Kohrt, W. M. *et al.* Timing of ibuprofen use and bone mineral density adaptations to exercise training. *J Bone Miner Res* **25**, 1415-1422 (2010).

24 Zelaya, C. E., Dahlhamer, J. M., Lucas, J. W. & Connor, E. M. *Chronic Pain and High-impact Chronic Pain Among U.S. Adults,* (2019). https://www.cdc.gov/nchs/products/databriefs/db390.htm

25 Tiwari, S. *et al.* Gender-specific changes in energy metabolism and protein degradation as major pathways affected in livers of mice treated with ibuprofen. *Sci Rep* **10**, 3386 (2020).

26 Kaufman, D. W. *et al.* Exceeding the daily dosing limit of nonsteroidal anti-inflammatory drugs among ibuprofen users. *Pharmacoepidemiol Drug Saf* **27**, 322-331 (2018).

27 Godersky, M. E., Vercammen, L. K., Ventura, A. S., Walley, A. Y. & Saitz, R. Identification of non-steroidal anti-inflammatory drug use disorder: A case report. *Addict Behav* **70**, 61-64 (2017).

28 Nieman, D. C. *et al.* Ibuprofen use, endotoxemia, inflammation, and plasma cytokines during ultramarathon competition. *Brain Behav Immun* **20**, 578-584 (2006).

29 Lipman, G. S. *et al.* 340 Ibuprofen Versus Placebo Effect on Acute Kidney Injury in Ultramarathon Runners. *Annals of Emergency Medicine* **68**, S130 (2016).

30 Irazabal, M. V. & Torres, V. E. Reactive Oxygen Species and Redox Signaling in Chronic Kidney Disease. *Cells* **9,** 1342 (2020).

31 Angadi, S. S. & Karn, A. Ibuprofen induced Stevens-Johnson syndrome - toxic epidermal necrolysis in Nepal. *Asia Pac Allergy* **6**, 70-73 (2016).

32 Hongo, T. *et al.* A rare case of Reye's syndrome induced by influenza A virus with use of ibuprofen in an adult. *Acute Med Surg* **7**, e457 (2020).

33 Alhatemi, A. Q. M., Hashim, H. T., Al-Tarbosh, M. A. S., Abdulhussain, R. & Hashim, A. T. Single-dose ibuprofen induced Stevens-Johnson Syndrome. *Clin Case Rep* **12**, e8574 (2024).

34 Gomez Garcia, E. B., Ruitenberg, A., Madretsma, G. S. & Hintzen, R. Q. Hyponatraemic coma induced by desmopressin and ibuprofen in a woman with von Willebrand's disease. *Haemophilia* **9**, 232-234 (2003).

35 Hall, A. H. *et al.* Ibuprofen overdose: 126 cases. *Ann Emerg Med* **15**, 1308-1313 (1986).

36 *Prescribers' Digital Reference. Ibuprofen drug summary: storage,* https://www.pdr.net/drug-summary/?drugLabelId=Ibuprofen-Tablets-ibuprofen-2618

37 Kumar, G. K. *Ibuprofen (Advil, Motrin, Caldolor) - Uses, Side Effects, and More,* (2024). https://www.webmd.com/drugs/2/drug-5166-9368/ibuprofen-oral/ibuprofen-oral/details

38 Archibald, T. & Brown, S. Monitoring Commercial Ibuprofen Potency Changes Over 1 Year When Stored in a Household Setting. *J Pharm Technol* **36**, 16-21 (2020).

39 Bennani, I. *et al.* The Influence of the coating on the release of Ibuprofen from the Tablet: Comparative Dissolution Study of the different types of coating. *Research Journal of Pharmacy and Technology* **14**, 5912-5914 (2023).

40 Lanza, F. L. *et al.* A double-blind placebo-controlled comparison of the efficacy and safety of 50, 100, and 200 micrograms of misoprostol QID in the prevention of ibuprofen-induced gastric and duodenal mucosal lesions and symptoms. *Am J Gastroenterol* **84**, 633-636 (1989).

41 Moghadamnia, Y. *et al.* New formulation of ibuprofen on absorption-rate: A comparative bioavailability study in healthy volunteers. *Caspian J Intern Med* **10**, 150-155 (2019).

42 Jan, S. U., Khan, G. M. & Hussain, I. Formulation development and investigation of ibuprofen controlled release tablets with hydrophilic polymers and the effect of co-excipients on drug release patterns. *Pak J Pharm Sci* **25**, 751-756 (2012).

43 Mandal, T. K. Effect of tablet integrity on the dissolution rate of sustained-release preparations. *J Clin Pharm Ther* **21**, 155-157 (1996).

44 Crushing tablets or opening capsules: many uncertainties, some established dangers. *Prescrire Int* **23**, 209-211, 213-204 (2014).

45 Meaidi, A. *et al.* Venous thromboembolism with use of hormonal contraception and non-steroidal anti-inflammatory drugs: nationwide cohort study. *BMJ* **382**, e074450 (2023).

46 Marasco, W. A. *et al.* Ibuprofen-associated renal dysfunction. Pathophysiologic mechanisms of acute renal failure, hyperkalemia, tubular necrosis, and proteinuria. *Arch Intern Med* **147**, 2107-2116 (1987).

47 Bird, S. T. *et al.* The association between drospirenone and hyperkalemia: a comparative-safety study. *BMC Clin Pharmacol* **11**, 23 (2011).

48 Allen, R. H. Combined estrogen-progestin oral contraceptives: patient selection, counseling, and use. *UpToDate, Waltham, MA.*(2023).

49 Thammineni, N., Kathi, P. R., Sharma, A. & Jawed, A. Ibuprofen Overuse Leading to Life-threatening Hypokalemia Associated with Renal Tubular Acidosis in Two Patients. *Cureus* **11**, e6404 (2019).

50 Back, D. J. & Orme, M. L. Pharmacokinetic drug interactions with oral contraceptives. *Clin Pharmacokinet* **18**, 472-484 (1990).

51 Bushra, R. & Aslam, N. An overview of clinical pharmacology of Ibuprofen. *Oman Med J* **25**, 155-1661 (2010).

52 *Ibuprofen*, (2024). https://pubchem.ncbi.nlm.nih.gov/compound/3672

53 Tan, S. C., Patel, B. K., Jackson, S. H., Swift, C. G. & Hutt, A. J. Influence of age on the enantiomeric disposition of ibuprofen in healthy volunteers. *Br J Clin Pharmacol* **55**, 579-587 (2003).

54 Narang, A. P., Datta, D. V. & Mathur, V. S. Impairment of drug elimination in patients with liver disease. *Int J Clin Pharmacol Ther Toxicol* **23**, 28-32 (1985).

55 Scott, C. S. *et al.* The pharmacokinetics of ibuprofen suspension, chewable tablets, and tablets in children with cystic fibrosis. *J Pediatr-Us* **134**, 58-63 (1999).

56 Lawati, H. A. & Jamali, F. Onset of Action and Efficacy of Ibuprofen Liquigel as Compared to Solid Tablets: A Systematic Review and Meta-Analysis. *J Pharm Pharm Sci* **19**, 301-311 (2016).

57 Beaver, W. T. Review of the analgesic efficacy of ibuprofen. *Int J Clin Pract Suppl*, 13-17 (2003).

58 Reker, D. *et al.* "Inactive" ingredients in oral medications. *Sci Transl Med* **11** (2019).

59 Streit, L. *What Is Lactose Monohydrate, and How Is It Used?*, (2020). https://www.healthline.com/nutrition/lactose-monohydrate

60 Bischoff, N. S. *et al.* Possible Adverse Effects of Food Additive E171 (Titanium Dioxide) Related to Particle Specific Human Toxicity, Including the Immune System. *Int J Mol Sci* **22** (2020).

61 Moore, N. Ibuprofen: a journey from prescription to over-the-counter use. *J R Soc Med* **100 Suppl 48**, 2-6 (2007).

62 Schwier, N. & Tran, N. Non-Steroidal Anti-Inflammatory Drugs and Aspirin Therapy for the Treatment of Acute and Recurrent Idiopathic Pericarditis. *Pharmaceuticals (Basel)* **9** (2016).

63 Dunayer, E. Ibuprofen toxicosis in dogs, cats, and ferrets. *Vet Med-Us* **99**, 580-+ (2004).

64 Kore, A. M. Toxicology of nonsteroidal antiinflammatory drugs. *Vet Clin North Am Small Anim Pract* **20**, 419-430 (1990).

65 Jones, R. D., Baynes, R. E. & Nimitz, C. T. Nonsteroidal anti-inflammatory drug toxicosis in dogs and cats: 240 cases (1989-1990). *J Am Vet Med Assoc* **201**, 475-477 (1992).

66 Cathers, T. E., Isaza, R. & Oehme, F. Acute ibuprofen toxicosis in a ferret. *J Am Vet Med Assoc* **216**, 1426-1428, 1412 (2000).

67 Cuthbert, R., Parry-Jones, J., Green, R. E. & Pain, D. J. NSAIDs and scavenging birds: potential impacts beyond Asia's critically endangered vultures. *Biol Lett* **3**, 90-93 (2007).

68 Giri, S. N. & Hyde, D. M. Increases in severity of lung damage and mortality by treatment with cyclo and lipoxygenase inhibitors in bleomycin and hyperoxia model of lung injury in hamsters. *Pathology* **19**, 150-158 (1987).

69 Ting, A. K. Y., Tay, V. S. Y., Chng, H. T. & Xie, S. A Critical Review on the Pharmacodynamics and Pharmacokinetics of Non-steroidal Anti-inflammatory Drugs and Opioid Drugs Used in Reptiles. *Vet Anim Sci* **17**, 100267 (2022).

70 Hovda, T. *Toxicoses From Human Analgesics in Animals*, (2025). https://www.merckvetmanual.com/toxicology/toxicoses-from-human-analgesics/toxicoses-from-human-analgesics-in-animals

71 Warden, S. J. Prophylactic use of NSAIDs by athletes: a risk/benefit assessment. *Phys Sportsmed* **38**, 132-138 (2010).

72 American Chemical Society. *Ibuprofen*, (2018). https://www.acs.org/molecule-of-the-week/archive/i/ibuprofen.html

73 Johnson, C. H. *et al.* NMR spectroscopic studies on the in vitro acyl glucuronide migration kinetics of Ibuprofen ((+/-)-(R,S)-2-(4-isobutylphenyl) propanoic acid), its metabolites, and analogues. *Anal Chem* **79**, 8720-8727 (2007).

74 Bennett, M. J., Sherwood, W. G., Bhala, A. & Hale, D. E. Identification of urinary metabolites of (+/-)-2-(p-isobutylphenyl)propionic acid (Ibuprofen) by routine organic acid screening. *Clin Chim Acta* **210**, 55-62 (1992).

75 *Ibuprofen*, (2004) https://pubchem.ncbi.nlm.nih.gov/#query=ibuprofen

76 Halford, G. M., Lordkipanidze, M. & Watson, S. P. 50th anniversary of the discovery of ibuprofen: an interview with Dr Stewart Adams. *Platelets* **23**, 415-422 (2012).

77 Rainsford, K. D. Ibuprofen: from invention to an OTC therapeutic mainstay. *Int J Clin Pract Suppl*, 9-20 (2013).

78 Rainsford, K. D. Fifty years since the discovery of ibuprofen. *Inflammopharmacology* **19**, 293-297 (2011).

79 *WHO Model List of Essential Medicines*, (2021). https://www.who.int/publications/i/item/WHO-MHP-HPS-EML-2021.02

80 *Ibuprofen*, https://list.essentialmeds.org/medicines/14

81 Varrassi, G., Pergolizzi, J. V., Dowling, P. & Paladini, A. Ibuprofen Safety at the Golden Anniversary: Are all NSAIDs the Same? A Narrative Review. *Adv Ther* **37**, 61-82 (2020).

82 Eccles, R. Efficacy and safety of over-the-counter analgesics in the treatment of common cold and flu. *J Clin Pharm Ther* **31**, 309-319 (2006).

83 Winther, B. & Mygind, N. The therapeutic effectiveness of ibuprofen on the symptoms of naturally acquired common colds. *Am J Rhinol* **15**, 239-242 (2001).

84 Melis, R. Ibuprofen and/or acetaminophen: what price for "euthermia"? *J Pediatr* **131** (1997).

85 McCarberg, B. & D'Arcy, Y. Target pain with topical peripheral analgesics. *Nurse Pract* **32**, 44-49 (2007).

86 Stanos, S. P. & Galluzzi, K. E. Topical therapies in the management of chronic pain. *Postgrad Med* **125**, 25-33 (2013).

87 Moore, N. & Scheiman, J. M. Gastrointestinal safety and tolerability of oral non-aspirin over-the-counter analgesics. *Postgrad Med* **130**, 188-199 (2018).

88 Fletcher, G., Ryan, D. K. & Bunker, C. B. Association between Stevens-Johnson syndrome and toxic epidermal necrolysis with ibuprofen: A pharmacovigilance study in the UK Yellow Card scheme and systematic review of case reports. *medRxiv*, 2023.2012.2005.23299283 (2023). https://doi.org/10.1101/2023.12.05.23299283

89 Ershad, M., Ameer, M. A., Chen, R. J. & Vearrier, D. *Ibuprofen Toxicity*, (2024). https://www.ncbi.nlm.nih.gov/books/NBK526078/

90 Cryer, B., Barnett, M. A., Wagner, J. & Wilcox, C. M. Overuse and Misperceptions of Nonsteroidal Anti-inflammatory Drugs in the United States. *Am J Med Sci* **352**, 472-480 (2016).

91 Rampal, P. *et al.* Gastrointestinal tolerability of ibuprofen compared with paracetamol and aspirin at over-the-counter doses. *J Int Med Res* **30**, 301-308 (2002).

92 Rainsford, K. D. Ibuprofen: pharmacology, efficacy and safety. *Inflammopharmacology* **17**, 275-342 (2009).

93 Lanza, F. L., Collaku, A. & Liu, D. J. Endoscopic comparison of gastroduodenal injury with over-the-counter doses of new fast-dissolving ibuprofen and paracetamol formulations: a randomized, placebo-controlled, 4-way crossover clinical trial. *Clin Exp Gastroenterol* **11**, 169-177 (2018).

94 Kelly, T., Conn, K. M. & Zak, M. Evaluation of Over-the-Counter Medication Knowledge and Literacy in Adolescent Students. *Acad Pediatr* **18**, 556-562 (2018).

95 Young, E. *et al.* Trends in diversity-related learning among secondary schools in 35 US states, 2014-2018. *Health Educ J* **83**, 52-64 (2024).

96 Rosenbloom, C. J., Morley, F. L., Ahmed, I. & Cox, A. R. Oral non-steroidal anti-inflammatory drug use in recreational runners participating in Parkrun UK: Prevalence of use and awareness of risk. *Int J Pharm Pract* **28**, 561-568 (2020).

97 Ulrich, A. *Ibuprofen Dosages for Adults: Your GoodRx Guide*, (2024). https://www.goodrx.com/ibuprofen/dosage

98 *Ibuprofen Dosage*, (2023). https://www.drugs.com/dosage/ibuprofen.html

99 *Ibuprofen dosing for children*, https://www.mountsinai.org/health-library/selfcare-instructions/ibuprofen-dosing-for-children

100 Gulzar, A. *Ibuprofen Dosage: A Guide on How Much to Take*, (2024). https://www.verywellhealth.com/ibuprofen-dosage-how-much-you-can-safely-take-8646449#citation-6

101 Schmitt, B. D. *Ibuprofen - Advil Motrin etc - Dosage Table* https://www.uhhospitals.org/rainbow/health-information/health-and-wellness-library/pediatric-drug-dosage-information/ibuprofen-advil-motrin-etc-dosage-table

102 *Ibuprofen (oral route)*, https://www.mayoclinic.org/drugs-supplements/ibuprofen-oral-route/description/drg-20070602?utm_source=chatgpt.com

103 Kuptniratsaikul, V. *et al.* Efficacy and safety of Curcuma domestica extracts compared with ibuprofen in patients with knee osteoarthritis: a multicenter study. *Clin Interv Aging* **9**, 451-458 (2014).

104 *Common questions about ibuprofen for adults*, (2021). https://www.nhs.uk/medicines/ibuprofen-for-adults/common-questions-about-ibuprofen-for-adults/?utm_source=chatgpt.com

105 Leverrier-Penna, S. *et al.* Ibuprofen is deleterious for the development of first trimester human fetal ovary ex vivo. *Hum Reprod* **33**, 482-493 (2018).

106 Sherif, B. Q., Al-Zohyri, A. M. & Shihab, S. S. Effects of Some Non Steroidal Anti-inflammatory Drugs on Ovulation in Women with Mild Musculoskeletal Pain (A Clinical Study). *IOSR Journal of Pharmacy and Biological Sciences* **9**, 43-44 (2014).

107 Morris, P. E., Promes, J. T., Guntupalli, K. K., Wright, P. E. & Arons, M. M. A multi-center, randomized, double-blind, parallel, placebo-controlled trial to evaluate the efficacy, safety, and pharmacokinetics of intravenous ibuprofen for the treatment of fever in critically ill and non-critically ill adults. *Crit Care* **14**, R125 (2010).

108 Khalil, S. N. *et al.* A multicenter, randomized, open-label, active-comparator trial to determine the efficacy, safety, and pharmacokinetics of intravenous ibuprofen for treatment of fever in hospitalized pediatric patients. *BMC Pediatr* **17**, 42 (2017).

109 Joseph, L., Goldberg, S., Cohen, S. & Picard, E. Ibuprofen does not prevent postbronchoscopy fever in children undergoing broncho-alveolar lavage. *Pediatr Pulmonol* **55**, 2737-2741 (2020).

110 Apfelbaum, J. L., Chen, C., Mehta, S. S. & Gan, T. J. Postoperative pain experience: results from a national survey suggest postoperative pain continues to be undermanaged. *Anesth Analg* **97**, 534-540 (2003).

111 Ilyas, A. M., Miller, A. J., Graham, J. G. & Matzon, J. L. Pain Management After Carpal Tunnel Release Surgery: A Prospective Randomized Double-Blinded Trial Comparing Acetaminophen, Ibuprofen, and Oxycodone. *J Hand Surg Am* **43**, 913-919 (2018).

112 Gozeler, M. S. *et al.* Does a single-dose preemptive intravenous ibuprofen have an effect on postoperative pain relief after septorhinoplasty? *Am J Otolaryngol* **39**, 726-730 (2018).

113 Liu, X. *et al.* A prospective, randomized, double-blind, placebo-controlled trial of acute postoperative pain treatment using opioid analgesics with intravenous ibuprofen after radical cervical cancer surgery. *Sci Rep* **8**, 10161 (2018).

114 Ngo, V. T. H. & Bajaj, T. Ibuprofen. in *StatPearls* (2025).

115 Feldman, C. A. *et al.* Nonopioid vs opioid analgesics after impacted third-molar extractions: The Opioid Analgesic Reduction Study randomized clinical trial. *J Am Dent Assoc* **156**, 110-123 e119 (2025).

116 Ryan, J. L. *et al.* Gender differences in analgesia for endodontic pain. *J Endod* **34**, 552-556 (2008).

117 Hersh, E. V. *et al.* Ibuprofen liquigel for oral surgery pain. *Clin Ther* **22**, 1306-1318 (2000).

118 Marjoribanks, J., Ayeleke, R. O., Farquhar, C. & Proctor, M. Nonsteroidal anti-inflammatory drugs for dysmenorrhoea. *Cochrane Database Syst Rev* **2015**, CD001751 (2015).

119 Donmez, S., Şener, A., Erdem, A. B., Çetin, Ç. & Ç.elik, G. K. Analgesic Efficacy of Ibuprofen in Dysmenorrhea. *Bezmialem Science* **11**, 163-169 (2023).

120 Codispoti, J. R., Prior, M. J., Fu, M., Harte, C. M. & Nelson, E. B. Efficacy of nonprescription doses of ibuprofen for treating migraine headache. a randomized controlled trial. *Headache* **41**, 665-679 (2001).

121 Dieppe, P. A. & Lohmander, L. S. Pathogenesis and management of pain in osteoarthritis. *Lancet* **365**, 965-973 (2005).

122 Adatia, A., Rainsford, K. D. & Kean, W. F. Osteoarthritis of the knee and hip. Part II: therapy with ibuprofen and a review of clinical trials. *J Pharm Pharmacol* **64**, 626-636 (2012).

123 Bannuru, R. R. *et al.* Comparative effectiveness of pharmacologic interventions for knee osteoarthritis: a systematic review and network meta-analysis. *Ann Intern Med* **162**, 46-54 (2015).

124 Moore, R. A., Derry, S., Wiffen, P. J., Straube, S. & Aldington, D. J. Overview review: Comparative efficacy of oral ibuprofen and paracetamol (acetaminophen) across acute and chronic pain conditions. *Eur J Pain* **19**, 1213-1223 (2015).

125 Fendrick, A. M. & Greenberg, B. P. A review of the benefits and risks of nonsteroidal anti-inflammatory drugs in the management of mild-to-moderate osteoarthritis. *Osteopath Med Prim Care* **3**, 1 (2009).

126 Ngo, V. T. H. & Bajaj, T. Ibuprofen in *StatPearls* (2024).

127 Pirmohamed, M. *et al.* Adverse drug reactions as cause of admission to hospital: prospective analysis of 18 820 patients. *BMJ* **329**, 15-19 (2004).

128 Curtis, J. R. & Singh, J. A. Use of biologics in rheumatoid arthritis: current and emerging paradigms of care. *Clin Ther* **33**, 679-707 (2011).

129 Riley, T. R. & George, M. D. Risk for infections with glucocorticoids and DMARDs in patients with rheumatoid arthritis. *RMD Open* **7** (2021).

130 Allen, A., Carville, S., McKenna, F. & Grp, G. D. Diagnosis and management of rheumatoid arthritis in adults: summary of updated NICE guidance. *Bmj-Brit Med J* **362** (2018).

131 Belbasis, L., Dosis, V. & Evangelou, E. Elucidating the environmental risk factors for rheumatic diseases: An umbrella review of meta-analyses. *Int J Rheum Dis* **21**, 1514-1524 (2018).

132 Lindqvist, E., Saxne, T., Geborek, P. & Eberhardt, K. Ten year outcome in a cohort of patients with early rheumatoid arthritis: health status, disease process, and damage. *Ann Rheum Dis* **61**, 1055-1059 (2002).

133 Smolen, J. S., Aletaha, D. & McInnes, I. B. Rheumatoid arthritis. *Lancet* **388**, 2023-2038 (2016).

134 Smolen, J. S. *et al.* EULAR recommendations for the management of rheumatoid arthritis with synthetic and biological disease-modifying antirheumatic drugs: 2019 update. *Ann Rheum Dis* **79**, 685-699 (2020).

135 Jorizzo, J. L. *et al.* Immunologic safety of ibuprofen in rheumatoid arthritis: preliminary evidence. *Clin Exp Rheumatol* **2**, 253-257 (1984).

136 Bancos, S., Bernard, M. P., Topham, D. J. & Phipps, R. P. Ibuprofen and other widely used non-steroidal anti-inflammatory drugs inhibit antibody production in human cells. *Cell Immunol* **258**, 18-28 (2009).

137 Coxib *et al.* Vascular and upper gastrointestinal effects of non-steroidal anti-inflammatory drugs: meta-analyses of individual participant data from randomised trials. *Lancet* **382**, 769-779 (2013).

138 Bergstra, S. A. *et al.* Efficacy, duration of use and safety of glucocorticoids: a systematic literature review informing the 2022 update of the EULAR recommendations for the management of rheumatoid arthritis. *Ann Rheum Dis* **82**, 81-94 (2023).

139 da Costa, B. R. *et al.* Effectiveness of non-steroidal anti-inflammatory drugs for the treatment of pain in knee and hip osteoarthritis: a network meta-analysis. *Lancet* **390**, e21-e33 (2017).

140 Derry, S., Conaghan, P., Da Silva, J. A., Wiffen, P. J. & Moore, R. A. Topical NSAIDs for chronic musculoskeletal pain in adults. *Cochrane Database Syst Rev* **4**, CD007400 (2016). https://doi.org/10.1002/14651858.CD007400.pub3

141 Fidahic, M., Jelicic Kadic, A., Radic, M. & Puljak, L. Celecoxib for rheumatoid arthritis. *Cochrane Database Syst Rev* **6**, CD012095 (2017).

142 Hazlewood, G., van der Heijde, D. M. & Bombardier, C. Paracetamol for the management of pain in inflammatory arthritis: a systematic literature review. *J Rheumatol Suppl* **90**, 11-16 (2012).

143 McWilliams, D. F. *et al.* The efficacy of systemic glucocorticosteroids for pain in rheumatoid arthritis: a systematic literature review and meta-analysis. *Rheumatology (Oxford)* **61**, 76-89 (2021).

144 Sohail, R. *et al.* Effects of Non-steroidal Anti-inflammatory Drugs (NSAIDs) and Gastroprotective NSAIDs on the Gastrointestinal Tract: A Narrative Review. *Cureus* **15**, e37080 (2023).

145 Pannunzio, A. & Coluccia, M. Cyclooxygenase-1 (COX-1) and COX-1 Inhibitors in Cancer: A Review of Oncology and Medicinal Chemistry Literature. *Pharmaceuticals (Basel)* **11** (2018).

146 Konstan, M. W., Byard, P. J., Hoppel, C. L. & Davis, P. B. Effect of high-dose ibuprofen in patients with cystic fibrosis. *N Engl J Med* **332**, 848-854 (1995).

147 Zappavigna, S. *et al.* Anti-Inflammatory Drugs as Anticancer Agents. *Int J Mol Sci* **21** (2020).

148 Kolawole, O. R. & Kashfi, K. NSAIDs and Cancer Resolution: New Paradigms beyond Cyclooxygenase. *Int J Mol Sci* **23** (2022).

149 Andrews, J., Djakiew, D., Krygier, S. & Andrews, P. Superior effectiveness of ibuprofen compared with other NSAIDs for reducing the survival of human prostate cancer cells. *Cancer Chemother Pharmacol* **50**, 277-284 (2002).

150 Akrami, H., Aminzadeh, S. & Fallahi, H. Inhibitory effect of ibuprofen on tumor survival and angiogenesis in gastric cancer cell. *Tumour Biol* **36**, 3237-3243 (2015).

151 Gao, X. *et al.* Ibuprofen induces ferroptosis of glioblastoma cells via downregulation of nuclear factor erythroid 2-related factor 2 signaling pathway. *Anticancer Drugs* **31**, 27-34 (2020).

152 Ricciotti, E. & FitzGerald, G. A. Prostaglandins and inflammation. *Arterioscler Thromb Vasc Biol* **31**, 986-1000 (2011).

153 Caughey, G. E., Cleland, L. G., Penglis, P. S., Gamble, J. R. & James, M. J. Roles of cyclooxygenase (COX)-1 and COX-2 in prostanoid production by human endothelial cells: selective up-regulation of prostacyclin synthesis by COX-2. *J Immunol* **167**, 2831-2838 (2001).

154 Hunter, T. S., Robison, C. & Gerbino, P. P. Emerging evidence in NSAID pharmacology: important considerations for product selection. *Am J Manag Care* **21**, S139-147 (2015).

155 Warner, T. D. *et al.* Nonsteroid drug selectivities for cyclo-oxygenase-1 rather than cyclo-oxygenase-2 are associated with human gastrointestinal toxicity: a full in vitro analysis. *Proc Natl Acad Sci U S A* **96**, 7563-7568 (1999).

156 Orlando, B. J., Lucido, M. J. & Malkowski, M. G. The structure of ibuprofen bound to cyclooxygenase-2. *J Struct Biol* **189**, 62-66 (2015).

157 Kawahara, K., Hohjoh, H., Inazumi, T., Tsuchiya, S. & Sugimoto, Y. Prostaglandin E2-induced inflammation: Relevance of prostaglandin E receptors. *Biochim Biophys Acta* **1851**, 414-421 (2015).

158 Kozak, K. R., Rowlinson, S. W. & Marnett, L. J. Oxygenation of the endocannabinoid, 2-arachidonylglycerol, to glyceryl prostaglandins by cyclooxygenase-2. *J Biol Chem* **275**, 33744-33749 (2000).

159 Fowler, C. J. The potential of inhibitors of endocannabinoid metabolism as anxiolytic and antidepressive drugs–A practical view. *Eur Neuropsychopharmacol* **25**, 749-762 (2015).

160 Alhouayek, M. & Muccioli, G. G. COX-2-derived endocannabinoid metabolites as novel inflammatory mediators. *Trends Pharmacol Sci* **35**, 284-292 (2014).

161 Tallima, H. Clarification of Arachidonic Acid Metabolic Pathway Intricacies. *ACS Omega* **6**, 15559-15563 (2021).

162 Sejdiu, B. I. & Tieleman, D. P. COX-1 – lipid interactions: arachidonic acid, cholesterol, and phospholipid binding to the membrane binding domain of COX-1. *BioRxiv* (2020).

163 Vecchio, A. J., Simmons, D. M. & Malkowski, M. G. Structural basis of fatty acid substrate binding to cyclooxygenase-2. *J Biol Chem* **285**, 22152-22163 (2010).

164 Vecchio, A. J., Orlando, B. J., Nandagiri, R. & Malkowski, M. G. Investigating substrate promiscuity in cyclooxygenase-2: the role of Arg-120 and residues lining the hydrophobic groove. *J Biol Chem* **287**, 24619-24630 (2012).

165 Kozak, K. R., Prusakiewicz, J. J. & Marnett, L. J. Oxidative metabolism of endocannabinoids by COX-2. *Curr Pharm Des* **10**, 659-667 (2004).

166 Vecchio, A. J. & Malkowski, M. G. The structural basis of endocannabinoid oxygenation by cyclooxygenase-2. *J Biol Chem* **286**, 20736-20745 (2011).

167 Rainsford, K. D. Discovery, mechanisms of action and safety of ibuprofen. *Int J Clin Pract Suppl*, 3-8 (2003).

168 Gahbauer, S. *et al.* Docking for EP4R antagonists active against inflammatory pain. *Nat Commun* **14**, 8067 (2023).

169 Aronoff, D. M. & Neilson, E. G. Antipyretics: mechanisms of action and clinical use in fever suppression. *Am J Med* **111**, 304-315 (2001).

170 Plaisance, K. I. & Mackowiak, P. A. Antipyretic therapy: physiologic rationale, diagnostic implications, and clinical consequences. *Arch Intern Med* **160**, 449-456 (2000).

171 Young, P. J. & Saxena, M. Fever management in intensive care patients with infections. *Crit Care* **18**, 206 (2014).

172 Schafer, A. I. Effects of nonsteroidal antiinflammatory drugs on platelet function and systemic hemostasis. *J Clin Pharmacol* **35**, 209-219 (1995).

173 Morgan, T. & Anderson, A. The effect of nonsteroidal anti-inflammatory drugs on blood pressure in patients treated with different antihypertensive drugs. *J Clin Hypertens (Greenwich)* **5**, 53-57 (2003).

174 Chen, M. R. & Dragoo, J. L. The effect of nonsteroidal anti-inflammatory drugs on tissue healing. *Knee Surg Sports Traumatol Arthrosc* **21**, 540-549 (2013).

175 Paccani, S. R. *et al.* Nonsteroidal anti-inflammatory drugs suppress T-cell activation by inhibiting p38 MAPK induction. *J Biol Chem* **277**, 1509-1513 (2002).

176 Guindon, J., De Lean, A. & Beaulieu, P. Local interactions between anandamide, an endocannabinoid, and ibuprofen, a nonsteroidal anti-inflammatory drug, in acute and inflammatory pain. *Pain* **121**, 85-93 (2006).

177 Dongdem, J. T., Helegbe, G. K., Opare-Asamoah, K., Wezena, C. A. & Ocloo, A. Assessment of NSAIDs as potential inhibitors of the fatty acid amide hydrolase I (FAAH-1) using three different primary fatty acid amide substrates in vitro. *BMC Pharmacol Toxicol* **23**, 1 (2022).

178 Schlosburg, J. E., Kinsey, S. G. & Lichtman, A. H. Targeting fatty acid amide hydrolase (FAAH) to treat pain and inflammation. *AAPS J* **11**, 39-44 (2009).

179 Wilkinson, B. L. *et al.* Ibuprofen attenuates oxidative damage through NOX2 inhibition in Alzheimer's disease. *Neurobiol Aging* **33**, 197 e121-132 (2012).

180 Stratman, N. C., Carter, D. B. & Sethy, V. H. Ibuprofen: effect on inducible nitric oxide synthase. *Brain Res Mol Brain Res* **50**, 107-112 (1997).

181 Fiorucci, S., Antonelli, E., Burgaud, J. L. & Morelli, A. Nitric oxide-releasing NSAIDs: a review of their current status. *Drug Saf* **24**, 801-811 (2001).

182 Cyr, A. R., Huckaby, L. V., Shiva, S. S. & Zuckerbraun, B. S. Nitric Oxide and Endothelial Dysfunction. *Crit Care Clin* **36**, 307-321 (2020).

183 Varadi, G. *et al.* Randomized clinical trial evaluating transdermal Ibuprofen for moderate to severe knee osteoarthritis. *Pain Physician* **16**, E749-762 (2013).

184 Narumiya, S. & FitzGerald, G. A. Genetic and pharmacological analysis of prostanoid receptor function. *J Clin Invest* **108**, 25-30 (2001).

185 Tsuge, K., Inazumi, T., Shimamoto, A. & Sugimoto, Y. Molecular mechanisms underlying prostaglandin E2-exacerbated inflammation and immune diseases. *Int Immunol* **31**, 597-606 (2019).

186 Stitham, J., Midgett, C., Martin, K. A. & Hwa, J. Prostacyclin: an inflammatory paradox. *Front Pharmacol* **2**, 24 (2011).

187 Lau, K. E. & Lui, F. Physiology, Prostaglandin I2, in *StatPearls* (2024).

188 Dorris, S. L. & Peebles, R. S., Jr. PGI2 as a regulator of inflammatory diseases. *Mediators Inflamm* **2012**, 926968 (2012).

189 Norlander, A. E. *et al.* Prostaglandin I(2) Therapy Promotes Regulatory T Cell Generation in Patients with Pulmonary Arterial Hypertension. *Am J Respir Crit Care Med* **208**, 737-739 (2023).

190 *Cancer Statistics*, https://www.cancer.gov/about-cancer/understanding/statistics

191 Swanton, C. *et al.* Embracing cancer complexity: Hallmarks of systemic disease. *Cell* **187**, 1589-1616 (2024).

192 *What is Cancer?*, https://www.cancer.gov/about-cancer/understanding/what-is-cancer#:~:text=Cancer%20is%20a%20disease%20in,benign%20tumors%20in%20the%20brain.

193 Baris, D. *et al.* Nonsteroidal anti-inflammatory drugs and other analgesic use and bladder cancer in northern New England. *Int J Cancer* **132**, 162-173 (2013).

194 Harris, R. E., Beebe-Donk, J., Doss, H. & Burr Doss, D. Aspirin, ibuprofen, and other non-steroidal anti-inflammatory drugs in cancer prevention: a critical review of non-selective COX-2 blockade (review). *Oncol Rep* **13**, 559-583 (2005).

195 Schack, A., Fransgaard, T., Klein, M. F. & Gogenur, I. Perioperative Use of Nonsteroidal Anti-inflammatory Drugs Decreases the Risk of Recurrence of Cancer After Colorectal Resection: A Cohort Study Based on Prospective Data. *Ann Surg Oncol* **26**, 3826-3837 (2019).

196 Janssen, A. *et al.* Evidence of COX-2 independent induction of apoptosis and cell cycle block in human colon carcinoma cells after S- or R-ibuprofen treatment. *Eur J Pharmacol* **540**, 24-33 (2006).

197 Flausino, L. E., Ferreira, I. N., Tuan, W. J., Estevez-Diz, M. D. P. & Chammas, R. Association of COX-inhibitors with cancer patients' survival under chemotherapy and radiotherapy regimens: a real-world data retrospective cohort analysis. *Front Oncol* **14**, 1433497 (2024).

198 *Lung Cancer Risk Factors*, (2025). https://www.cdc.gov/lung-cancer/risk-factors/index.html

199 *Lung Cancer Risk Factors*, https://www.cancer.org/cancer/types/lung-cancer/causes-risks-prevention/risk-factors.html

200 *Cancer Facts & Figures 2024*, https://www.cancer.org/content/dam/cancer-org/research/cancer-facts-and-statistics/annual-cancer-facts-and-figures/2024/2024-cancer-facts-and-figures-acs.pdf

201 *Lung Cancer Risk Factors*, (2024). https://www.cdc.gov/lung-cancer/risk-factors/index.html#:~:text=People%20who%20smoke%20cigarettes%20are,the%20risk%20of%20lung%20cancer

202 Bittoni, M. A., Carbone, D. P. & Harris, R. E. Ibuprofen and fatal lung cancer: A brief report of the prospective results from the Third National Health and Nutrition Examination Survey (NHANES III). *Mol Clin Oncol* **6**, 917-920 (2017).

203 Endo, H., Yano, M., Okumura, Y. & Kido, H. Ibuprofen enhances the anticancer activity of cisplatin in lung cancer cells by inhibiting the heat shock protein 70. *Cell Death Dis* **5**, e1027 (2014).

204 Khusnurrokhman, G. & Wati, F. F. Tumor-promoting inflammation in lung cancer: A literature review. *Ann Med Surg (Lond)* **79**, 104022 (2022).

205 Stabile, L. P. *et al.* Preclinical Evidence for Combined Use of Aromatase Inhibitors and NSAIDs as Preventive Agents of Tobacco-Induced Lung Cancer. *J Thorac Oncol* **13**, 399-412 (2018).

206 Zhao, H. *et al.* Inflammation and tumor progression: signaling pathways and targeted intervention. *Signal Transduct Target Ther* **6**, 263 (2021).

207 Harris, R. E., Beebe-Donk, J. & Schuller, H. M. Chemoprevention of lung cancer by non-steroidal anti-inflammatory drugs among cigarette smokers. *Oncol Rep* **9**, 693-695 (2002).

208 Shen, W. *et al.* Ibuprofen mediates histone modification to diminish cancer cell stemness properties via a COX2-dependent manner. *Br J Cancer* **123**, 730-741 (2020).

209 Yurtdas-Kirimlioglu, G., Gorgulu, S. & Berkman, M. S. Novel approaches to cancer therapy with ibuprofen-loaded Eudragit((R)) RS 100 and/or octadecylamine-modified PLGA nanoparticles by assessment of their effects on apoptosis. *Drug Dev Ind Pharm* **46**, 1133-1149 (2020).

210 Zendehdel, A., Ansari, M., Khatami, F., Mansoursamaei, S. & Dialameh, H. The effect of vitamin D supplementation on the progression of benign prostatic hyperplasia: A randomized controlled trial. *Clin Nutr* **40**, 3325-3331 (2021).

211 Soucek, K., Lincova, E., Starsichova, A., Hofmanova, J. & Kozubik, A. Interaction between effects of vitamin D3 and nonsteroidal anti-inflammatory drugs in prostate and colon epithelial cells. *Cancer Research*, 3287 (2007).

212 Gavrilov, V., Steiner, M. & Shany, S. The combined treatment of 1,25-dihydroxyvitamin D3 and a non-steroid anti-inflammatory drug is highly effective in suppressing prostate cancer cell line (LNCaP) growth. *Anticancer Res* **25**, 3425-3429 (2005).

213 Barathan, M. *et al.* Viral Persistence and Chronicity in Hepatitis C Virus Infection: Role of T-Cell Apoptosis, Senescence and Exhaustion. *Cells* **7** (2018).

214 Arisan, E. D. *et al.* The molecular targets of diclofenac differs from ibuprofen to induce apoptosis and epithelial mesenchymal transition due to alternation on oxidative stress management p53 independently in PC3 prostate cancer cells. *Prostate Int* **7**, 156-165 (2019).

215 Wynne, S. & Djakiew, D. NSAID inhibition of prostate cancer cell migration is mediated by Nag-1 Induction via the p38 MAPK-p75(NTR) pathway. *Mol Cancer Res* **8**, 1656-1664 (2010).

216 John-Aryankalayil, M. *et al.* NS-398, ibuprofen, and cyclooxygenase-2 RNA interference produce significantly different gene expression profiles in prostate cancer cells. *Mol Cancer Ther* **8**, 261-273 (2009).

217 Bonelli, P. *et al.* Ibuprofen delivered by poly(lactic-co-glycolic acid) (PLGA) nanoparticles to human gastric cancer cells exerts antiproliferative activity at very low concentrations. *Int J Nanomedicine* **7**, 5683-5691 (2012).

218 Najafzadeh, M. *et al.* DNA Damage in Healthy Individuals and Respiratory Patients after Treating Whole Blood In vitro with the Bulk and Nano Forms of NSAIDs. *Front Mol Biosci* **3**, 50 (2016).

219 Guma, A. *et al.* Ex vivo/in vitro effects of aspirin and ibuprofen, bulk and nano forms, in peripheral lymphocytes of prostate cancer patients and healthy individuals. *Mutat Res Genet Toxicol Environ Mutagen* **861-862**, 503306 (2021).

220 Singer, E. A., Palapattu, G. S. & van Wijngaarden, E. Prostate-specific antigen levels in relation to consumption of nonsteroidal anti-inflammatory drugs and acetaminophen: results from the 2001-2002 National Health and Nutrition Examination Survey. *Cancer* **113**, 2053-2057 (2008).

221 *Key Statistics for Breast Cancer*, (2025). https://www.cancer.org/cancer/types/breast-cancer/about/how-common-is-breast-cancer.html#:~:text=Breast%20cancer%20is%20the%20most,will%20die%20from%20breast%20cancer

222 Kehm, R. D. *et al.* Regular use of aspirin and other non-steroidal anti-inflammatory drugs and breast cancer risk for women at familial or genetic risk: a cohort study. *Breast Cancer Res* **21**, 52 (2019). 223 Xu, X. C. COX-2 inhibitors in cancer treatment and prevention, a recent development. *Anticancer Drugs* **13**, 127-137 (2002).

224 Gandhi, J., Khera, L., Gaur, N., Paul, C. & Kaul, R. Role of Modulator of Inflammation Cyclooxygenase-2 in Gammaherpesvirus Mediated Tumorigenesis. *Front Microbiol* **8**, 538 (2017).

225 Marshall, S. F. *et al.* Nonsteroidal anti-inflammatory drug use and breast cancer risk by stage and hormone receptor status. *J Natl Cancer Inst* **97**, 805-812 (2005).

226 Dierssen-Sotos, T. *et al.* Use of non-steroidal anti-inflammatory drugs and risk of breast cancer: The Spanish Multi-Case-control (MCC) study. *BMC Cancer* **16**, 660 (2016).

227 Yang, Y. S., Kornelius, E., Lo, S. C., Wang, Y. H. & Huang, C. N. Aspirin and Risk of Specific Breast Cancer Subtype in Women with Diabetes. *J Womens Health (Larchmt)* **32**, 341-346 (2023).

228 Daugherty, S. E. *et al.* Nonsteroidal antiinflammatory drugs and bladder cancer: a pooled analysis. *Am J Epidemiol* **173**, 721-730 (2011).

229 Freedman, N. D., Silverman, D. T., Hollenbeck, A. R., Schatzkin, A. & Abnet, C. C. Association between smoking and risk of bladder cancer among men and women. *JAMA* **306**, 737-745 (2011).

230 Letasiova, S. *et al.* Bladder cancer, a review of the environmental risk factors. *Environ Health* **11 Suppl 1**, S11 (2012).

231 West, E. G., Lang, R., Sellers, D., Chess-Williams, R. & McDermott, C. Ibuprofen Decreases Spontaneous Activity and Enhances Nerve-Evoked Contractions to Minimize Mitomycin C-Induced Bladder Dysfunction. *J Pharmacol Exp Ther* **366**, 282-290 (2018).

232 Reagan-Shaw, S., Nihal, M. & Ahmad, N. Dose translation from animal to human studies revisited. *FASEB J* **22**, 659-661 (2008).

233 *What Is Colorectal Cancer?*, https://www.cancer.org/cancer/types/colon-rectal-cancer/about/what-is-colorectal-cancer.html#:~:text=Pathology%20Report:%20Polyps.-,How%20colorectal%20cancer%20spreads,staging%2C%20see%20Colorectal%20Cancer%20Stages.

234 Siegel, R. L., Wagle, N. S., Cercek, A., Smith, R. A. & Jemal, A. Colorectal cancer statistics, 2023. *CA Cancer J Clin* **73**, 233-254 (2023).

235 *Colorectal Cancer: Screening*, https://www.uspreventiveservicestaskforce.org/uspstf/recommendation/colorectal-cancer-screening (2021).

236 Chudy-Onwugaje, K. *et al.* Aspirin, ibuprofen, and reduced risk of advanced colorectal adenoma incidence and recurrence and colorectal cancer in the PLCO Cancer Screening Trial. *Cancer* **127**, 3145-3155 (2021).

237 Goncalves, V., Henriques, A. F. A., Matos, P. & Jordan, P. Ibuprofen disrupts a WNK1/GSK3beta/SRPK1 protein complex required for expression of tumor-related splicing variant RAC1B in colorectal cells. *Oncotarget* **11**, 4421-4437 (2020).

238 Bando, H., Ohtsu, A. & Yoshino, T. Therapeutic landscape and future direction of metastatic colorectal cancer. *Nat Rev Gastroenterol Hepatol* **20**, 306-322 (2023).

239 Pathak, P. S., Chan, G., Deming, D. A. & Chee, C. E. State-of-the-Art Management of Colorectal Cancer: Treatment Advances and Innovation. *Am Soc Clin Oncol Educ Book* **44**, e438466 (2024).

240 Zhao, K. *et al.* HSP70 Family in Cancer: Signaling Mechanisms and Therapeutic Advances. *Biomolecules* **13** (2023).

241 Fan, C. C. *et al.* EFHD2 contributes to non-small cell lung cancer cisplatin resistance by the activation of NOX4-ROS-ABCC1 axis. *Redox Biol* **34**, 101571 (2020).

242 Thun, M. J., Henley, S. J. & Patrono, C. Nonsteroidal anti-inflammatory drugs as anticancer agents: mechanistic, pharmacologic, and clinical issues. *J Natl Cancer Inst* **94**, 252-266 (2002).

243 Janelsins, M. C. *et al.* Nationwide phase II randomized controlled trial of low-dose ibuprofen vs placebo for cancer-related cognitive impairment (CRCI). *Journal of Clinical Oncology* **41** (2023).

244 Le, T. T. *et al.* Effect of Ibuprofen on BrainAGE: A Randomized, Placebo-Controlled, Dose-Response Exploratory Study. *Biol Psychiatry Cogn Neurosci Neuroimaging* **3**, 836-843 (2018).

245 *Brain health. World Health Organization*, (2021-2025). https://www.who.int/health-topics/brain-health#tab=tab_1

246 Collaborators, G. B. D. N. S. D. Global, regional, and national burden of disorders affecting the nervous system, 1990-2021: a systematic analysis for the Global Burden of Disease Study 2021. *Lancet Neurol* **23**, 344-381 (2024).

247 Durankus, F. *et al.* Beneficial Effects of Ibuprofen on Pentylenetetrazol-induced Convulsion. *Neurochem Res* **45**, 2409-2416 (2020).

248 Terzi, M. *et al.* The use of non-steroidal anti-inflammatory drugs in neurological diseases. *J Chem Neuroanat* **87**, 12-24 (2018).

249 Parepally, J. M., Mandula, H. & Smith, Q. R. Brain uptake of nonsteroidal anti-inflammatory drugs: ibuprofen, flurbiprofen, and indomethacin. *Pharm Res* **23**, 873-881 (2006).

250 Gao, X., Chen, H., Schwarzschild, M. A. & Ascherio, A. Use of ibuprofen and risk of Parkinson disease. *Neurology* **76**, 863-869 (2011).

251 Moore, A. H. *et al.* Non-Steroidal Anti-Inflammatory Drugs in Alzheimer's Disease and Parkinson's Disease: Reconsidering the Role of Neuroinflammation. *Pharmaceuticals (Basel)* **3**, 1812-1841 (2010).

252 Poduri, A. & Lowenstein, D. Epilepsy genetics–past, present, and future. *Curr Opin Genet Dev* **21**, 325-332 (2011).

253 *Epilepsy*, (2024). https://www.who.int/news-room/fact-sheets/detail/epilepsy

254 Gonzalez, H. F. J., Yengo-Kahn, A. & Englot, D. J. Vagus Nerve Stimulation for the Treatment of Epilepsy. *Neurosurg Clin N Am* **30**, 219-230 (2019).

255 Peng, J. *et al.* Effect of Ibuprofen on Autophagy of Astrocytes During Pentylenetetrazol-Induced Epilepsy and its Significance: An Experimental Study. *Neurochem Res* **44**, 2566-2576 (2019).

256 Liu, R. *et al.* Ibuprofen Exerts Antiepileptic and Neuroprotective Effects in the Rat Model of Pentylenetetrazol-Induced Epilepsy via the COX-2/NLRP3/IL-18 Pathway. *Neurochem Res* **45**, 2516-2526 (2020).

257 Zhao, J. *et al.* Activated astrocytes attenuate neocortical seizures in rodent models through driving Na(+)-K(+)-ATPase. *Nat Commun* **13**, 7136 (2022).

258 Hayatdavoudi, P., Hosseini, M., Hajali, V., Hosseini, A. & Rajabian, A. The role of astrocytes in epileptic disorders. *Physiol Rep* **10**, e15239 (2022).

259 Strengell, T. *et al.* Antipyretic agents for preventing recurrences of febrile seizures: randomized controlled trial. *Arch Pediatr Adolesc Med* **163**, 799-804 (2009).

260 Murphy, M. P. & LeVine, H., 3rd. Alzheimer's disease and the amyloid-beta peptide. *J Alzheimers Dis* **19**, 311-323 (2010).

261 Sastre, M. & Gentleman, S. M. NSAIDs: How they Work and their Prospects as Therapeutics in Alzheimer's Disease. *Front Aging Neurosci* **2**, 20 (2010).

262 Lichtenstein, M. P., Carriba, P., Masgrau, R., Pujol, A. & Galea, E. Staging anti-inflammatory therapy in Alzheimer's disease. *Front Aging Neurosci* **2**, 142 (2010).

263 Kuchibhotla, K. V. *et al.* Neurofibrillary tangle-bearing neurons are functionally integrated in cortical circuits in vivo. *Proc Natl Acad Sci U S A* **111**, 510-514 (2014).

264 Stewart, W. F., Kawas, C., Corrada, M. & Metter, E. J. Risk of Alzheimer's disease and duration of NSAID use. *Neurology* **48**, 626-632 (1997).

265 Van Dam, D., Coen, K. & De Deyn, P. P. Ibuprofen modifies cognitive disease progression in an Alzheimer's mouse model. *J Psychopharmacol* **24**, 383-388 (2010).

266 Zhang, C., Wang, Y., Wang, D., Zhang, J. & Zhang, F. NSAID Exposure and Risk of Alzheimer's Disease: An Updated Meta-Analysis From Cohort Studies. *Front Aging Neurosci* **10**, 83 (2018).

267 Rivers-Auty, J., Mather, A. E., Peters, R., Lawrence, C. B. & Brough, D. Anti-inflammatories in Alzheimer's disease-potential therapy or spurious correlate? *Brain Commun* **2**, fcaa109 (2020).

268 Szekely, C. A. *et al.* NSAID use and dementia risk in the Cardiovascular Health Study: role of APOE and NSAID type. *Neurology* **70**, 17-24 (2008).

269 Vlad, S. C., Miller, D. R., Kowall, N. W. & Felson, D. T. Protective effects of NSAIDs on the development of Alzheimer disease. *Neurology* **70**, 1672-1677 (2008).

270 DeSai, C. & Hays Shapshak, A. Cerebral Ischemia, in *StatPearls* (2024).

271 Iwata, Y., Nicole, O., Zurakowski, D., Okamura, T. & Jonas, R. A. Ibuprofen for neuroprotection after cerebral ischemia. *J Thorac Cardiovasc Surg* **139**, 489-493 (2010).

272 Zaminelli, T. *et al.* Antidepressant and antioxidative effect of Ibuprofen in the rotenone model of Parkinson's disease. *Neurotox Res* **26**, 351-362 (2014).

273 Grotemeyer, A., McFleder, R. L., Wu, J., Wischhusen, J. & Ip, C. W. Neuroinflammation in Parkinson's Disease - Putative Pathomechanisms and Targets for Disease-Modification. *Front Immunol* **13**, 878771 (2022).

274 Swiatkiewicz, M., Zaremba, M., Joniec, I., Czlonkowski, A. & Kurkowska-Jastrzebska, I. Potential neuroprotective effect of ibuprofen, insights from the mice model of Parkinson's disease. *Pharmacol Rep* **65**, 1227-1236 (2013).

275 Badawoud, A. M. *et al.* The relation between Parkinson's disease and non-steroidal anti-inflammatories; a systematic review and meta-analysis. *Front Pharmacol* **15**, 1434512 (2024).

276 Chen, H. *et al.* Nonsteroidal anti-inflammatory drugs and the risk of Parkinson disease. *Arch Neurol* **60**, 1059-1064 (2003).

277 San Luciano, M. *et al.* Nonsteroidal Anti-inflammatory Use and LRRK2 Parkinson's Disease Penetrance. *Mov Disord* **35**, 1755-1764 (2020).

278 Valkovic, P. *et al.* Pain in Parkinson's Disease: A Cross-Sectional Study of Its Prevalence, Types, and Relationship to Depression and Quality of Life. *PLoS One* **10**, e0136541 (2015).

279 Blanchet, P. J. & Brefel-Courbon, C. Chronic pain and pain processing in Parkinson's disease. *Prog Neuropsychopharmacol Biol Psychiatry* **87**, 200-206 (2018).

280 Cinar, E., Tel, B. C. & Sahin, G. Neuroinflammation in Parkinson's Disease and its Treatment Opportunities. *Balkan Med J* **39**, 318-333 (2022).

281 Lin, C. H., Wu, R. M., Chang, H. Y., Chiang, Y. T. & Lin, H. H. Preceding pain symptoms and Parkinson's disease: a nationwide population-based cohort study. *Eur J Neurol* **20**, 1398-1404 (2013).

282 Aisen, P. S. *et al.* Effects of rofecoxib or naproxen vs placebo on Alzheimer disease progression: a randomized controlled trial. *JAMA* **289**, 2819-2826 (2003).

283 Dill, J. *et al.* A molecular mechanism for ibuprofen-mediated RhoA inhibition in neurons. *J Neurosci* **30**, 963-972 (2010).

284 Casper, D., Yaparpalvi, U., Rempel, N. & Werner, P. Ibuprofen protects dopaminergic neurons against glutamate toxicity in vitro. *Neurosci Lett* **289**, 201-204 (2000).

285 de Martino, M., Chiarugi, A., Boner, A., Montini, G. & De' Angelis, G. L. Working Towards an Appropriate Use of Ibuprofen in Children: An Evidence-Based Appraisal. *Drugs* **77**, 1295-1311 (2017).

286 Wansink, B. & van Ittersum, K. Spoons systematically bias dosing of liquid medicine. *Ann Intern Med* **152**, 66-67 (2010).

287 van Ittersum, K. & Wansink, B. Stop spoon dosing: milliliter instructions reduce inclination to spoon dosing. *BMC Res Notes* **9**, 33 (2016).

288 Mayo Clinic. *Fever*, (2022). https://www.mayoclinic.org/diseases-conditions/fever/symptoms-causes/syc-20352759

289 Baxter, L. *et al.* The association between ibuprofen administration in children and the risk of developing or exacerbating asthma: a systematic review and meta-analysis. *BMC Pulm Med* **24**, 412 (2024).

290 Stehlin, F. *et al.* Guiding Drug Provocation Testing for Ibuprofen Hypersensitivity in a Pediatric Population: Development of the I3A Risk-Stratification Tool. *J Allergy Clin Immunol Pract* (2024).

291 Smith, M. D. *et al.* Out-of-hospital medication errors among young children in the United States, 2002-2012. *Pediatrics* **134**, 867-876 (2014).

292 Cheraghi, R., Elyaszadeh, S. & Alizadeh, M. Gastrointestinal Bleeding and Hepatotoxicity: Acetaminophen and Ibuprofen Home Medication Administration Errors in Fever Treatment of Children. *J Caring Sci* **13**, 146-147 (2024).

293 Li, S. F., Lacher, B. & Crain, E. F. Acetaminophen and ibuprofen dosing by parents. *Pediatr Emerg Care* **16**, 394-397 (2000).

294 in *Drugs and Lactation Database (LactMed(R))* (2006).

295 Kirby, B. J. & Unadkat, J. D. Grapefruit juice, a glass full of drug interactions? *Clin Pharmacol Ther* **81**, 631-633 (2007).

296 Banerjee, S. Interactions between Common Foods and Drugs - A Narrative Review *Asian Journal of Pharmaceutical Research* **10**, 188-194 (2020).

297 Perrott, D. A., Piira, T., Goodenough, B. & Champion, G. D. Efficacy and safety of acetaminophen vs ibuprofen for treating children's pain or fever: a meta-analysis. *Arch Pediatr Adolesc Med* **158**, 521-526 (2004).

298 Pierce, C. A. & Voss, B. *Efficacy and safety of ibuprofen and acetaminophen in children and adults: a meta-analysis and qualitative review*, (2010). https://www.ncbi.nlm.nih.gov/books/NBK79235/

299 Balestracci, A. *et al.* Ibuprofen-associated acute kidney injury in dehydrated children with acute gastroenteritis. *Pediatr Nephrol* **30**, 1873-1878 (2015).

300 Pierce, C. A. & Voss, B. Efficacy and safety of ibuprofen and acetaminophen in children and adults: a meta-analysis and qualitative review. *Ann Pharmacother* **44**, 489-506 (2010).

301 Tan, E., Braithwaite, I., McKinlay, C. J. D. & Dalziel, S. R. Comparison of Acetaminophen (Paracetamol) With Ibuprofen for Treatment of Fever or Pain in Children Younger Than 2 Years: A Systematic Review and Meta-analysis. *JAMA Netw Open* **3**, e2022398 (2020).

https://doi.org/10.1001/jamanetworkopen.2020.22398

302 De la Cruz-Mena, J. E. *et al.* Short-term Dual Therapy or Mono Therapy With Acetaminophen and Ibuprofen for Fever: A Network Meta-Analysis. *Pediatrics* **154** (2024).

303 Wade, K. C. & Mathis, C. Antipyretic Strategies: Is Fever Clearance Enough to Justify Dual Therapy? *Pediatrics* **154** (2024).

304 NIH. *Feverish Illness in Children: Assessment and Initial Management in Children Younger Than 5 Years National Institute for Health and Care Excellence: Guidelines* (2013).

305 Section on Clinical, P., Therapeutics, Committee on, D., Sullivan, J. E. & Farrar, H. C. Fever and antipyretic use in children. *Pediatrics* **127**, 580-587 (2011).

306 Wright, A. D. & Liebelt, E. L. Alternating antipyretics for fever reduction in children: an unfounded practice passed down to parents from pediatricians. *Clin Pediatr (Phila)* **46**, 146-150 (2007).

307 Mayoral, C. E., Marino, R. V., Rosenfeld, W. & Greensher, J. Alternating antipyretics: is this an alternative? *Pediatrics* **105**, 1009-1012 (2000).

308 Shortridge, L. & Harris, V. Alternating acetaminophen and ibuprofen. *Paediatr Child Health* **12**, 127-128 (2007).

309 Sarrell, E. M., Wielunsky, E. & Cohen, H. A. Antipyretic treatment in young children with fever: acetaminophen, ibuprofen, or both alternating in a randomized, double-blind study. *Arch Pediatr Adolesc Med* **160**, 197-202 (2006).

310 Hudson, J. B. J. *et al.* Use of NSAIDs and acetaminophen and risk of spontaneous intestinal perforations in premature infants: a systematic review and meta-analysis. *Front Pediatr* **12**, 1450121 (2024).

311 Smith, C. & Goldman, R. D. Alternating acetaminophen and ibuprofen for pain in children. *Can Fam Physician* **58**, 645-647 (2012).

312 Saleh, E., Swamy, G. K., Moody, M. A. & Walter, E. B. Parental Approach to the Prevention and Management of Fever and Pain Following Childhood Immunizations: A Survey Study. *Clin Pediatr (Phila)* **56**, 435-442 (2017).

313 *Preventing pediatric medication errors*, (2021). https://www.jointcommission.org/-/media/tjc/documents/resources/patient-safety-topics/sentinel-event/sea-39-ped-med-errors-rev-final-4-14-21.pdf

314 Moore, N., Carleton, B., Blin, P., Bosco-Levy, P. & Droz, C. Does Ibuprofen Worsen COVID-19? *Drug Safety* **43**, 611-614 (2020). 315 Valenzuela, R. *et al.* Interactions between ibuprofen, ACE2, renin-angiotensin system, and spike protein in the lung. Implications for COVID-19. *Clin Transl Med* **11** (2021).

316 Rinott, E., Kozer, E., Shapira, Y., Bar-Haim, A. & Youngster, I. Ibuprofen use and clinical outcomes in COVID-19 patients. *Clin Microbiol Infec* **26** (2020).

317 Kragholm, K. *et al.* Association Between Prescribed Ibuprofen and Severe COVID-19 Infection: A Nationwide Register-Based Cohort Study. *Cts-Clin Transl Sci* **13**, 1103-1107 (2020).

318 Xie, J. *et al.* Risk of COVID-19 Diagnosis and Hospitalisation in Patients with Osteoarthritis or Back Pain Treated with Ibuprofen Compared to Other NSAIDs or Paracetamol: A Network Cohort Study. *Drugs* **83**, 249-263 (2023).

319 Drake, T. M. *et al.* Non-steroidal anti-inflammatory drug use and outcomes of COVID-19 in the ISARIC Clinical Characterisation Protocol UK cohort: a matched, prospective cohort study. *Lancet Rheumatol* **3**, e498-e506 (2021).

320 Althubaiti, A. Information bias in health research: definition, pitfalls, and adjustment methods. *J Multidiscip Healthc* **9**, 211-217 (2016).

321 Faber, J. & Fonseca, L. M. How sample size influences research outcomes. *Dental Press J Orthod* **19**, 27-29 (2014).

322 Kutti Sridharan, G. *et al.* COVID-19 and Avoiding Ibuprofen. How Good Is the Evidence? *Am J Ther* **27**, e400-e402 (2020).

323 Laughey, W. *et al.* Ibuprofen, other NSAIDs and COVID-19: a narrative review. *Inflammopharmacology* **31**, 2147-2159 (2023).

324 Kang, D. O. *et al.* Cardiovascular and Bleeding Risks Associated With Nonsteroidal Anti-Inflammatory Drugs After Myocardial Infarction. *J Am Coll Cardiol* **76**, 518-529 (2020).

325 Thai, P. N. *et al.* Chronic Diclofenac Exposure Increases Mitochondrial Oxidative Stress, Inflammatory Mediators, and Cardiac Dysfunction. *Cardiovasc Drugs Ther* **37**, 25-37 (2023).

326 Grosser, T., Fries, S. & FitzGerald, G. A. Biological basis for the cardiovascular consequences of COX-2 inhibition: therapeutic challenges and opportunities. *J Clin Invest* **116**, 4-15 (2006).

327 Patrono, C. & Baigent, C. Nonsteroidal anti-inflammatory drugs and the heart. *Circulation* **129**, 907-916 (2014).

328 Patrono, C. Cardiovascular effects of cyclooxygenase-2 inhibitors: a mechanistic and clinical perspective. *Br J Clin Pharmacol* **82**, 957-964 (2016).

329 Trelle, S. *et al.* Cardiovascular safety of non-steroidal anti-inflammatory drugs: network meta-analysis. *BMJ* **342**, c7086 (2011).

330 Kearney, P. M. *et al.* Do selective cyclo-oxygenase-2 inhibitors and traditional non-steroidal anti-inflammatory drugs increase the risk of atherothrombosis? Meta-analysis of randomised trials. *BMJ* **332**, 1302-1308 (2006).

331 Graham, D. J. *et al.* Risk of acute myocardial infarction and sudden cardiac death in patients treated with cyclo-oxygenase 2 selective and non-selective non-steroidal anti-inflammatory drugs: nested case-control study. *Lancet* **365**, 475-481 (2005).

332 Curfman, G. *FDA strengthens warning that NSAIDs increase heart attack and stroke risk*, https://www.health.harvard.edu/blog/fda-strengthens-warning-that-nsaids-increase-heart-attack-and-stroke-risk-201507138138 (2019).

333 Wong, M., Chowienczyk, P. & Kirkham, B. Cardiovascular issues of COX-2 inhibitors and NSAIDs. *Aust Fam Physician* **34**, 945-948 (2005).

334 *COX-2 Selective (includes Bextra, Celebrex, and Vioxx) and Non-Selective Non-Steroidal Anti-Inflammatory Drugs (NSAIDs)*, https://www.fda.gov/drugs/postmarket-drug-safety-information-patients-and-providers/cox-2-selective-includes-bextra-celebrex-and-vioxx-and-non-selective-non-steroidal-anti-inflammatory

335 FDA. FDA Drug Safety Communication: FDA strengthens warning that non-aspirin nonsteroidal anti-inflammatory drugs (NSAIDs) can cause heart attacks or strokes. (2015).

336 Ghosh, R., Alajbegovic, A. & Gomes, A. V. NSAIDs and Cardiovascular Diseases: Role of Reactive Oxygen Species. *Oxid Med Cell Longev* **2015**, 536962 (2015).

337 Mitchell, J. A. *et al.* Cyclooxygenases and the cardiovascular system. *Pharmacol Ther* **217**, 107624 (2021).

338 Ghosh, R., Hwang, S. M., Cui, Z., Gilda, J. E. & Gomes, A. V. Different effects of the nonsteroidal anti-inflammatory drugs meclofenamate sodium and naproxen sodium on proteasome activity in cardiac cells. *J Mol Cell Cardiol* **94**, 131-144 (2016).

339 Ghosh, R., Goswami, S. K., Feitoza, L., Hammock, B. & Gomes, A. V. Diclofenac induces proteasome and mitochondrial dysfunction in murine cardiomyocytes and hearts. *Int J Cardiol* **223**, 923-935 (2016).

340 Juan, C. A., Perez de la Lastra, J. M., Plou, F. J. & Perez-Lebena, E. The Chemistry of Reactive Oxygen Species (ROS) Revisited: Outlining Their Role in Biological Macromolecules (DNA, Lipids and Proteins) and Induced Pathologies. *Int J Mol Sci* **22** (2021).

341 Zhou, B. & Tian, R. Mitochondrial dysfunction in pathophysiology of heart failure. *J Clin Invest* **128**, 3716-3726 (2018).

342 Chen, Q., Wang, Q., Zhu, J., Xiao, Q. & Zhang, L. Reactive oxygen species: key regulators in vascular health and diseases. *Br J Pharmacol* **175**, 1279-1292 (2018).

343 Batty, M., Bennett, M. R. & Yu, E. The Role of Oxidative Stress in Atherosclerosis. *Cells* **11** (2022).

344 Schulz, E., Gori, T. & Munzel, T. Oxidative stress and endothelial dysfunction in hypertension. *Hypertens Res* **34**, 665-673 (2011).

345 Incalza, M. A. *et al.* Oxidative stress and reactive oxygen species in endothelial dysfunction associated with cardiovascular and metabolic diseases. *Vascul Pharmacol* **100**, 1-19 (2018).

346 Zhang, Q. *et al.* Signaling pathways and targeted therapy for myocardial infarction. *Signal Transduct Target Ther* **7**, 78 (2022).

347 Ross, J. M., Olson, L. & Coppotelli, G. Mitochondrial and Ubiquitin Proteasome System Dysfunction in Ageing and Disease: Two Sides of the Same Coin? *Int J Mol Sci* **16**, 19458-19476 (2015).

348 Rasheed Sule, Shuchita Tiwari, Gabriela Rivera, a. & Gomes, A. Ibuprofen causes mitochondrial and proteasome dysfunction in murine hearts. *American Physiological Society* **38** (2023).

349 Stepanova, A. *et al.* The dependence of brain mitochondria reactive oxygen species production on oxygen level is linear, except when inhibited by antimycin A. *J Neurochem* **148**, 731-745 (2019).

350 Maharjan, S., Oku, M., Tsuda, M., Hoseki, J. & Sakai, Y. Mitochondrial impairment triggers cytosolic oxidative stress and cell death following proteasome inhibition. *Sci Rep* **4**, 5896 (2014).

351 Aiken, C. T., Kaake, R. M., Wang, X. & Huang, L. Oxidative stress-mediated regulation of proteasome complexes. *Mol Cell Proteomics* **10**, R110 006924 (2011).

352 Driver, B., Marks, D. C. & van der Wal, D. E. Not all (N)SAID and done: Effects of nonsteroidal anti-inflammatory drugs and paracetamol intake on platelets. *Res Pract Thromb Haemost* **4**, 36-45 (2020).

353 Goldenberg, N. A., Jacobson, L. & Manco-Johnson, M. J. Brief communication: duration of platelet dysfunction after a 7-day course of Ibuprofen. *Ann Intern Med* **142**, 506-509 (2005).

354 Adler, Y. *et al.* 2015 ESC Guidelines for the diagnosis and management of pericardial diseases: The Task Force for the Diagnosis and Management of Pericardial Diseases of the European Society of Cardiology (ESC)Endorsed by: The European Association for Cardio-Thoracic Surgery (EACTS). *Eur Heart J* **36**, 2921-2964 (2015).

355 Eika, J. K. *et al.* Ibuprofen for Acute Pericarditis and Associated Cardiovascular Risks: A Danish Nationwide, Population-Based Cohort Study. *Clin Epidemiol* **16**, 793-802 (2024).

356 De Caterina, R., Ruigomez, A. & Rodriguez, L. A. Long-term use of anti-inflammatory drugs and risk of atrial fibrillation. *Arch Intern Med* **170**, 1450-1455 (2010).

357 Yang, Z. F. *et al.* Possible arrhythmiogenic mechanism produced by ibuprofen. *Acta Pharmacol Sin* **29**, 421-429 (2008).

358 Douglas, R. J. Palpitations following regular ibuprofen dosing in a 13-year-old girl: a case report. *J Med Case Rep* **4**, 76 (2010).

359 Ruppert, S., Vormberge, T., Igl, B. W. & Hoffmann, M. ECG telemetry in conscious guinea pigs. *J Pharmacol Toxicol Methods* **81**, 88-98 (2016).

360 Heist, E. K. & Ruskin, J. N. Drug-induced arrhythmia. *Circulation* **122**, 1426-1435 (2010).

361 Farkouh, M. E. *et al.* Cardiovascular outcomes in high risk patients with osteoarthritis treated with ibuprofen, naproxen or lumiracoxib. *Ann Rheum Dis* **66**, 764-770 (2007).

362 Radack, K. L., Deck, C. C. & Bloomfield, S. S. Ibuprofen interferes with the efficacy of antihypertensive drugs. A randomized, double-blind, placebo-controlled trial of ibuprofen compared with acetaminophen. *Ann Intern Med* **107**, 628-635 (1987).

363 Ruschitzka, F. *et al.* Differential blood pressure effects of ibuprofen, naproxen, and celecoxib in patients with arthritis: the PRECISION-ABPM (Prospective Randomized Evaluation of Celecoxib Integrated Safety Versus Ibuprofen or Naproxen Ambulatory Blood Pressure Measurement) Trial. *Eur Heart J* **38**, 3282-3292 (2017).

364 Salort-Llorca, C., Minguez-Serra, M. P. & Silvestre-Donat, F. J. Interactions between ibuprofen and antihypertensive drugs: incidence and clinical relevance in dental practice. *Med Oral Patol Oral Cir Bucal* **13**, E717-721 (2008).

365 Sondergaard, K. B. *et al.* Non-steroidal anti-inflammatory drug use is associated with increased risk of out-of-hospital cardiac arrest: a nationwide case-time-control study. *Eur Heart J Cardiovasc Pharmacother* **3**, 100-107 (2017).

366 Devarbhavi, H. *et al.* Global burden of liver disease: 2023 update. *J Hepatol* **79**, 516-537 (2023).

367 Asrani, S. K., Devarbhavi, H., Eaton, J. & Kamath, P. S. Burden of liver diseases in the world. *J Hepatol* **70**, 151-171 (2019).

368 Mayo_Clinic_Staff. *Liver Disease at Mayo Clinic* https://www.mayoclinic.org/diseases-conditions/liver-problems/symptoms-causes/syc-20374502

369 National_Institute_of_Diabetes_and_Digestive_and_Kidney_Diseases. Symptoms & Causes of Cirrhosis.

370 Francis, P. & Navarro, V. J. Drug-Induced Hepatotoxicity, in *StatPearls* (2024).

371 Sriuttha, P., Sirichanchuen, B. & Permsuwan, U. Hepatotoxicity of Nonsteroidal Anti-Inflammatory Drugs: A Systematic Review of Randomized Controlled Trials. *Int J Hepatol* **2018**, 5253623 (2018).

372 Zoubek, M. E., Lucena, M. I., Andrade, R. J. & Stephens, C. Systematic review: ibuprofen-induced liver injury. *Aliment Pharmacol Ther* **51**, 603-611 (2020).

373 Bjornsson, E. S. Drug-induced liver injury: an overview over the most critical compounds. *Arch Toxicol* **89**, 327-334 (2015).

374 Zoubek, M. E. *et al.* High Prevalence of Ibuprofen Drug-Induced Liver Injury in Spanish and Latin-American Registries. *Clin Gastroenterol Hepatol* **16**, 292-294 (2018).

375 Devarbhavi, H. *et al.* Single-center experience with drug-induced liver injury from India: causes, outcome, prognosis, and predictors of mortality. *Am J Gastroenterol* **105**, 2396-2404 (2010).

376 Escalera, Á. Common over-the-counter tablets in Spain now only available on prescription. (2022).

377 Chandok, N. & Watt, K. D. Pain management in the cirrhotic patient: the clinical challenge. *Mayo Clin Proc* **85**, 451-458 (2010).

378 Lee, C. Y. & Finkler, A. Acute intoxication due to ibuprofen overdose. *Arch Pathol Lab Med* **110**, 747-749 (1986).

379 Shahnazarian, V., Ramai, D. & Reddy, M. A Rare Case of Ibuprofen-induced Acute Liver Injury. *Cureus* **10**, e3225 (2018).

380 Laurent, S., Rahier, J., Geubel, A. P., Lerut, J. & Horsmans, Y. Subfulminant hepatitis requiring liver transplantation following ibuprofen overdose. *Liver* **20**, 93-94 (2000).

381 Tiwari, S. *et al.* Ibuprofen alters epoxide hydrolase activity and epoxy-oxylipin metabolites associated with different metabolic pathways in murine livers. *Sci Rep* **11**, 7042 (2021).

382 Cousins, K., Chen, C. C., Sehanobish, E. & Jerschow, E. The role of oxylipins in NSAID-exacerbated respiratory disease (N-ERD). *Adv Pharmacol* **97**, 423-444 (2023).

383 Schuck, R. N. *et al.* Cytochrome P450-derived eicosanoids and vascular dysfunction in coronary artery disease patients. *Atherosclerosis* **227**, 442-448 (2013).

384 Cho, C., Aliwarga, T., Wiley, A. M. & Totah, R. A. Cardioprotective mechanisms of cytochrome P450 derived oxylipins from omega-3 and omega-6 PUFAs. *Adv Pharmacol* **97**, 201-227 (2023).

385 Morisseau, C. *et al.* Relative Importance of Soluble and Microsomal Epoxide Hydrolases for the Hydrolysis of Epoxy-Fatty Acids in Human Tissues. *Int J Mol Sci* **22** (2021).

386 Morisseau, C. & Hammock, B. D. Impact of soluble epoxide hydrolase and epoxyeicosanoids on human health. *Annu Rev Pharmacol Toxicol* **53**, 37-58 (2013).

387 Walker, J. S. & Carmody, J. J. Experimental pain in healthy human subjects: gender differences in nociception and in response to ibuprofen. *Anesth Analg* **86**, 1257-1262 (1998).

388 Morgan, J. *et al.* Sex and gender differences in pain perception and management in clinical settings. *All Life* **17**, 2357421 (2024).

389 O'Gorman, D. M., O'Carroll, C. & Carmody, R. J. Evidence that marine-derived, multi-mineral, Aquamin inhibits the NF-kappaB signaling pathway in vitro. *Phytother Res* **26**, 630-632 (2012).

390 Ait Abdellah, S., Gal, C., Leblanc, A., Trouvin, A. P. & Perrot, S. Clusters of Responders and Predictive Factors for Response to Supplementation with Boswellia, Turmeric, and Red Algae Extracts in Painful Knee Osteoarthritis: A Prospective Observational Study Using an Arsenal of Patient-Centered Measures. *Open Access Rheumatol* **13**, 1-13 (2021).

391 Wu, D. & Cederbaum, A. I. Alcohol, oxidative stress, and free radical damage. *Alcohol Res Health* **27**, 277-284 (2003).

392 Kim, M., Lee, E. J. & Lim, K. M. Ibuprofen Increases the Hepatotoxicity of Ethanol through Potentiating Oxidative Stress. *Biomol Ther (Seoul)* **29**, 205-210 (2021).

393 Roujeau, J. C. & Stern, R. S. Severe adverse cutaneous reactions to drugs. *N Engl J Med* **331**, 1272-1285 (1994).

394 Gui, M. Z., Ni, M., Yin, X. D., Zhang, T. & Li, Z. L. Ibuprofen induced Stevens-Johnson syndrome and liver injury in children: a case report. *Transl Pediatr* **10**, 1737-1742 (2021).

395 Devarbhavi, H. *et al.* Drug-induced liver injury associated with Stevens-Johnson syndrome/toxic epidermal necrolysis: Patient characteristics, causes, and outcome in 36 cases. *Hepatology* **63**, 993-999 (2016).

396 *Ibuprofen*, (2018). https://www.ncbi.nlm.nih.gov/books/NBK547845/

397 Ogobuiro, I., Gonzales, J., Shumway, K. R. & Tuma, F. Physiology, Gastrointestinal, in *StatPearls* (2024).

398 Tai, F. W. D. & McAlindon, M. E. Non-steroidal anti-inflammatory drugs and the gastrointestinal tract. *Clin Med (Lond)* **21**, 131-134 (2021).

399 McEvoy, L., Carr, D. F. & Pirmohamed, M. Pharmacogenomics of NSAID-Induced Upper Gastrointestinal Toxicity. *Front Pharmacol* **12**, 684162 (2021).

400 Laine, L. GI risk and risk factors of NSAIDs. *J Cardiovasc Pharmacol* **47 Suppl 1**, S60-66 (2006).

401 Sostres, C., Gargallo, C. J. & Lanas, A. Nonsteroidal anti-inflammatory drugs and upper and lower gastrointestinal mucosal damage. *Arthritis Res Ther* **15 Suppl 3**, S3 (2013).

402 Jones, R. H. & Tait, C. L. Gastrointestinal side-effects of NSAIDs in the community. *Br J Clin Pract* **49**, 67-70 (1995).

403 Goddard, A. F., James, M. W., McIntyre, A. S., Scott, B. B. & British Society of, G. Guidelines for the management of iron deficiency anaemia. *Gut* **60**, 1309-1316 (2011).

404 *Gastritis*, (2024). https://www.mayoclinic.org/diseases-conditions/gastritis/symptoms-causes/syc-20355807#:~:text=Regular%20use%20of%20pain%20relievers,may%20damage%20the%20stomach%20lining

405 White, A., Litten, R. Z., Kwako, L. E. & Gardner, M. B. *Alcohol-Medication Interactions: Potentially Dangerous Mixes*, (2025). https://www.niaaa.nih.gov/health-professionals-communities/core-resource-on-alcohol/alcohol-medication-interactions-potentially-dangerous-mixes#:~:text=Nonsteroidal%20anti%2Dinflammatory%20drugs%20(NSAIDs,alcohol%20significantly%20increases%20the%20risk

406 Scheiman, J. M. The use of proton pump inhibitors in treating and preventing NSAID-induced mucosal damage. *Arthritis Res Ther* **15 Suppl 3**, S5 (2013).

407 van de Laar, M., Schofl, R., Prevoo, M. & Jastorff, J. Predictive value of gastrointestinal symptoms and patient risk factors for NSAID-associated gastrointestinal ulcers defined by endoscopy? Insights from a pooled analysis of two naproxen clinical trials. *PLoS One* **18**, e0284358 (2023).

408 Silverstein, F. E. *et al.* Gastrointestinal toxicity with celecoxib vs nonsteroidal anti-inflammatory drugs for osteoarthritis and rheumatoid arthritis: the CLASS study: A randomized controlled trial. Celecoxib Long-term Arthritis Safety Study. *JAMA* **284**, 1247-1255 (2000).

409 Watson, D. J. *et al.* Gastrointestinal tolerability of the selective cyclooxygenase-2 (COX-2) inhibitor rofecoxib compared with nonselective COX-1 and COX-2 inhibitors in osteoarthritis. *Arch Intern Med* **160**, 2998-3003 (2000).

410 Kaewput, W., Disorn, P. & Satirapoj, B. Selective cyclooxygenase-2 inhibitor use and progression of renal function in patients with chronic kidney disease: a single-center retrospective cohort study. *Int J Nephrol Renovasc Dis* **9**, 273-278 (2016).

411 Mukherjee, D., Nissen, S. E. & Topol, E. J. Risk of cardiovascular events associated with selective COX-2 inhibitors. *JAMA* **286**, 954-959 (2001).

412 Maseda, D. & Ricciotti, E. NSAID-Gut Microbiota Interactions. *Front Pharmacol* **11**, 1153 (2020).

413 Wang, X. *et al.* Gut Microbiota in NSAID Enteropathy: New Insights From Inside. *Front Cell Infect Microbiol* **11**, 679396 (2021).

414 Robert, A. & Asano, T. Resistance of germfree rats to indomethacin-induced intestinal lesions. *Prostaglandins* **14**, 333-341 (1977).

415 Rogers, M. A. M. & Aronoff, D. M. The influence of non-steroidal anti-inflammatory drugs on the gut microbiome. *Clin Microbiol Infect* **22**, 178 e171-178 e179 (2016).

416 Tang, Q. *et al.* Current Sampling Methods for Gut Microbiota: A Call for More Precise Devices. *Front Cell Infect Microbiol* **10**, 151 (2020).

417 Verhaegh, B. P. *et al.* High risk of drug-induced microscopic colitis with concomitant use of NSAIDs and proton pump inhibitors. *Aliment Pharmacol Ther* **43**, 1004-1013 (2016).

418 Bonderup, O. K., Nielsen, G. L., Dall, M., Pottegard, A. & Hallas, J. Significant association between the use of different proton pump inhibitors and microscopic colitis: a nationwide Danish case-control study. *Aliment Pharmacol Ther* **48**, 618-625 (2018).

419 Tarar, Z. I. *et al.* Are Drugs Associated with Microscopic Colitis? A Systematic Review and Meta-Analysis. *Diseases* **11** (2022).

420 Jaynes, M. & Kumar, A. B. The risks of long-term use of proton pump inhibitors: a critical review. *Ther Adv Drug Saf* **10**, 2042098618809927 (2019).

421 Hernandez-Diaz, S. & Rodriguez, L. A. Association between nonsteroidal anti-inflammatory drugs and upper gastrointestinal tract bleeding/perforation: an overview of epidemiologic studies published in the 1990s. *Arch Intern Med* **160**, 2093-2099 (2000).

422 Chi, T. Y., Zhu, H. M. & Zhang, M. Risk factors associated with nonsteroidal anti-inflammatory drugs (NSAIDs)-induced gastrointestinal bleeding resulting on people over 60 years old in Beijing. *Medicine (Baltimore)* **97**, e0665 (2018).

423 *Harmful Interactions. Mixing Alcohol With Medicines*, (2014). https://www.niaaa.nih.gov/publications/brochures-and-fact-sheets/harmful-interactions-mixing-alcohol-with-medicines

424 Al-Saeed, A. Gastrointestinal and Cardiovascular Risk of Nonsteroidal Anti-inflammatory Drugs. *Oman Med J* **26**, 385-391 (2011).

425 Hemarajata, P. & Versalovic, J. Effects of probiotics on gut microbiota: mechanisms of intestinal immunomodulation and neuromodulation. *Therap Adv Gastroenterol* **6**, 39-51 (2013).

426 *Nonsteroidal Anti-Inflammatory Drugs (NSAIDs)*, (2024). https://healthy.kaiserpermanente.org/health-wellness/health-encyclopedia/he.nonsteroidal-anti-inflammatory-drugs-nsaids.sid7998

427 Horl, W. H. Nonsteroidal Anti-Inflammatory Drugs and the Kidney. *Pharmaceuticals (Basel)* **3**, 2291-2321 (2010).

428 Gunaydin, C. & Bilge, S. S. Effects of Nonsteroidal Anti-Inflammatory Drugs at the Molecular Level. *Eurasian J Med* **50**, 116-121 (2018).

429 Bouck, Z. *et al.* Frequency and Associations of Prescription Nonsteroidal Anti-inflammatory Drug Use Among Patients With a Musculoskeletal Disorder and Hypertension, Heart Failure, or Chronic Kidney Disease. *JAMA Intern Med* **178**, 1516-1525 (2018).

430 Nelson, D. A., Marks, E. S., Deuster, P. A., O'Connor, F. G. & Kurina, L. M. Association of Nonsteroidal Anti-inflammatory Drug Prescriptions With Kidney Disease Among Active Young and Middle-aged Adults. *JAMA Netw Open* **2**, e187896 (2019).

431 Zhang, X., Donnan, P. T., Bell, S. & Guthrie, B. Non-steroidal anti-inflammatory drug induced acute kidney injury in the community dwelling general population and people with chronic kidney disease: systematic review and meta-analysis. *BMC Nephrol* **18**, 256 (2017).

432 Hsu, C. C. *et al.* Use of Nonsteroidal Anti-Inflammatory Drugs and Risk of Chronic Kidney Disease in Subjects With Hypertension: Nationwide Longitudinal Cohort Study. *Hypertension* **66**, 524-533 (2015).

433 Roche, C., Ragot, C., Moalic, J. L., Simon, F. & Oliver, M. Ibuprofen can induce syndrome of inappropriate diuresis in healthy young patients. *Case Rep Med* **2013**, 167267 (2013).

434 Su, L. *et al.* Association of Ibuprofen Prescription With Acute Kidney Injury Among Hospitalized Children in China. *JAMA Netw Open* **4**, e210775 (2021).

435 Brater, D. C. Renal effects of cyclooxygenase-2-selective inhibitors. *J Pain Symptom Manage* **23**, S15-20; discussion S21-13 (2002).

436 Dixit, M., Doan, T., Kirschner, R. & Dixit, N. Significant Acute Kidney Injury Due to Non-steroidal Anti-inflammatory Drugs: Inpatient Setting. *Pharmaceuticals (Basel)* **3**, 1279-1285 (2010).

437 Kim, G. H. Renal effects of prostaglandins and cyclooxygenase-2 inhibitors. *Electrolyte Blood Press* **6**, 35-41 (2008).

438 Chopra, S. & Kumar, D. Ibuprofen as an emerging organic contaminant in environment, distribution and remediation. *Heliyon* **6** (2020).

439 Heberer, T. Occurrence, fate, and removal of pharmaceutical residues in the aquatic environment: a review of recent research data. *Toxicol Lett* **131**, 5-17 (2002).

440 Pal, A., Gin, K. Y. H., Lin, A. Y. C. & Reinhard, M. Impacts of emerging organic contaminants on freshwater resources: Review of recent occurrences, sources, fate and effects. *Sci Total Environ* **408**, 6062-6069 (2010).

441 Ashfaq, M. *et al.* Ecological risk assessment of pharmaceuticals in the receiving environment of pharmaceutical wastewater in Pakistan. *Ecotox Environ Safe* **136**, 31-39 (2017).

442 Wu, C. X., Witter, J. D., Spongberg, A. L. & Czajkowski, K. P. Occurrence of selected pharmaceuticals in an agricultural landscape, western Lake Erie basin. *Water Res* **43**, 3407-3416 (2009).

443 Peng, X. Z. *et al.* Occurrence of steroid estrogens, endocrine-disrupting phenols, and acid pharmaceutical residues in urban riverine water of the Pearl River Delta, South China. *Sci Total Environ* **397**, 158-166 (2008).

444 Madikizela, L. M. & Chimuka, L. Occurrence of naproxen, ibuprofen, and diclofenac residues in wastewater and river water of KwaZulu-Natal Province in South Africa. *Environ Monit Assess* **189** (2017).

445 Luo, Y. L. *et al.* A review on the occurrence of micropollutants in the aquatic environment and their fate and removal during wastewater treatment. *Sci Total Environ* **473**, 619-641 (2014).

446 Buser, H. R., Poiger, T. & Muller, M. D. Occurrence and environmental behavior of the chiral pharmaceutical drug ibuprofen in surface waters and in wastewater. *Environ Sci Technol* **33**, 2529-2535 (1999).

447 Jan-Roblero, J. & Cruz-Maya, J. A. Ibuprofen: Toxicology and Biodegradation of an Emerging Contaminant. *Molecules* **28** (2023).

448 Placova, K., Halfar, J., Brozova, K., & Heviankova, S. Issues of Non-Steroidal Anti-Inflammatory Drugs in Aquatic Environments: A Review Study. *Engineering Proceedings* **57**, 13 (2023).

449 Pomati, F. *et al.* Effects of a complex mixture of therapeutic drugs at environmental levels on human embryonic cells. *Environ Sci Technol* **40**, 2442-2447 (2006).

450 Galus, M. *et al.* Chronic, low concentration exposure to pharmaceuticals impacts multiple organ systems in zebrafish. *Aquat Toxicol* **132**, 200-211 (2013).

451 Ogunwole, G. A. & Saliu, J. K. Seasonal Occurrence of Ibuprofen in Sediment, Water, and Biota in River Owena and Ogbese, and its Ecological Risk Assessment. *Annals of Science and Technology* **5**, 11-19 (2020).

452 Kristensen, D. M. *et al.* Ibuprofen alters human testicular physiology to produce a state of compensated hypogonadism (vol 115, pg E715, 2018). *P Natl Acad Sci USA* **115**, E4143-E4143 (2018).

453 Stocco, C. Tissue physiology and pathology of aromatase. *Steroids* **77**, 27-35 (2012).

454 Xia, L., Zheng, L. & Zhou, J. L. Effects of ibuprofen, diclofenac and paracetamol on hatch and motor behavior in developing zebrafish. *Chemosphere* **182**, 416-425 (2017).

455 De Lange, H. J., Noordoven, W., Murk, A. J., Lürling, M. & Peeters, E. T. H. M. Behavioural responses of (Crustacea, Amphipoda) to low concentrations of pharmaceuticals. *Aquat Toxicol* **78**, 209-216 (2006).

456 Ji, K. *et al.* Effects of non-steroidal anti-inflammatory drugs on hormones and genes of the hypothalamic-pituitary-gonad axis, and reproduction of zebrafish. *J Hazard Mater* **254**, 242-251 (2013).

457 Liu, S. *et al.* Shifts of bacterial community and molecular ecological network in activated sludge system under ibuprofen stress. *Chemosphere* **295**, 133888 (2022).

458 Ellepola, N. *et al.* A toxicological study on photo-degradation products of environmental ibuprofen: Ecological and human health implications. *Ecotoxicol Environ Saf* **188**, 109892 (2020).

459 Wijaya, L. *et al.* Ecotoxicological Effects of Ibuprofen on Plant Growth of Vigna unguiculata L. *Plants (Basel)* **9**, 1473 (2020).

460 He, Y. *et al.* Metabolism of Ibuprofen by Phragmites australis: Uptake and Phytodegradation. *Environ Sci Technol* **51**, 4576-4584 (2017).

461 Vellinga, A. *et al.* Public practice regarding disposal of unused medicines in Ireland. *Sci Total Environ* **478**, 98-102 (2014).

462 Kanyari, S. S., Senapati, T. R. & Kar, A. Disposal Practices of Unused and Expired Medicines Among the General Public and Pharmacies: A Mixed-Method Study in the Odisha State of Eastern India. *Cureus J Med Science* **16** (2024).

463 Toe, J., Orok, E. & Erah, P. Assessment of knowledge and disposal practices of unused and expired household medicines in a community in Liberia. *Explor Res Clin Soc* **12** (2023).

464 FDA. *Drug Disposal: Drug Take-Back Options*, (2024). https://www.fda.gov/drugs/disposal-unused-medicines-what-you-should-know/drug-disposal-drug-take-back-options

465 FDA. *Disposal of Unused Medicines: What You Should Know*, https://www.fda.gov/drugs/safe-disposal-medicines/disposal-unused-medicines-what-you-should-know

466 *National Prescription Drug Take Back Day*, https://www.deadiversion.usdoj.gov/drug_disposal/takeback/takeback.html

467 *Dispose Safely: Help prevent poisoning, misuse, and overdose*, https://safe.pharmacy/drug-disposal/

468 EPA. *Household Hazardous Waste (HHW)*,(2024). https://www.epa.gov/hw/household-hazardous-waste-hhw

469 *Ibuprofen*, (2023). https://medlineplus.gov/druginfo/meds/a682159.html

470 *Ibuprofen poisoning in dogs and cats*, (2023). https://www.pdsa.org.uk/pet-help-and-advice/pet-health-hub/conditions/ibuprofen-poisoning-in-dogs-and-cats

471 *PROPRINAL- ibuprofen tablet, sugar coated* (2025).

472 Enteric coating of ibuprofen tablets (200 mg) using an aqueous dispersion system. *Braz. J. Pharm. Sci.* **46**, 99-107 (2010).

473 Schulze, J. D. *et al.* Concentration-dependent effects of polyethylene glycol 400 on gastrointestinal transit and drug absorption. *Pharm Res* **20**, 1984-1988 (2003).

474 van Spronsen, F. J. *et al.* Phenylketonuria. *Nat Rev Dis Primers* **7**, 36 (2021).

475 *Tainted Arthritis / Pain Products*, (2024). https://www.fda.gov/drugs/medication-health-fraud/tainted-arthritis-pain-products

476 *Tapee Tea contains hidden drug ingredients*, (2023). https://www.fda.gov/drugs/medication-health-fraud/tapee-tea-contains-hidden-drug-ingredients

477 *Public Notification: Arth-Q Contains Hidden Drug Ingredient*, (2014). https://www.fda.gov/drugs/medication-health-fraud/public-notification-arth-q-contains-hidden-drug-ingredient

478 *Public Notification: Dream Body Extreme Gold contains hidden drug ingredients*, (2016). https://www.fda.gov/drugs/medication-health-fraud/public-notification-dream-body-extreme-gold-contains-hidden-drug-ingredients

479 Al-Waeli, H. *et al.* Chronotherapy of Non-Steroidal Anti-Inflammatory Drugs May Enhance Postoperative Recovery. *Sci Rep* **10**, 468 (2020).

480 Nuelle, J. A. V. *et al.* Effect of NSAID Use on Bone Healing in Pediatric Fractures: A Preliminary, Prospective, Randomized, Blinded Study. *J Pediatr Orthop* **40**, e683-e689 (2020).

481 Chuang, P. Y., Yang, T. Y., Tsai, Y. H. & Huang, K. C. Do NSAIDs affect bone healing rate, delay union, or cause non-union: an updated systematic review and meta-analysis. *Front Endocrinol (Lausanne)* **15**, 1428240 (2024).

482 Koenigsknecht, M. J. *et al.* In Vivo Dissolution and Systemic Absorption of Immediate Release Ibuprofen in Human Gastrointestinal Tract under Fed and Fasted Conditions. *Mol Pharm* **14**, 4295-4304 (2017).

483 Lee, J. H., Kuhar, S., Seo, J. H., Pasricha, P. J. & Mittal, R. Computational modeling of drug dissolution in the human stomach: Effects of posture and gastroparesis on drug bioavailability. *Phys Fluids (1994)* **34**, 081904 (2022).

484 Enthoven, W. T., Roelofs, P. D., Deyo, R. A., van Tulder, M. W. & Koes, B. W. Non-steroidal anti-inflammatory drugs for chronic low back pain. *Cochrane Database Syst Rev* **2**, CD012087 (2016).

485 Parisien, M. *et al.* Acute inflammatory response via neutrophil activation protects against the development of chronic pain. *Sci Transl Med* **14**, eabj9954 (2022).

486 Bjordal, J. M., Ljunggren, A. E., Klovning, A. & Slordal, L. Non-steroidal anti-inflammatory drugs, including cyclo-oxygenase-2 inhibitors, in osteoarthritic knee pain: meta-analysis of randomised placebo controlled trials. *BMJ* **329**, 1317 (2004).

487 Salis, Z. & Sainsbury, A. Association of long-term use of non-steroidal anti-inflammatory drugs with knee osteoarthritis: a prospective multi-cohort study over 4-to-5 years. *Sci Rep* **14**, 6593 (2024).

488 Wang, X. *et al.* Ibuprofen enhances recovery from spinal cord injury by limiting tissue loss and stimulating axonal growth. *J Neurotrauma* **26**, 81-95 (2009).

489 Zhou, Y. *et al.* Nonsteroidal anti-inflammatory drugs can lower amyloidogenic Abeta42 by inhibiting Rho. *Science* **302**, 1215-1217 (2003).

490 Lambrechts, M. J. & Cook, J. L. Nonsteroidal Anti-Inflammatory Drugs and Their Neuroprotective Role After an Acute Spinal Cord Injury: A Systematic Review of Animal Models. *Global Spine J* **11**, 365-377 (2021).

491 Meyer, H. C. Alopecia associated with ibuprofen. *JAMA* **242**, 142 (1979).

492 Hwang, J. H., Chu, H., Ahn, Y., Kim, J. & Kim, D. Y. HMGB1 promotes hair growth via the modulation of prostaglandin metabolism. *Sci Rep* **9**, 6660 (2019).

493 Shin, D. W. The physiological and pharmacological roles of prostaglandins in hair growth. *Korean J Physiol Pharmacol* **26**, 405-413 (2022).

494 Sciorati, C. *et al.* Co-administration of ibuprofen and nitric oxide is an effective experimental therapy for muscular dystrophy, with immediate applicability to humans. *Br J Pharmacol* **160**, 1550-1560 (2010).

495 Rigamonti, E. *et al.* Requirement of inducible nitric oxide synthase for skeletal muscle regeneration after acute damage. *J Immunol* **190**, 1767-1777 (2013).

496 Nair, A. B. & Jacob, S. A simple practice guide for dose conversion between animals and human. *J Basic Clin Pharm* **7**, 27-31 (2016).

497 Collier, A. F. *et al.* Effect of Ibuprofen on Skeletal Muscle of Dysferlin-Null Mice. *J Pharmacol Exp Ther* **364**, 409-419 (2018).

498 Curhan, S. G., Glicksman, J., Wang, M., Eavey, R. D. & Curhan, G. C. Longitudinal Study of Analgesic Use and Risk of Incident Persistent Tinnitus. *J Gen Intern Med* **37**, 3653-3662 (2022).

499 Dogan, S. *et al.* Assessment of pediatric patients with suspected nonsteroidal anti-inflammatory drug hypersensitivity. *Allergy Asthma Proc* **45**, e81-e86 (2024).

500 Sipahi Cimen, S. *et al.* Hypersensitivity to Ibuprofen: Real-Life Experience in Children with History of Suspected Immediate Reactions. *Int Arch Allergy Immunol* **184**, 33-42 (2023).

501 Boizet-Bonhoure, B., Dejardin, S., Rossitto, M., Poulat, F. & Philibert, P. Using Experimental Models to Decipher the Effects of Acetaminophen and NSAIDs on Reproductive Development and Health. *Front Toxicol* **4**, 835360 (2022).

502 Nezvalova-Henriksen, K., Spigset, O. & Nordeng, H. Effects of ibuprofen, diclofenac, naproxen, and piroxicam on the course of pregnancy and pregnancy outcome: a prospective cohort study. *BJOG* **120**, 948-959 (2013).

503 Sordillo, J. E. *et al.* Prenatal and infant exposure to acetaminophen and ibuprofen and the risk for wheeze and asthma in children. *J Allergy Clin Immunol* **135**, 441-448 (2015).

504 Petersen, T. G. *et al.* Use of paracetamol, ibuprofen or aspirin in pregnancy and risk of cerebral palsy in the child. *Int J Epidemiol* **47**, 121-130 (2018).

505 Rifas-Shiman, S. L. *et al.* Associations of prenatal or infant exposure to acetaminophen or ibuprofen with mid-childhood executive function and behaviour. *Paediatr Perinat Epidemiol* **34**, 287-298 (2020).

506 *FDA recommends avoiding use of NSAIDs in pregnancy at 20 weeks or later because they can result in low amniotic fluid*, (2020).

507 Li, D. K., Ferber, J. R., Odouli, R. & Quesenberry, C. Use of nonsteroidal antiinflammatory drugs during pregnancy and the risk of miscarriage. *Am J Obstet Gynecol* **219**, 275 e271-275 e278 (2018).

508 Mayoral Andrade, G. *et al.* Molecules and Prostaglandins Related to Embryo Tolerance. *Front Immunol* **11**, 555414 (2020).

509 Markovic, M. *et al.* Prenatal exposure to non-steroidal anti-inflammatory drugs (NSAIDs) and neurodevelopmental outcomes in children. *Pharmacoepidemiol Drug Saf* **28**, 452-459 (2019).

510 Kristensen, D. M. *et al.* Ibuprofen alters human testicular physiology to produce a state of compensated hypogonadism. *Proc Natl Acad Sci U S A* **115**, E715-E724 (2018).

511 Banihani, S. A. Effect of ibuprofen on semen quality. *Andrologia* **51**, e13228 (2019).

512 Pallangyo, P. *et al.* A community-based study on prevalence and correlates of erectile dysfunction among Kinondoni District Residents, Dar Es Salaam, Tanzania. *Reprod Health* **13**, 140 (2016).

513 Shiri, R. *et al.* Effect of nonsteroidal anti-inflammatory drug use on the incidence of erectile dysfunction. *J Urol* **175**, 1812-1815; discussion 1815-1816 (2006).

514 Vandivier, R. W. *et al.* Down-regulation of nitric oxide production by ibuprofen in human volunteers. *J Pharmacol Exp Ther* **289**, 1398-1403 (1999).

515 Patel, D. P. *et al.* Non-steroidal anti-inflammatory drug (NSAID) use is not associated with erectile dysfunction risk: results from the Prostate Cancer Prevention Trial. *BJU Int* **117**, 500-506 (2016).

516 Kujan, O. *et al.* An unusual side effect of Ibuprofen post dental therapy: increased erectile and libido activity. *J Int Oral Health* **6**, 94-95 (2014).

517 Murphy, P. J., Badia, P., Myers, B. L., Boecker, M. R. & Wright, K. P., Jr. Nonsteroidal anti-inflammatory drugs affect normal sleep patterns in humans. *Physiol Behav* **55**, 1063-1066 (1994).

518 Gengo, F. Effects of ibuprofen on sleep quality as measured using polysomnography and subjective measures in healthy adults. *Clin Ther* **28**, 1820-1826 (2006).

519 Hayaishi, O. Molecular mechanisms of sleep-wake regulation: roles of prostaglandins D2 and E2. *FASEB J* **5**, 2575-2581 (1991).

520 Browning, C. H. Nonsteroidal anti-inflammatory drugs and severe psychiatric side effects. *Int J Psychiatry Med* **26**, 25-34 (1996).

521 Fitton, R., Sweetman, J., Heseltine-Carp, W. & van der Feltz-Cornelis, C. Anti-inflammatory medications for the treatment of mental disorders: A scoping review. *Brain Behav Immun Health* **26**, 100518 (2022).

522 Kari, H., Nurminen, F., Ratto, H. & Koskinen, H. Non-dispensed prescriptions - A nationwide descriptive study. *Explor Res Clin Soc Pharm* **16**, 100541 (2024).

523 Wallum, M., Vakkalanka, J. P., Krispin, S. & McCabe, D. J. Risk of mortality among adolescents and young adults following hospitalization from an intentional overdose. *Am J Emerg Med* **88**, 140-144 (2024).

524 Fitzpatrick, D., Leckie, T., Heine, G. & Hodgson, L. The use of pain killers (NSAIDs) in athletes: How large is the risk? *J Sci Med Sport* (2024).

525 Stuart, M., Kwon, Y. I. & Rhie, S. J. Pharmacy services at the PyeongChang 2018 Olympic and Paralympic Winter Games. *Br J Sports Med* **53**, 1105-1110 (2019).

526 Kasashi, K. *et al.* The Tokyo 2020 Olympic and Paralympic pharmacy services during the COVID-19 pandemic. *J Am Pharm Assoc (2003)* **63**, 1156-1161 (2023).

527 Tscholl, P. M., Vaso, M., Weber, A. & Dvorak, J. High prevalence of medication use in professional football tournaments including the World Cups between 2002 and 2014: a narrative review with a focus on NSAIDs. *Br J Sports Med* **49**, 580-582 (2015).

528 Tso, J. *et al.* Nonsteroidal Anti-inflammatory Drugs and Cardiovascular Risk in American Football. *Med Sci Sports Exerc* **52**, 2522-2528 (2020).

529 Rudgard, W. E., Hirsch, C. A., Rosenbloom, C. & Cox, A. R. Amateur endurance athletes' use of non-steroidal anti-inflammatory drugs: a cross-sectional survey. *Int J Pharm Pract* **27**, 105-107 (2019).

530 Goldfarb, S. *Investigation of Non-Steroidal Anti-Inflammatory Drug (NSAID) Prevalence and Education in DIII College Athletes*, (2023). https://www.professionalpt.com/investigation-of-non-steroidal-anti-inflammatory-drug-nsaid-prevalence-and-education-in-diii-college-athletes/

531 Cohen, R. A. & Mykyta, L. *QuickStats: Percentage of Adults Aged ≥18 Years Who Took Prescription Medication During the Past 12 Months,† by Sex and Age Group — National Health Interview Survey, United States*, (2021, 2023).

532 Qiuping, G., Dillon, C. F. & Burt, V. L. Prescription Drug Use Continues to Increase: U.S. Prescription Drug Data for 2007-2008. *NCHS Data Brief* (2010).

533 Malhi, G. S., Tanious, M., Das, P. & Berk, M. The science and practice of lithium therapy. *Aust N Z J Psychiatry* **46**, 192-211 (2012).

534 Raza, S., Doumas, S. & Afzal, S. Lithium: Past, Present, and Future. *Psychiatric Times* **40** (2023).

535 Nunes, R. P. Lithium interactions with non-steroidal anti-inflammatory drugs and diuretics - A Review. *Archives of Clinical Psychiatry (Sao Paulo)* **45** (2018).

536 Ragheb, M. The clinical significance of lithium-nonsteroidal anti-inflammatory drug interactions. *J Clin Psychopharmacol* **10**, 350-354 (1990).

537 Ragheb, M. Ibuprofen can increase serum lithium level in lithium-treated patients. *J Clin Psychiatry* **48**, 161-163 (1987).

538 Hedya, S. A., Avula, A. & Swoboda, H. D. Lithium Toxicity, in *StatPearls* (2024).

539 Schulman, S. & Henriksson, K. Interaction of ibuprofen and warfarin on primary haemostasis. *Br J Rheumatol* **28**, 46-49 (1989).

540 Hamid, S. J. & Salih, T. Design, Synthesis, and Anti-Inflammatory Activity of Some Coumarin Schiff Base Derivatives: In silico and in vitro Study. *Drug Des Devel Ther* **16**, 2275-2288 (2022).

541 Loncar, M. *et al.* Coumarins in Food and Methods of Their Determination. *Foods* **9**, 645 (2020).

542 MacDonald, T. M. & Wei, L. Effect of ibuprofen on cardioprotective effect of aspirin. *Lancet* **361**, 573-574 (2003).

543 *How Ibuprofen (Advil; Motrin) Inhibits the Antithrombotic Activity of Aspirin*, (2015). https://www.ebmconsult.com/articles/how-does-ibuprofen-aspirin-drug-interaction-thrombotic-effect

544 Garcia Rodriguez, L. A. & Hernandez-Diaz, S. The risk of upper gastrointestinal complications associated with nonsteroidal anti-inflammatory drugs, glucocorticoids, acetaminophen, and combinations of these agents. *Arthritis Res* **3**, 98-101 (2001).

545 Grennan, D. M., Ferry, D. G., Ashworth, M. E., Kenny, R. E. & Mackinnon, M. The aspirin-ibuprofen interaction in rheumatoid arthritis. *Br J Clin Pharmacol* **8**, 497-503 (1979).

546 Garcia Rodriguez, L. A. & Jick, H. Risk of upper gastrointestinal bleeding and perforation associated with individual non-steroidal anti-inflammatory drugs. *Lancet* **343**, 769-772 (1994).

547 Leete, J., Wang, C., Lopez-Hernandez, F. J. & Layton, A. T. Determining risk factors for triple whammy acute kidney injury. *Math Biosci* **347**, 108809 (2022).

548 Greer, R. C. *et al.* Potassium-Enriched Salt Substitutes as a Means to Lower Blood Pressure: Benefits and Risks. *Hypertension* **75**, 266-274 (2020).

549 *How and when to take or use ibuprofen*, (2021). https://www.nhs.uk/medicines/ibuprofen-for-adults/how-and-when-to-take-ibuprofen/#:~:text=Take%20ibuprofen%20tablets%2C%20capsules%2C%20granules,take%20longer%20to%20start%20working

550 Moore, R. A., Derry, S., Wiffen, P. J. & Straube, S. Effects of food on pharmacokinetics of immediate release oral formulations of aspirin, dipyrone, paracetamol and NSAIDs - a systematic review. *Br J Clin Pharmacol* **80**, 381-388 (2015).

551 Golovachevam, V. A. & Golovacheva, A. A. B vitamins and nonsteroidal anti-inflammatory drugs: the efficacy of the combination for nonspecific back pain. *Nevrologiya, neiropsikhiatriya, psikhosomatika = Neurology, Neuropsychiatry, Psychosomatics* **12** (2020).

552 Kim, S. & Joo, K. W. Electrolyte and Acid-base disturbances associated with non-steroidal anti-inflammatory drugs. *Electrolyte Blood Press* **5**, 116-125 (2007).

553 Derry, S., Wiffen, P. J. & Moore, R. A. Single dose oral ibuprofen plus caffeine for acute postoperative pain in adults. *Cochrane Database Syst Rev* **2015**, CD011509 (2015).

554 Kondal, A. & Garg, S. K. Influence of acidic beverage (Coca-Cola) on pharmacokinetics of ibuprofen in healthy rabbits. *Indian J Exp Biol* **41**, 1322-1324 (2003).

555 Weiser, T., Schepers, C., Muck, T. & Lange, R. Pharmacokinetic Properties of Ibuprofen (IBU) From the Fixed-Dose Combination IBU/Caffeine (400/100 mg; FDC) in Comparison With 400 mg IBU as Acid or Lysinate Under Fasted and Fed Conditions-Data From 2 Single-Center, Single-Dose, Randomized Crossover Studies in Healthy Volunteers. *Clin Pharmacol Drug Dev* **8**, 742-753 (2019).

556 Abebe, W. Herbal medication: potential for adverse interactions with analgesic drugs. *J Clin Pharm Ther* **27**, 391-401 (2002).

557 Sun, C. K. & Tsai, T. H. Pharmacokinetic and pharmacodynamic herb-drug interactions of common over-the-counter pain medications. *Biomed Chromatogr* **37**, e5591 (2023).

558 Meisel, C., Johne, A. & Roots, I. Fatal intracerebral mass bleeding associated with Ginkgo biloba and ibuprofen. *Atherosclerosis* **167**, 367 (2003).

559 Bell, E. C., Ravis, W. R., Lloyd, K. B. & Stokes, T. J. Effects of St. John's wort supplementation on ibuprofen pharmacokinetics. *Ann Pharmacother* **41**, 229-234 (2007).

560 Bent, S., Goldberg, H., Padula, A. & Avins, A. L. Spontaneous bleeding associated with ginkgo biloba: a case report and systematic review of the literature: a case report and systematic review of the literature. *J Gen Intern Med* **20**, 657-661 (2005).

561 Marrone, C. M. Safety issues with herbal products. *Ann Pharmacother* **33**, 1359-1362 (1999).

562 Niu, J., Straubinger, R. M. & Mager, D. E. Pharmacodynamic Drug-Drug Interactions. *Clin Pharmacol Ther* **105**, 1395-1406 (2019).

563 Jiang, H. *et al.* Adverse drug reactions and correlations with drug-drug interactions: A retrospective study of reports from 2011 to 2020. *Front Pharmacol* **13**, 923939 (2022).

564 *Ibuprofen Interactions*, https://www.drugs.com/drug-interactions/ibuprofen.html

565 Kraus, V. B. *et al.* Effects of Physical Activity in Knee and Hip Osteoarthritis: A Systematic Umbrella Review. *Med Sci Sports Exerc* **51**, 1324-1339 (2019).

566 Veronese, N., Ragusa, F. S., Dominguez, L. J., Cusumano, C. & Barbagallo, M. Mediterranean diet and osteoarthritis: an update. *Aging Clin Exp Res* **36**, 231 (2024).

567 Babyak, M. *et al.* Exercise treatment for major depression: maintenance of therapeutic benefit at 10 months. *Psychosom Med* **62**, 633-638 (2000).

568 *Can diet heal chronic pain?*, (2021). https://www.health.harvard.edu/pain/can-diet-heal-chronic-pain

569 Geneen, L. J. *et al.* Physical activity and exercise for chronic pain in adults: an overview of Cochrane Reviews. *Cochrane Database Syst Rev* **4**, CD011279 (2017).

570 Ambrose, K. R. & Golightly, Y. M. Physical exercise as non-pharmacological treatment of chronic pain: Why and when. *Best Pract Res Clin Rheumatol* **29**, 120-130 (2015).

571 Skou, S. T., Pedersen, B. K., Abbott, J. H., Patterson, B. & Barton, C. Physical Activity and Exercise Therapy Benefit More Than Just Symptoms and Impairments in People With Hip and Knee Osteoarthritis. *J Orthop Sports Phys Ther* **48**, 439-447 (2018).

572 Zhao, Y. Editorial: Exercise and chronic disease. *Front Public Health* **12**, 1375156 (2024).

573 Heijnen, S., Hommel, B., Kibele, A. & Colzato, L. S. Neuromodulation of Aerobic Exercise-A Review. *Front Psychol* **6**, 1890 (2015).

574 Peterson, M. D., Rhea, M. R. & Alvar, B. A. Applications of the dose-response for muscular strength development: a review of meta-analytic efficacy and reliability for designing training prescription. *J Strength Cond Res* **19**, 950-958 (2005).

575 Behm, D. G. & Chaouachi, A. A review of the acute effects of static and dynamic stretching on performance. *Eur J Appl Physiol* **111**, 2633-2651 (2011).

576 Huang, H., Wolf, S. L. & He, J. Recent developments in biofeedback for neuromotor rehabilitation. *J Neuroeng Rehabil* **3**, 11 (2006).

577 Katzman, W. B. *et al.* Targeted spine strengthening exercise and posture training program to reduce hyperkyphosis in older adults: results from the study of hyperkyphosis, exercise, and function (SHEAF) randomized controlled trial. *Osteoporos Int* **28**, 2831-2841 (2017).

578 Alnawwar, M. A. *et al.* The Effect of Physical Activity on Sleep Quality and Sleep Disorder: A Systematic Review. *Cureus* **15**, e43595 (2023).

579 Finan, P. H., Goodin, B. R. & Smith, M. T. The association of sleep and pain: an update and a path forward. *J Pain* **14**, 1539-1552 (2013).

580 Runge, N. *et al.* The bidirectional relationship between sleep problems and chronic musculoskeletal pain: a systematic review with meta-analysis. *Pain* **165**, 2455-2467 (2024).

581 *Global recommendations on physical activity for health*, (2010). https://www.who.int/publications/i/item/9789241599979

582 Fransen, M. *et al.* Exercise for osteoarthritis of the knee: a Cochrane systematic review. *Br J Sports Med* **49**, 1554-1557 (2015).

583 Bull, F. C. *et al.* World Health Organization 2020 guidelines on physical activity and sedentary behaviour. *Br J Sports Med* **54**, 1451-1462 (2020).

584 Wu, M. *et al.* Potential mechanisms of exercise for relieving inflammatory pain: a literature review of animal studies. *Front Aging Neurosci* **16**, 1359455 (2024).

585 Harris, P. L. The future of vascular surgery. *Br J Surg* **80**, 943-944 (1993).

586 Mousavi-Shirazi-Fard, Z., Mazloom, Z., Izadi, S. & Fararouei, M. The effects of modified anti-inflammatory diet on fatigue, quality of life, and inflammatory biomarkers in relapsing-remitting multiple sclerosis patients: a randomized clinical trial. *Int J Neurosci* **131**, 657-665 (2021).

587 Buck, A. N. *et al.* Evidence-Based Dietary Practices to Improve Osteoarthritis Symptoms: An Umbrella Review. *Nutrients* **15** (2023).

588 Itsiopoulos, C., Mayr, H. L. & Thomas, C. J. The anti-inflammatory effects of a Mediterranean diet: a review. *Curr Opin Clin Nutr Metab Care* **25**, 415-422 (2022).

589 Aleksandrova, K., Koelman, L. & Rodrigues, C. E. Dietary patterns and biomarkers of oxidative stress and inflammation: A systematic review of observational and intervention studies. *Redox Biol* **42**, 101869 (2021).

590 Thomas, M. S., Calle, M. & Fernandez, M. L. Healthy plant-based diets improve dyslipidemias, insulin resistance, and inflammation in metabolic syndrome. A narrative review. *Adv Nutr* **14**, 44-54 (2023).

591 Gunes-Bayir, A., Mendes, B. & Dadak, A. The Integral Role of Diets Including Natural Products to Manage Rheumatoid Arthritis: A Narrative Review. *Curr Issues Mol Biol* **45**, 5373-5388 (2023).

592 Scotece, M. *et al.* New drugs from ancient natural foods. Oleocanthal, the natural occurring spicy compound of olive oil: a brief history. *Drug Discov Today* **20**, 406-410 (2015).

593 Tessier, A. J. *et al.* Consumption of Olive Oil and Diet Quality and Risk of Dementia-Related Death. *JAMA Netw Open* **7**, e2410021 (2024).

594 Cusimano, A. *et al.* Oleocanthal exerts antitumor effects on human liver and colon cancer cells through ROS generation. *Int J Oncol* **51**, 533-544 (2017).

595 Khaki Vaighan, M. *et al.* Ameliorative Effects of Ginger on Allergic Diseases: An Updated Review. *Mol Nutr Food Res* **68**, e2300899 (2024).

596 Mathieu, S. *et al.* A Meta-Analysis of the Impact of Nutritional Supplementation on Osteoarthritis Symptoms. *Nutrients* **14** (2022).

597 Zahedi, E. *et al.* Ginger Extract Improves Cognitive Dysfunction via Modulation of Gut Microbiota-Derived Short-Chain Fatty Acids in D-Galactose/Ovariectomy-Induced Alzheimer-Like Disease. *Mol Neurobiol* (2024).

598 Yang, C. S., Lambert, J. D. & Sang, S. Antioxidative and anti-carcinogenic activities of tea polyphenols. *Arch Toxicol* **83**, 11-21 (2009).

599 Hashempur, M. H., Sadrneshin, S., Mosavat, S. H. & Ashraf, A. Green tea (Camellia sinensis) for patients with knee osteoarthritis: A randomized open-label active-controlled clinical trial. *Clin Nutr* **37**, 85-90 (2018).

600 Ma, X., Zhao, W., Yang, F. & Chin, K. Y. Efficacy and mechanisms of curcumin in the treatment of osteoarthritis: A scoping review. *Biomol Biomed* (2024).

601 Dubey, V., Kheni, D. & Sureja, V. Efficacy evaluation of standardized Boswellia serrata extract (Aflapin(®)) in osteoarthritis: A systematic review and sub-group meta-analysis study. *Explore (NY)* **20**, 102983 (2024).

602 Steptoe, A. & Kivimaki, M. Stress and cardiovascular disease: an update on current knowledge. *Annu Rev Public Health* **34**, 337-354 (2013).

603 Leigh, S. J. *et al.* The impact of acute and chronic stress on gastrointestinal physiology and function: a microbiota-gut-brain axis perspective. *J Physiol* **601**, 4491-4538 (2023).

604 Fischer, S. *et al.* Stress exacerbates pain in the everyday lives of women with fibromyalgia syndrome–The role of cortisol and alpha-amylase. *Psychoneuroendocrinology* **63**, 68-77 (2016).

605 Worku, B., Alishetti, S. & Ramasubbu, K. Stress kills. *J Card Surg* **36**, 770-771 (2021).

606 Gu, Q., Hou, J. C. & Fang, X. M. Mindfulness Meditation for Primary Headache Pain: A Meta-Analysis. *Chin Med J (Engl)* **131**, 829-838 (2018).

607 Petrucci, G. *et al.* Psychological Approaches for the Integrative Care of Chronic Low Back Pain: A Systematic Review and Metanalysis. *Int J Environ Res Public Health* **19** (2021).

608 Russell, G. & Lightman, S. The human stress response. *Nat Rev Endocrinol* **15**, 525-534 (2019).

609 Adler-Neal, A. L. *et al.* The Role of Heart Rate Variability in Mindfulness-Based Pain Relief. *J Pain* **21**, 306-323 (2020).

610 Wipplinger, F. *et al.* Meditation as an Adjunct to the Management of Acute Pain. *Curr Pain Headache Rep* **27**, 209-216 (2023).

611 Zeidan, F. *et al.* Brain mechanisms supporting the modulation of pain by mindfulness meditation. *J Neurosci* **31**, 5540-5548 (2011).

612 Zeidan, F., Grant, J. A., Brown, C. A., McHaffie, J. G. & Coghill, R. C. Mindfulness meditation-related pain relief: evidence for unique brain mechanisms in the regulation of pain. *Neurosci Lett* **520**, 165-173 (2012).

613 Hilton, L. *et al.* Mindfulness Meditation for Chronic Pain: Systematic Review and Meta-analysis. *Ann Behav Med* **51**, 199-213 (2017).

614 Paschali, M. *et al.* Mindfulness-based Interventions for Chronic Low Back Pain: A Systematic Review and Meta-analysis. *Clin J Pain* **40**, 105-113 (2024).

615 Adler-Neal, A. L. & Zeidan, F. Mindfulness Meditation for Fibromyalgia: Mechanistic and Clinical Considerations. *Curr Rheumatol Rep* **19**, 59 (2017).

616 Zeidan, F. & Vago, D. R. Mindfulness meditation-based pain relief: a mechanistic account. *Ann N Y Acad Sci* **1373**, 114-127 (2016).

617 *Mindfulness Techniques For Pain Management*, https://www.physio-pedia.com/Mindfulness_Techniques_For_Pain_Management

618 Ma, X. *et al.* The Effect of Diaphragmatic Breathing on Attention, Negative Affect and Stress in Healthy Adults. *Front Psychol* **8**, 874 (2017).

619 Brandel, M. G. *et al.* Mindfulness Meditation in the Treatment of Chronic Pain. *Neurosurg Clin N Am* **33**, 275-279 (2022).

620 Connolly, D. A., McHugh, M. P., Padilla-Zakour, O. I., Carlson, L. & Sayers, S. P. Efficacy of a tart cherry juice blend in preventing the symptoms of muscle damage. *Br J Sports Med* **40**, 679-683; discussion 683 (2006).

621 Kuehl, K. S., Perrier, E. T., Elliot, D. L. & Chesnutt, J. C. Efficacy of tart cherry juice in reducing muscle pain during running: a randomized controlled trial. *J Int Soc Sports Nutr* **7**, 17 (2010).

622 Hooper, D. R. *et al.* Broad Spectrum Polyphenol Supplementation from Tart Cherry Extract on Markers of Recovery from Intense Resistance Exercise. *J Int Soc Sports Nutr* **18**, 47 (2021).

623 Chai, S. C., Jerusik, J., Davis, K., Wright, R. S. & Zhang, Z. Effect of Montmorency tart cherry juice on cognitive performance in older adults: a randomized controlled trial. *Food Funct* **10**, 4423-4431 (2019).

624 Martin, K. R. & Coles, K. M. Consumption of 100% Tart Cherry Juice Reduces Serum Urate in Overweight and Obese Adults. *Curr Dev Nutr* **3**, nzz011 (2019).

625 *Tart Cherry - Uses, Side Effects, and More* (2024). https://www.webmd.com/vitamins/ai/ingredientmono-771/tart-cherry

626 Kelley, D. S., Rasooly, R., Jacob, R. A., Kader, A. A. & Mackey, B. E. Consumption of Bing sweet cherries lowers circulating concentrations of inflammation markers in healthy men and women. *J Nutr* **136**, 981-986 (2006).

627 Seeram, N. P., Momin, R. A., Nair, M. G. & Bourquin, L. D. Cyclooxygenase inhibitory and antioxidant cyanidin glycosides in cherries and berries. *Phytomedicine* **8**, 362-369 (2001).

628 Zhang, Y. *et al.* Cherry consumption and decreased risk of recurrent gout attacks. *Arthritis Rheum* **64**, 4004-4011 (2012).

629 Collins, M. W., Saag, K. G. & Singh, J. A. Is there a role for cherries in the management of gout? *Ther Adv Musculoskelet Dis* **11**, 1759720X19847018 (2019).

630 Laurindo, L. F. *et al.* Acai (Euterpe oleracea Mart.) in Health and Disease: A Critical Review. *Nutrients* **15** (2023).

631 Kim, H. *et al.* Acai (Euterpe oleracea Mart.) beverage consumption improves biomarkers for inflammation but not glucose- or lipid-metabolism in individuals with metabolic

syndrome in a randomized, double-blinded, placebo-controlled clinical trial. *Food Funct* **9**, 3097-3103 (2018).

632 Kolehmainen, M. *et al.* Bilberries reduce low-grade inflammation in individuals with features of metabolic syndrome. *Mol Nutr Food Res* **56**, 1501-1510 (2012).

633 McAnulty, L. S. *et al.* Effect of blueberry ingestion on natural killer cell counts, oxidative stress, and inflammation prior to and after 2.5 h of running. *Appl Physiol Nutr Metab* **36**, 976-984 (2011).

634 Sarikaya, B., Kolay, E., Guney-Coskun, M., Yigit-Ziolkowski, A. & Aktac, S. The Effect of Black Chokeberry (Aronia melanocarpa) on Human Inflammation Biomarkers and Antioxidant Enzymes: A Systematic Review of Randomized Controlled Trials. *Nutr Rev* 83,1083-1098 (2025).

635 Hernandez, C. A., Nicolas, J. C., Fernandez, J. & Pizarro, P. Determination of plasma trypsin-like activity in healthy subjects, patients with mild to moderate alcoholic chronic pancreatitis, and patients with nonjaundice pancreatic cancer. *Dig Dis Sci* **50**, 2165-2169 (2005).

636 Mohseni, S. *et al.* Curcumin for the clinical treatment of inflammatory bowel diseases: a systematic review and meta-analysis of placebo-controlled randomized clinical trials. *Front Nutr* **12**, 1494351 (2025).

637 Mali, A. M., Behal, R. & Gilda, S. S. Comparative evaluation of 0.1% turmeric mouthwash with 0.2% chlorhexidine gluconate in prevention of plaque and gingivitis: A clinical and microbiological study. *J Indian Soc Periodontol* **16**, 386-391 (2012).

638 Bai, K. Y. *et al.* 12-week curcumin supplementation may relieve postexercise muscle fatigue in adolescent athletes. *Front Nutr* **9**, 1078108 (2022).

639 Siddiqui, M. Z. Boswellia serrata, a potential antiinflammatory agent: an overview. *Indian J Pharm Sci* **73**, 255-261 (2011).

640 Ammon, H. P. Boswellic Acids and Their Role in Chronic Inflammatory Diseases. *Adv Exp Med Biol* **928**, 291-327 (2016).

641 Yu, G. *et al.* Effectiveness of Boswellia and Boswellia extract for osteoarthritis patients: a systematic review and meta-analysis. *BMC Complement Med Ther* **20**, 225 (2020).

642 Monteiro, E. M. *et al.* Antinociceptive and anti-inflammatory activities of the sesame oil and sesamin. *Nutrients* **6**, 1931-1944 (2014).

643 Helli, B., Shahi, M. M., Mowla, K., Jalali, M. T. & Haghighian, H. K. A randomized, triple-blind, placebo-controlled clinical trial, evaluating the sesamin supplement effects on proteolytic enzymes, inflammatory markers, and clinical indices in women with rheumatoid arthritis. *Phytother Res* **33**, 2421-2428 (2019).

644 Gholami, M. *et al.* Effects of Topical Sesame Oil Extracted from Tahini (Ardeh) on Pain Severity in Trauma Patients: A Randomized Double-Blinded Placebo-Controlled Clinical Trial. *Bull Emerg Trauma* **8**, 179-185 (2020).

645 O'Gorman, D. M., Tierney, C. M., Brennan, O. & O'Brien, F. J. The marine-derived, multi-mineral formula, Aquamin, enhances mineralisation of osteoblast cells in vitro. *Phytother Res* **26**, 375-380 (2012).

646 Frestedt, J. L., Walsh, M., Kuskowski, M. A. & Zenk, J. L. A natural mineral supplement provides relief from knee osteoarthritis symptoms: a randomized controlled pilot trial. *Nutr J* **7**, 9 (2008).

647 Frestedt, J. L., Kuskowski, M. A. & Zenk, J. L. A natural seaweed derived mineral supplement (Aquamin F) for knee osteoarthritis: a randomised, placebo controlled pilot study. *Nutr J* **8**, 7 (2009).

648 Malhotra, R. Understanding migraine: Potential role of neurogenic inflammation. *Ann Indian Acad Neurol* **19**, 175-182 (2016).

649 Cohen, F. *et al.* Prevalence and burden of migraine in the United States: A systematic review. *Headache* **64**, 516-532 (2024).

650 *Economic Impact of Migraines*, (2020). https://www.ajmc.com/view/economic-impact-of-migraines

651 Sasannejad, P. *et al.* Lavender essential oil in the treatment of migraine headache: a placebo-controlled clinical trial. *Eur Neurol* **67**, 288-291 (2012).

652 Rodenak-Kladniew, B., Castro, M. A., Crespo, R., Galle, M. & Garcia de Bravo, M. Anti-cancer mechanisms of linalool and 1,8-cineole in non-small cell lung cancer A549 cells. *Heliyon* **6**, e05639 (2020).

653 Ahmadifard, M. *et al.* The Efficacy of Topical Basil Essential Oil on Relieving Migraine Headaches: A Randomized Triple-Blind Study. *Complement Med Res* **27**, 310-318 (2020).

654 Maghbooli, M., Golipour, F., Moghimi Esfandabadi, A. & Yousefi, M. Comparison between the efficacy of ginger and sumatriptan in the ablative treatment of the common migraine. *Phytother Res* **28**, 412-415 (2014).

655 Martins, L. B. *et al.* Double-blind placebo-controlled randomized clinical trial of ginger (Zingiber officinale Rosc.) addition in migraine acute treatment. *Cephalalgia* **39**, 68-76 (2019).

656 Rudrappa, G. H., Chakravarthi, P. T. & Benny, I. R. Efficacy of high-dissolution turmeric-sesame formulation for pain relief in adult subjects with acute musculoskeletal pain compared to acetaminophen: A randomized controlled study. *Medicine (Baltimore)* **99**, e20373 (2020).

657 Chen, T. *et al.* Cooling Blankets in Hospitalized Patients: Time to Reevaluate. *Am J Med Sci* **362**, 601-605 (2021).

658 *Global ibuprofen market size, share, trends, global growth & forecast. Straits Research*, (2023).

659 Derry, S., Karlin, S. M. & Moore, R. A. Single dose oral ibuprofen plus codeine for acute postoperative pain in adults. *Cochrane Database Syst Rev* **2015**, CD010107 (2015).

660 Panbachi, S., Beranek, J. & Kuentz, M. Abiraterone acetate fixed-dosed combinations with ibuprofen-based therapeutic eutectic and deep eutectic solvents. *Int J Pharm* **671**, 125279 (2025).

661 Qi, Q. M. & Mitragotri, S. Mechanistic study of transdermal delivery of macromolecules assisted by ionic liquids. *J Control Release* **311-312**, 162-169 (2019).

662 Boscariol, R., Oliveira Junior, J. M., Baldo, D. A., Balcao, V. M. & Vila, M. Transdermal permeation of curcumin promoted by choline geranate ionic liquid: Potential for the treatment of skin diseases. *Saudi Pharm J* **30**, 382-397 (2022).

663 Gholizadeh, H. *et al.* Smart thermosensitive chitosan hydrogel for nasal delivery of ibuprofen to treat neurological disorders. *Expert Opin Drug Deliv* **16**, 453-466 (2019).

664 Yenigun, V. B., Yenigun, A., Sagiroglu, A. A., Kocyigit, A. & Ozturan, O. Formulation of nasal analgesic sprays with diclofenac sodium, ibuprofen, paracetamol, and evaluation of in vitro toxicity. *Sci Prog* **107**, 368504241304200 (2024).

665 Anjani, Q. K., Sabri, A. H. B., Utomo, E., Dominguez-Robles, J. & Donnelly, R. F. Elucidating the Impact of Surfactants on the Performance of Dissolving Microneedle Array Patches. *Mol Pharm* **19**, 1191-1208 (2022).

666 Sandoval-Acuna, C., Lopez-Alarcon, C., Aliaga, M. E. & Speisky, H. Inhibition of mitochondrial complex I by various non-steroidal anti-inflammatory drugs and its protection by quercetin via a coenzyme Q-like action. *Chem Biol Interact* **199**, 18-28 (2012).

667 Chen, X. *et al.* Vascular and pulmonary effects of ibuprofen on neonatal lung development. *Respir Res* **24**, 39 (2023).

668 Casmir, O. E., Chiazor, U. P., Eze, E. C. & al, e. The protective role of α-tocopherol, vitamin C and quercetin against ibuprofen-induced liver damage in male Wistar rats. *GSC Biological and Pharmaceutical Sciences,* **24**, 170–184 (2023).

669 Laine, L. *et al.* Double-blind randomized trials of single-tablet ibuprofen/high-dose famotidine vs. ibuprofen alone for reduction of gastric and duodenal ulcers. *Am J Gastroenterol* **107**, 379-386 (2012).

670 Gholami, M. *et al.* Radioprotective Effects of Vitamin C, Cimetidine, and Famotidine on Lipid Peroxidase and Hepatic Glutathione Levels in Mouse Liver. *Int J Cell Biol* **2025**, 1106920 (2025).

671 Agundez, J. A. G. *et al.* Editorial: NSAIDs Pharmacogenomics. *Front Pharmacol* **12**, 798447 (2021).

672 do Couto, M. L. F., Fonseca, S. & Pozza, D. H. Pharmacogenetic Approaches in Personalized Medicine for Postoperative Pain Management. *Biomedicines* **12** (2024).

673 Bagher, A. M. Association of CYP2C9 *3 and CYP2C8 *3 Non-Functional Alleles with Ibuprofen-Induced Upper Gastrointestinal Toxicity in a Saudi Patient. *Case Rep Med* **2023**, 6623269 (2023).

674 Zajic, S. C. *et al.* Individuals with CYP2C8 and CYP2C9 reduced metabolism haplotypes self-adjusted ibuprofen dose in the Coriell Personalized Medicine Collaborative. *Pharmacogenet Genomics* **29**, 49-57 (2019).

675 Acetti, D., Brenna, E., Fronza, G. & Fuganti, C. Monitoring the synthetic procedures of commercial drugs by H NMR spectroscopy:: The case of ibuprofen and naproxen. *Talanta* **76**, 651-655 (2008).

676 Ha, M. W. & Paek, S. M. Recent Advances in the Synthesis of Ibuprofen and Naproxen. *Molecules* **26** (2021).

677 Agee, B. M., Mullins, G. & Swartling, D.J. Progress towards a more sustainable synthetic pathway to ibuprofen through the use of solar heating. *Sustain Chem Process* **4** (2016).

https://sustainablechemicalprocesses.springeropen.com/articles/10.1186/s40508-016-0052-y

678 *A behind-the-scenes tour of BASF's ibuprofen plant in Bishop, Texas*, (2021). https://pharma.basf.com/learning-center/videos/watch/a-behind-the-scenes-tour-of-basfs-ibuprofen-plant-in-bishop-texas

679 Bodach, A. *et al.* Scalability of Pharmaceutical Co-Crystal Formation by Mechanochemistry in Batch. *ChemSusChem* **17**, e202301220 (2024).

680 Thakur, S. *et al.* Novel drug delivery systems for NSAIDs in management of rheumatoid arthritis: An overview. *Biomed Pharmacother* **106**, 1011-1023 (2018).

681 Myburgh, J., Liebenberg, W., Willers, C., Dube, A. & Gerber, M. Investigation and Evaluation of the Transdermal Delivery of Ibuprofen in Various Characterized Nano-Drug Delivery Systems. *Pharmaceutics* **15** (2023).

682 Khan, D. *et al.* Development of an intelligent, stimuli-responsive transdermal system for efficient delivery of Ibuprofen against rheumatoid arthritis. *Int J Pharmaceut* **610** (2021).

683 Khan, S. & Minhas, M. U. Microarray patch assisted transdermal delivery of high dose, ibuprofen sodium using thermoresponsive sodium alginate/poly (vinylcaprolactam) in situ gels depot. *Int J Biol Macromol* **252** (2023).

684 Duan, Y. *et al.* A brief review on solid lipid nanoparticles: part and parcel of contemporary drug delivery systems. *RSC Adv* **10**, 26777-26791 (2020).

685 Miranda, G. M. *et al.* Inclusion Complexes of Non-Steroidal Anti-Inflammatory Drugs with Cyclodextrins: A Systematic Review. *Biomolecules* **11** (2021).

686 Perehudoff, K. Universal access to essential medicines as part of the right to health: a cross-national comparison of national laws, medicines policies, and health system indicators. *Global Health Action* **13** (2020). *USDAnalytics*, (2024). https://www.usdanalytics.com/industry-reports/ibuprofen-market

688 Safe and Effective Medicines for Children: Pediatric Studies Conducted Under the Best Pharmaceuticals for Children Act and the Pediatric Research Equity Act, (2012). https://www.ncbi.nlm.nih.gov/books/NBK202037/

689 Carvalho, A. S. *et al.* Ethical decision making in pain management: a conceptual framework. *J Pain Res* **11**, 967-976 (2018).

690 Limbu, Y. B. & Huhmann, B. A. Ethical Issues in Pharmaceutical Marketing: A Systematic Review and Future Research Agenda. *Journal of Global Marketing* **35**, 1–20 (2021).

691 *Tris Pharma Issues Voluntary Nationwide Recall of Infants' Ibuprofen Concentrated Oral Suspension, USP (NSAID) 50 mg per 1.25 mL, Due to Potential Higher Concentrations of Ibuprofen*, (2018). https://www.fda.gov/safety/recalls-market-withdrawals-safety-alerts/tris-pharma-issues-voluntary-nationwide-recall-infants-ibuprofen-concentrated-oral-suspension-usp

692 Lima, A. O. D. *et al.* Safety considerations during prescription of non-steroidal anti-inflammatory drugs (NSAIDs), through a review of systematic reviews. *An Sist Sanit Navar* **44**, 261-273 (2021).

693 Fu, L. S., Lin, C. C., Wei, C. Y., Lin, C. H. & Huang, Y. C. Risk of acute exacerbation between acetaminophen and ibuprofen in children with asthma. *PeerJ* **7**, e6760 (2019).

694 Schneider, V., Levesque, L. E., Zhang, B., Hutchinson, T. & Brophy, J. M. Association of selective and conventional nonsteroidal antiinflammatory drugs with acute renal failure: A population-based, nested case-control analysis. *Am J Epidemiol* **164**, 881-889 (2006).

695 *Risk Factors for Chronic Kidney Disease*, (2024). https://www.cdc.gov/kidney-disease/risk-factors/index.html

696 Eisenstein, A. *et al.* Activation of the transcription factor NRF2 mediates the anti-inflammatory properties of a subset of over-the-counter and prescription NSAIDs. *Immunity* **55**, 1082-1095 e1085 (2022).

697 *FDA Approves Novel Non-Opioid Treatment for Moderate to Severe Acute Pain*, (2025). https://www.fda.gov/news-events/press-announcements/fda-approves-novel-non-opioid-treatment-moderate-severe-acute-pain

698 Straube, S., Tramer, M. R., Moore, R. A., Derry, S. & McQuay, H. J. Mortality with upper gastrointestinal bleeding and perforation: effects of time and NSAID use. *BMC Gastroenterol* **9**, 41 (2009).

Index

Made in the USA
Monee, IL
12 September 2026

62980098R00226